Drying Technologies for Biotechnology and Pharmaceutical Applications

Drying Technologies for Biotechnology and Pharmaceutical Applications

Edited by

Satoshi Ohtake
Ken-ichi Izutsu
David Lechuga-Ballesteros

WILEY-VCH

Editors

Dr. Satoshi Ohtake
Pfizer, Inc.
Pharmaceutical R&D
875 Chesterfield Parkway West
MO 63017
United States

Dr. Ken-ichi Izutsu
National Institute of Health Sciences
Division of Drugs
Tonomachi 3-25-26
Kawasaki 2109501
Kanagawa
Japan

Dr. David Lechuga-Ballesteros
AstraZeneca Pharmaceuticals, LP
Pharmaceutical Technology and Development
121 Oyster Point Boulevard, South San Francisco
CA 94080
United States

Cover
Cover Images: A multicolored powder explosion © Jag_cz/iStock.com, Vaccination © AlexRaths/iStock.com, Ceramic powder © aytacbicer/iStock.com

Library of Congress Card No.:
applied for

British Library Cataloguing-in-Publication Data
A catalogue record for this book is available from the British Library.

Bibliographic information published by the Deutsche Nationalbibliothek
The Deutsche Nationalbibliothek lists this publication in the Deutsche Nationalbibliografie; detailed bibliographic data are available on the Internet at <http://dnb.d-nb.de>.

Print ISBN: 978-3-527-34112-2
ePDF ISBN: 978-3-527-80209-8
ePub ISBN: 978-3-527-80211-1
oBook ISBN: 978-3-527-80210-4

Typesetting SPi Global, Chennai, India
Printing and Binding Markono Print Media Pte Ltd, Singapore
Printed on acid-free paper

10 9 8 7 6 5 4 3 2 1

Contents

1

Introduction

Alex Langford[1], Satoshi Ohtake[1], David Lechuga-Ballesteros[2], and Ken-ichi Izutsu[3]

[1] *Pfizer BioTherapeutics, Pharmaceutical Sciences, 875 Chesterfield Parkway West, Chesterfield, MO 63017, USA*
[2] *AstraZeneca Pharmaceuticals LP, Pharmaceutical Technology and Development, 121 Oyster Point Boulevard, South San Francisco, CA 94080, USA*
[3] *National Institute of Health Sciences, Division of Drugs, Tonomachi 3-25-26, Kawasaki 2109501, Kanagawa, Japan*

Succeeding the inception of recombinant DNA technology in the 1970s [1], the pharmaceutical industry observed a significant shift from chemically synthesized drugs toward biologics. Biopharmaceuticals or biologics, distinct from small molecule drugs, include a wide variety of therapeutic products derived from living organisms or produced using biotechnology, e.g. recombinant proteins, vaccines, blood components, cellular therapies, and gene therapies. Biopharmaceuticals are characterized by a composition containing biological components or subunits including peptides, proteins, nucleic acids, and cells [2].

Since the US Food and Drug Administration (FDA) approved the first recombinant protein-based biologic in 1982 (recombinant insulin, Humulin®, Eli Lilly and Co., Indianapolis, IN, USA) [3] and monoclonal antibody-based therapy in 1986 [4], there has been continual growth in the number of biopharmaceuticals on the market. There were only nine biopharmaceutical approvals prior to 1990; however, since the mid-1990s, the United States and European Union have seen a combined average of more than 10 new approvals each year (based on Figure 1b of [5]). A survey of biopharmaceuticals published by Walsh [5] in 2014 reported that there were 212 approved biopharmaceutical products on the market in the United States and European Union with biopharmaceuticals making up an estimated 26% of all new drug approvals. The annual sales value of biopharmaceuticals in 2013 was reported to be US$140 billion, a value noted to be greater than the gross domestic product (GDP) of 156 of 214 countries listed in the World Bank GDP database. In 2017, the highest selling biologic was adalimumab (Humira, AbbVie Inc., North Chicago, IL, USA) at over US$18 billion in annual sales [6].

In more recent years, the diversity and complexity of the biopharmaceuticals in development has continued to increase. Protein-based therapeutics remain common, but the breadth of compounds the industry is currently faced with manufacturing has expanded significantly. Some examples of the products currently in development and on the market include antibody drug conjugates (ADCs),

Drying Technologies for Biotechnology and Pharmaceutical Applications, First Edition.
Edited by Satoshi Ohtake, Ken-ichi Izutsu, and David Lechuga-Ballesteros.

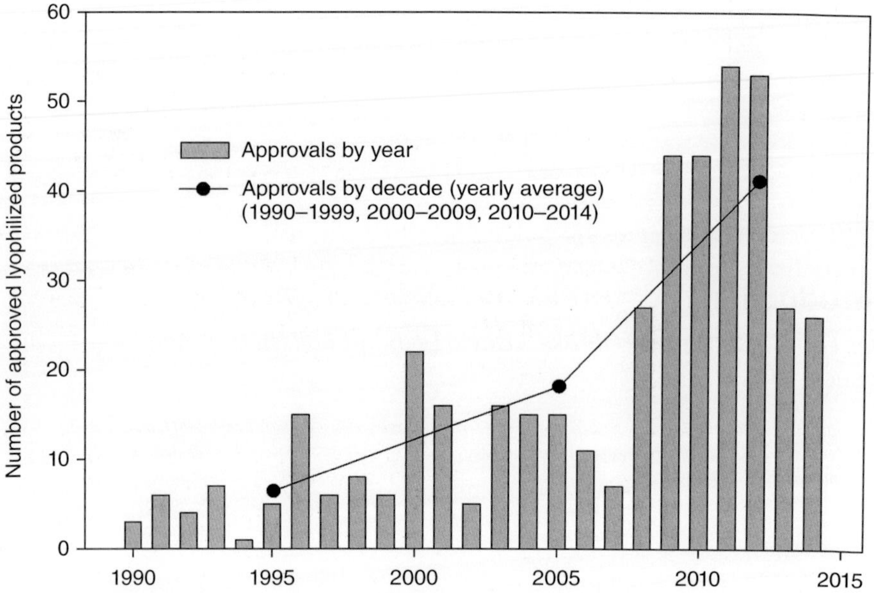

Figure 1.1 Number of FDA-approved lyophilized drugs by year and decade of approval. Source: Adapted with permission from Ref. [8].

multivalent polysaccharide conjugate vaccines, live attenuated vaccines, cellular therapies, and gene therapies.

As the biopharmaceutical industry continues to evolve, advances in technologies will be required to address the challenges of speed to market, reducing developmental costs, improving storage stability, maintaining high product quality, and enhancing end-user convenience. The dehydration of material provides advantages that are able to address some of these challenges. While many biological materials contain high water content (typically ≥80%, w/w), the removal of water confers benefits such as ease of handling and storage, reduction in transportation costs, and improved stability [7]. For these reasons, the number of approved pharmaceutical products requiring lyophilization has significantly increased over the last two decades, as demonstrated by the increasing number of FDA-approved products that are freeze-dried (Figure 1.1). Furthermore, it was reported that the percentage of all approved injectable/infusible drugs that were lyophilized increased from only 12% between 1990 and 1998 to greater than 50% between 2013 and 2015 [8]. An increase in the number of biological therapy approvals by the FDA has been accompanied with a parallel increase in the overall number of approved drugs.

Whether it is the ancient use of sun and air drying as a means of food preservation, a primitive form of lyophilization used by the Incan Empire centuries ago using radiation from the sun and reduced pressure at high altitudes [9], or any advanced drying technology used in modern manufacturing processes across the globe, the basic principles of drying remain the same. Drying is the process of dehydration or the removal of water from a solution or suspension to form a solid. During the drying process, an energy source transfers heat to the solution through conduction, convection, and/or radiation to vaporize water. An aqueous solution is dried by two fundamental processes to remove either bound or unbound water (i.e. bulk water). The first process is the evaporation of surface moisture from the transfer of heat, or other forms of energy, to the wet feed. The second process is the transfer of internal moisture to the product surface where it can then evaporate following the first process [10]. Chapter 2 expands on the various ways in which these principles have been applied throughout history.

Since the dawn of modern engineering, drying has continued to mature, and now hundreds of dryer types are available for industrial applications. Chapter 2 provides a review of the current applications of drying technologies in industries other than pharmaceuticals, such as the food, agriculture, and textile industries. While many drying technologies in these industries are considered well established, the need for significant improvements to existing processes remains with respect to efficiency and control. The process efficiency of dryers has been reported to range from under 5% to approximately 35% on the high side due to (i) the high latent heat of vaporization of water and (ii) the inefficient heat transfer of convection (a common method of heat transfer in industrial dryers) [10]. The rate of drying is largely based on the amount of heat transferred to the wet feed through conduction, convection, and/or radiation. Additionally, it can be altered by changing factors such as the type of energy source used and/or application of forced air or a vacuum.

Traditional methods of commercial drying are limited either by their high production costs (e.g. freeze-drying) or severe reduction in product quality due to long exposure times at high temperatures (e.g. hot air drying). For biopharmaceuticals, the maintenance of high product quality is a crucial consideration for an optimized drying process. In general, a higher drying temperature will negatively impact product quality though reduce overall processing time. Often, loss of a drug substance and/or drug product batch has such a significant impact on developmental cost and/or clinical timelines that very conservative drying temperatures (i.e. lower temperatures) are utilized early in development. These lower drying temperatures often maintain product quality but require significantly longer processing time. In addition, a greater deviation of the processing temperature from ambient typically requires greater energy consumption. Thus, finding the optimum drying temperature is the most common problem encountered in developing an efficient drying process.

Historically within the pharmaceutical industry, engineers and scientists have been very limited in their use of drying technologies. The need to preserve high product quality of labile biomolecules and maintain aseptic processing has severely reduced the number of methods used in the industry. The gold standard for the drying of biopharmaceuticals is freeze-drying as evidenced by the significant number of freeze-dried biomolecule products on the market [11]. Due to its prominence in the field, the first drying technology to be reviewed in this book is freeze-drying (Chapter 6). In addition, there are several supplemental resources on this topic recommended for further reading [12–14]. Even though the freeze-drying process is common and relatively well established, it has several shortcomings, including high energy consumption, long drying times, low process efficiency, formulation limitations (i.e. challenges with low collapse temperature excipients such as salts), and incompatibility with continuous manufacturing. The efficiency of fully loaded laboratory- and production-scale lyophilizers was reported to range from 1.5% to 2% as calculated by Alexeenko [15]. While higher process efficiency is possible through other drying technologies, consideration of alternative drying methods depends on several factors such as the physical properties of the product, application of the product, type of energy source available, container closure system, and scalability of the equipment. Chapter 12 reviews the desired characteristics of a novel drying technology and requirements for implementation into the current manufacturing environment.

As mentioned above, drying can provide significant benefits to the stabilization of labile biomolecules. A liquid drug product formulation is often preferred due to reduced manufacturing costs and end-user convenience (i.e. no reconstitution required); however, sufficient stabilization in the liquid state often cannot be achieved. In an aqueous solution, water serves as a medium that results in significant molecular mobility and conformational perturbations and acts as a catalyst for chemical degradation that can promote instability during storage and shipping [16]. The removal of water through drying significantly retards water-mediated degradation. An early-stage clinical development strategy may be to proceed with a dried formulation as a means of quickly achieving adequate product stability without needing to develop a liquid formulation. This may be a preferred approach since many products do not make it to approval based on clinical results and the consequential reduction of up-front resources may help to reduce the company's developmental costs. That being said, smaller organizations may benefit from developing a stable liquid dosage form due to the increased cost of manufacturing a freeze-dried product. Chapter 13 presents additional details on relevant challenges in the development of liquid dosage forms and the benefits of solid-state stabilization. A drying process cannot be designed as a stand-alone entity, and the characteristics of the molecule to be processed must be considered. Chapters 3, 4, and 5 review the unique considerations when applying drying processes to small molecule active pharmaceutical ingredient (API), proteins, and vaccines, respectively.

Even though a well-designed drying procedure can often sufficiently stabilize biomolecules, drying induces new stresses to a product that are not present in a liquid formulation. From a freeze-drying perspective, these stresses include the ice–water interface, low temperature, cryo-concentration [17], freezing-induced pH shifts [18], and the removal of bulk and bound water during drying [14, 19]. It has been widely reported that the degradation of biomolecules, such as monoclonal antibodies, caused by some of these stresses can be overcome by the use of stabilizing excipients, such as disaccharides [16, 17]. Chapter 13 presents the primary considerations when developing a stable solid-state formulation in addition to discussing the key role of water in the final product. Looking toward the future, as biomolecules continue to increase in complexity (e.g. mammalian cell-based therapies), these drying-induced stresses may prove to be more problematic, and stabilizing excipients alone may not be sufficient to adequately stabilize dried formulations. The formulation scientist may have to consider the unique benefits of next-generation drying technologies to overcome such challenges [20].

Next-generation drying technologies for biological materials include but are not limited to spray freeze-drying (Chapter 8) [21, 22], microwave drying (Chapter 9) [23, 24], foam drying (Chapter 10) [25, 26], and the use of electromagnetic/magnetic waves on freeze-drying (Chapter 11) [27]. While these "novel" drying techniques currently have limited application in the biopharmaceutical industry, many are commonly used in other industries. Benefits such as improved stabilization of biomolecules, compatibility with continuous manufacturing, and improved process efficiency compared with freeze-drying are potential reasons to evaluate these technologies. Microwave-assisted freeze-drying is an example of utilizing a hybrid of two drying methods to significantly reduce drying process time [24, 28]. For these reasons, this book will veer away from established biopharmaceutical development approaches and conventional drying processes, such as freeze-drying and spray drying (Chapter 7), to discuss and evaluate these promising next-generation technologies. Chapter 14 reviews the challenges and considerations for implementing these new technologies into the current manufacturing environment as well as discusses the potential synergy with process analytical technologies (PAT). These novel techniques are presented to the reader in hope that they will consider how to utilize them to overcome new problems and inefficiencies they encounter.

Several resources are currently available to engineers, scientists, and academics that review the fundamentals of drying and its application to various industries. However, there is currently no book that focuses solely on the application of a variety of drying technologies to biopharmaceuticals. The aim of this book is to fill this void by providing a comprehensive resource reviewing the current state and future direction of drying technologies for biopharmaceutical applications. The authors hope that this book will serve scientists and engineers in the pharmaceutical industry as well as academics, particularly in chemical engineering and pharmaceutical sciences, as a single source of information related to pharmaceutical drying technologies. Since this book presents the latest developments related to drying technologies in the field, senior leaders in the industry may find it useful for identifying improvements to current and/or new technologies to implement into their current manufacturing environment. The authors hope that the specific focus of this book on biopharmaceutical applications will enhance its effectiveness in providing a clear vision of the current and future (Chapter 15) landscape of drying in the pharmaceutical industry.

Acknowledgement

The authors along with the other contributors of the book would like to acknowledge the contributions made by Professor Michael J. Pikal to advance our understanding of and technical capability of various drying processes. He sadly passed away prior to the completion of the book and we dedicate this book to Prof. Pikal, who was our friend, colleague, and mentor.

References

1 Berg, P. and Mertz, J.E. (2010). Personal reflections on the origins and emergence of recombinant DNA technology. *Genetics* 184 (1): 9–17.

2 Shih, H.H., Miller, P., and Harnish, D.C. (2010). An overview of the discovery and development process for biologics. In: *Pharmaceutical Sciences Encyclopedia* (ed. S.C. Gad). New York, NY: Wiley.

3 Altman, L.K. (1982). A new insulin given approval for use in the U.S. *The New York Times* (30 October).

4 Goswami, S., Wang, W., Arakawa, T., and Ohtake, S. (2013). Developments and challenges for mAb-based therapeutics. *Antibodies* 2 (3): 452–500.

5 Walsh, G. (2014). Biopharmaceutical benchmarks 2014. *Nature Biotechnology* 32 (10): 992–1000.

6 AbbVie Inc. (2018). AbbVie reports full-year and fourth-quarter 2017 financial results. Press release (26 January).

7 Walters, R.H., Bhatnagar, B., Tchessalov, S. et al. (2014). Next-generation drying technologies for pharmaceutical applications. *Journal of Pharmaceutical Sciences* 103 (9): 2673–2695.

8 Arduini, M. (2016). *Freeze Drying Market Analysis*. Amherst, NY: Aseptic Processing Symposium.

9 Rey, L. (2004). Glimpses into the realm of freeze-drying: fundamental issues. In: *Freeze-Drying/Lyophilization of Pharmaceutical and Biological Products*, 2e (eds. L. Rey and J.C. May), 1–32. New York, NY: Marcel Dekker, Inc.

10 Mujumdar, A.S. (2006). Principles, classification, and selection of dryers. In: *Handbook of Industrial Drying*, 3e (ed. A.S. Mujumdar). Cleveland, OH: CRC Press LLC.

11 Gokarn, Y.R., Kosky, A., Kras, E. et al. (2006). Excipients for protein drugs. In: *Excipient Development for Pharmaceutical, Biotechnology, and Drug Delivery Systems* (eds. A. Katdare and M.V. Chaubal). Cleveland, OH: CRC Press LLC.

12 Carpenter, J.F., Pikal, M.J., Chang, B.S., and Randolph, T.W. (1997). Rational design of stable lyophilized protein formulations: some practical advice. *Pharmaceutical Research* 14 (8): 969–975.

13 Pikal, M.J. (2006). Freeze drying. In: *Encyclopedia of Pharmaceutical Technology* (ed. J. Swarbrick), 1807–1833. New York, NY: Informa Healthcare.

14 Bhatnagar, B.S., Tchessalov, S., Lewis, L.M., and Johnson, R. (2013). Freeze drying of biologics. In: *Encyclopedia of Pharmaceutical Science and Technology*, 4e (ed. J. Swarbrick), 1673–1722. Cleveland, OH: CRC Press LLC.

15 Alexeenko, A. (2011). Controlling the freeze-drying process: simulations and modeling. World Lyophilization Summit, Boston, MA.

16 Carpenter, J.F. and Chang, B.S. (1996). Lyophilization of protein pharmaceuticals. In: *Biotechnology and Biopharmaceutical Manufacturing, Processing, and Preservation* (eds. K.E. Avis and V.L. Wu), 199–264. Cleveland, OH: CRC Press LLC.

17 Bhatnagar, B.S., Bogner, R.H., and Pikal, M.J. (2007). Protein stability during freezing: separation of stresses and mechanisms of protein stabilization. *Pharmaceutical Development and Technology* 12 (5): 505–523.

18 Kolhe, P., Amend, E., and Singh, S.K. (2010). Impact of freezing on pH of buffered solutions and consequences for monoclonal antibody aggregation. *Biotechnology Progress* 26 (3): 727–733.

19 Luthra, S., Obert, J.-P., Kalonia, D.S., and Pikal, M.J. (2007). Investigation of drying stresses on proteins during lyophilization: differentiation between primary and secondary-drying stresses on lactate dehydrogenase using a humidity controlled mini freeze-dryer. *Journal of Pharmaceutical Sciences* 96 (1): 61–70.

20 Langford, A., Bhatnagar, B., Walters, R. et al. (2018). Drying technologies for biopharmaceutical applications: recent developments and future direction. *Drying Technology* 36 (6): 677–684.

21 Leuenberger, H., Prasch, A., and Luy, B. (2001). Method for producing particulate goods. WO2001063191, filed 2001 and issued 2001.

22 Randolph, T.W., Seid, R., Truong-Le, V. et al. (2003). Spray freeze dry of compositions for intranasal administration. WO2003086443, filed 2003 and issued 2003.

23 Durance, T.D., Yaghmaee, P., Ahmad, S., and Zhang, G. (2007). Method of drying biological materials. WO2008092228, filed 2007 and issued 2008.

24 Gitter, J.H., Geidobler, R., Presser, I., and Winter, G. (2018). Significant drying time reduction using microwave-assisted freeze-drying for a monoclonal antibody. *Journal of Pharmaceutical Sciences* 107 (10): 2538–2543.

25 Truong-Le, V. (2003). Preservation of bioactive materials by freeze dried foams. WO2003087327, filed 2003 and issued 2003.

26 Vehring, R. and Ao, Y. (2008). Preservation of bioactive materials by freeze dried foam. WO2008143782, filed 2008 and issued 2008.

27 Woo, M.W. and Mujumdar, A.S. (2010). Effects of electric and magnetic field on freezing and possible relevance in freeze drying. *Drying Technology* 28 (4): 433–443.

28 Duan, X., Zhang, M., and Mujumdar, A.S. (2007). Studies on the microwave freeze drying technique and sterilization characteristics of cabbage. *Drying Technology* 25 (10): 1725–1731.

2

A Concise History of Drying

Sakamon Devahastin[1,2] *and Maturada Jinorose*[3]

[1] *King Mongkut's University of Technology Thonburi, Advanced Food Processing Research Laboratory, Department of Food Engineering, Faculty of Engineering, Bangkok 10140, Thailand*
[2] *The Royal Society of Thailand, The Academy of Science, Dusit, Bangkok 10300, Thailand*
[3] *King Mongkut's Institute of Technology Ladkrabang, Department of Food Engineering, Faculty of Engineering, Bangkok 10520, Thailand*

2.1 Introduction

Drying has been conducted since time immemorial with the main purpose of preserving food and agricultural produce. Although the main objective of drying has not changed since its first application, drying is also used nowadays for a number of other equally important purposes. Among such purposes is the use of drying to produce products that cannot be obtained by other processing means. These range from such ubiquitous products as instant milk, coffee, and other beverages to some household products such as detergent powder to some advanced materials, including pharmaceutical products.

As far as 20 000 BC, humans started to dry meat via the method of sun drying. Some 10 000 years later, fish was noted to be dried in France, while some grains and legumes were dried in the Middle and Near East. Around 9000 BC, salt was made by drying seawater, but it was only 1500 years ago in India that sugar was first dried into a solid form [1]. Development of most drying techniques that are widely in use today started only in the nineteenth century. Around 1800, a dryer made of brick, which can probably be regarded as an early version of a mechanical dryer, was constructed and used to dry grains.

In 1856, Gail Borden Jr., based on his earlier experience producing the so-called meat biscuit [2, 3], which was a dehydrated meat mixed with flour, patented a process for concentrating and preserving milk (Figure 2.1) by "coagulating and rearranging the albuminous particles in combination with the evaporation of the fluid in vacuo." This represents an early attempt to develop a water-removal process under vacuum. Many other patents on the production of various dried products have been filed afterward. For example, in 1865, Charles A. La Mont patented a process to manufacture dried egg [4]. This probably represents the first attempt to spray-dry a product as the egg can be forced "by means of a powerful blast of air, into a thin spray, which is made to fall through a current of

Drying Technologies for Biotechnology and Pharmaceutical Applications, First Edition.
Edited by Satoshi Ohtake, Ken-ichi Izutsu, and David Lechuga-Ballesteros.

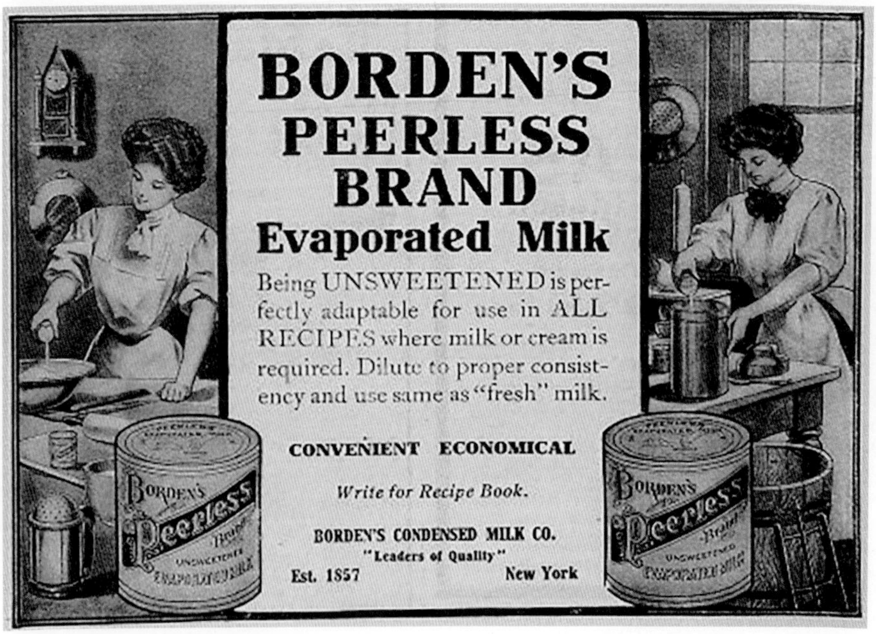

Figure 2.1 Advertisement of an earlier version of evaporated milk. Source: https://tshaonline.org/handbook/online/articles/fbo24 (accessed 1 April 2018).

heated air, as aforesaid, and dry in small, fine particles," among other possible alternatives. Samuel R. Percy, however, was the one credited for the invention of modern spray drying. He was granted in 1872 a patent on the method to improve atomizing and drying liquid substances by the process of atomization [5]. Several advanced designs of spray dryer have emerged during the twentieth century [1, 6]. Some investigator has even declared that it was the invention and continuous development of spray drying that ultimately helped advance the manufacturing technology for solubilizing drug molecules [7].

Another important drying technology, especially for such highly heat-sensitive materials as pharmaceutical products, is freeze drying. A technique similar to freeze drying was first noted to be used by the Peruvian Incas to dry potatoes and other crops and by Japanese monks living on a mountain to dry tofu. In such cases, drying materials were carried high into the mountains where temperatures descended below the freezing point of water; atmospheric pressure was also low due to the high altitudes, resulting in the removal of water within the materials [8]. Modern-day freeze drying, however, started only in the late nineteenth century, with Richard Altman in 1890 drying pieces of frozen tissues by placing them in a vacuum desiccator at −20 °C. Freeze drying became more popular during World War II as a means to preserve blood plasma and eventually vaccines and many other biological molecules [9].

In addition to the developments in drying equipment, theoretical developments have also flourished since the beginning of the twentieth century. Warren K. Lewis and Thomas K. Sherwood (of the well-known Sherwood number) were among the first who laid the foundations of modern-day theoretical study of drying [10–12]. Throughout the century, progress has significantly been made by a large number of fine individuals working in both academia and industry. Freeze drying of pharmaceuticals, for example, has been well studied by the late Prof. Michael J. Pikal, to whom this book is dedicated, along with many other researchers.

The history of drying would not be complete without the mentioning of the journal devoted solely to the science and engineering of drying. *Drying Technology*, which was launched in 1983 under the editorship of the late Prof. Carl W. Hall, now (2019) publishes 16 issues per annum under the editorship of Prof. Arun S. Mujumdar; drying of pharmaceuticals is of course one of the main themes of the journal. Prof. Mujumdar also launched another important knowledge dissemination outlet in 1978 in the form of the *International Drying Symposium*, which has since uninterruptedly held on a biennial basis and already celebrated its 40th anniversary at the 21st symposium in Valencia, Spain, in 2018. Coincidently or not, it is interesting to note that Prof. Mujumdar started the important aforementioned activity while at McGill University in Canada, the institution where Prof. Sherwood received his first degree in chemical engineering in 1923.

In the next section, a concise history of drying of pharmaceutical products is provided. Brief histories of some popular drying techniques for drugs and other relevant molecules will also be given.

2.2 History of Drying of Pharmaceutical Products

Pharmaceutical products have been dried for millennia, starting in the form of herbs and other medicinal natural products. In fact, the word "drug" is derived from French "drogue," which means dried herb [13].

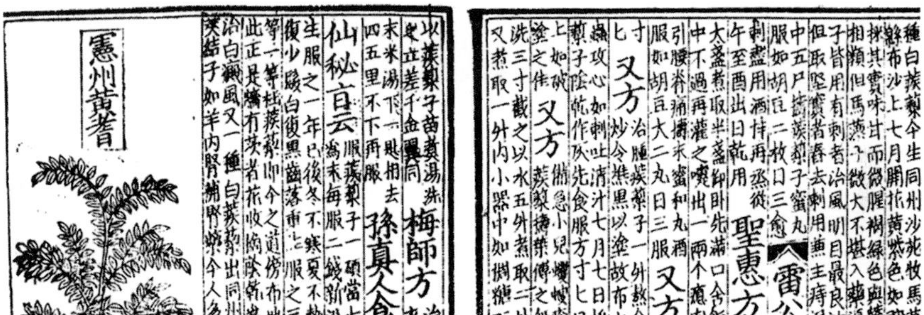

Figure 2.2 Sample page of Pen T'Sao. Source: https://commons.wikimedia.org/wiki/File:Pen_ts%27ao,_woodblock_book_1249-ce.png (accessed 1 April 2018).

The Chinese book on roots and grasses *Pen T'Sao* (Figure 2.2), written by Emperor Shen Nung as early as 2500 BC, mentioned as many as 365 drugs obtained from dried parts of medicinal plants, many of which are still in use even today such as *Rhei rhizoma*, camphor, *Theae folium*, *Podophyllum*, ginseng, jimson weed, cinnamon bark, and ephedra [14]. Since then a large number of books describing a very wide array of aromatic plants, spices, and plant drugs have been written in other parts of the world, including Egypt, India, the Middle East, and different parts of Asia and Europe. Later, between the sixteenth and eighteenth centuries, compound drugs, which consisted of medicinal plants along with drugs of plant and animal origins, started to receive more attention. From today's technological point of view, this represents more challenges for drying to retain bioactivities of the drugs. These challenges might nevertheless not be well recognized some five centuries ago.

One important dried pharmaceutical product of the eighteenth century was the so-called Dover's powder (Figure 2.3), which was introduced by Thomas Dover. The powder was prescribed as diaphoretics but was aimed for the treatment of gout. The powder was prepared and used, as stated in the section on gout in Dover's book *The Ancient Physician's Legacy to his Country,*[1] by "Tak(ing)e Opium one ounce, Salt-Petre and Tartar vitriolated each four ounces, Ipocacuana one ounce. Put the Salt-Petre and Tartar into a red-hot mortar, stirring them with a spoon until they have done flaming. Then powder them very fine; after that slice in your opium, grind them to a powder, and then mix the other powders with these. Dose from forty to sixty or seventy grains in a glass of white wine Posset, going to bed; covering up warm, and drinking a quart or three pints of the Posset –

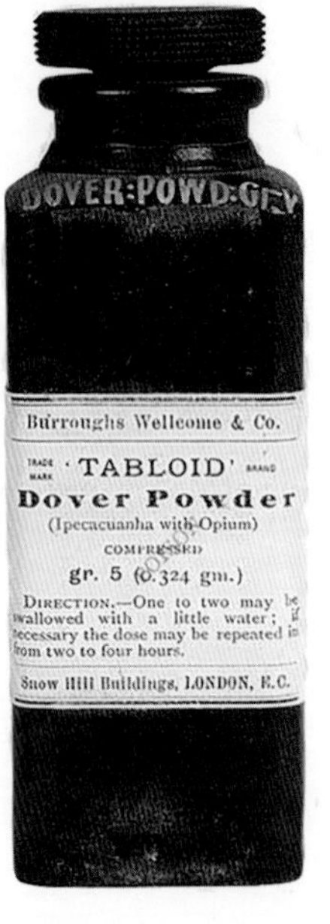

Figure 2.3 Dover's powder. Source: https://commons.wikimedia.org/wiki/File:Bottle_of_Dover_Powder_Wellcome_L0047580.jpg (accessed 30 March 2018).

1 The last name was, for some reason, spelled as "Dovar" on the cover of the book.

Drink while sweating." The compound had become the most widely used opium preparation for the next 150 years [15, 16].

The importance of drying on the drug activities was revisited in the late nineteenth century when various investigators started to note that the healing effect of medicinal plants depended on the mode of drying. On a side note, drying was used in 1884 as a means to attenuate the rabies virus by Louis Pasteur; drying of viral infected tissues was noted to help weaken the virus [17]. In the early twentieth century, stabilization methods for fresh medicinal plants started to be proposed. Significant effort has since been made to study the effects of manufacturing conditions on the activities of medicinal plants and drugs. Extensive literature on drying of pharmaceutical and related products has been produced [18, 19], making the field expand very rapidly.

2.3 History of Selected Drying Technologies

2.3.1 Freeze Drying

As mentioned earlier, a process that can be more or less qualified as freeze drying has started to be practiced by the South American natives some centuries ago. Tubers of frost-resistant potato varieties are frozen overnight and later warmed in indirect sun. In this way, the ice is removed by sublimation. The semi-dried product is trampled to remove the skins and eliminate the residual water, which allow for further freezing and drying. The so-called white chuño (or tunta) is made by soaking the partially dried tubers in water for a week (or even several weeks in some cases) prior to sun drying. Black chuño is, on the other hand, obtained from tubers subjected directly to sun drying without prior soaking or washing [20, 21]. Note that white chuño is covered during sun drying by blankets to avoid direct exposure to sunlight; this results in the different appearance of the two chuño (Figure 2.4). As a dried product, chuño has extended shelf life in comparison with unprocessed tubers. Chuño possesses higher contents of some minerals, including calcium and iron, than its unprocessed counterpart. However, chuño has lower contents of phosphorus, potassium, magnesium, and zinc as well as some antioxidants (e.g. phenolic compounds) than unprocessed tubers. This is particularly true in the case of white chuño due to its long exposure to water during processing [22, 23].

In the pharmaceutical industry, freeze drying (or lyophilization) is among the most widely and successfully utilized methods for transforming a wide range of aqueous and nonaqueous solutions of bioactive substances, including antibiotics, bacteria, sera, vaccines, diagnostic medications, protein-containing and biotechnological products, cells and tissues, and chemicals, into a solid, stable state [24].

The development of freeze drying can be traced back to as early as 1811 when Sir John Leslie first demonstrated the process of ice sublimation [25]. Later in 1813, William H. Wollaston, in his lecture to the Royal Society of London, defined such a process in which a solid (ice) is converted into a gaseous state and then recondensed as a solid, thereby completely avoiding the intervention of a liquid state during the process [21]. Neither Leslie nor Wollaston seemed to use

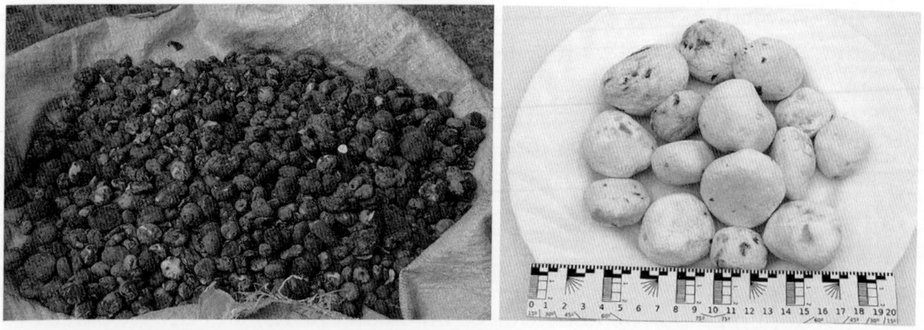

Figure 2.4 Black chuño (left) and white chuño (right). Source: Black Chuno: https://commons.wikimedia.org/wiki/File:Chu%C3%B1o.jpg and White Chuno: https://commons.wikimedia.org/wiki/File:Tunta-02.jpg (accessed 1 April 2018).

the process of sublimation for drying, however. The actual freeze-drying process was first tested by Richard Altman in Leipzig in 1890 for drying pieces of frozen tissues. Later in 1903, Vansteenberghe freeze-dried rabies virus, and in 1906, Jacques-Arsene d'Arsonval removed water at a lower temperature for distillation [26]. The first patent for freeze drying was issued to a French inventor Henri Tival in 1927. Later in 1934, William Elser received a patent for a freeze-drying apparatus that did not supply heat (but rather employed the so-called solid carbon dioxide cold trap) for sublimation [27]. In fact, all related works conducted up to this point involved the use of no heat for drying. Test materials were either vacuum-insulated from the atmosphere or the whole apparatus was placed in a cold room [28].

In 1935, Earl W. Flosdorf and Stuart Mudd were the first to use a high-temperature source to perform freeze drying; human blood serum and plasma were dried for clinical use [28]. Their subsequent efforts led to commercial freeze-drying applications in the United States. Application of the process to food (fruit juices and milk) started in 1935, and a British patent was issued to Franklin Kidd in 1941 for the freeze drying of foods [26, 29]. Due to technological restrictions, however, the process was not often used and was difficult to replicate.

Freeze drying became of practical importance during World War II. Many blood supplies being sent to Europe from the United States for medical treatment spoiled before reaching their destination. Freeze drying, through the research of Flosdorf and Mudd, was then used to produce blood that was chemically stable and viable without requiring refrigeration. Shortly thereafter, the process was also applied to penicillin and bone [30]. At about the same time, freeze-drying applications were developed under the leadership of Ronald I. N. Greaves of Cambridge University, first also to dry blood and later as a means to alleviate the food crisis during World War II. In 1951, the British Ministry of Food Research was established in Aberdeen, Scotland, where a vacuum contact plate freeze dryer that improved the product quality and reduced the time required for rehydration was developed. A continuous process for freeze drying was eventually developed by Greaves in 1960 [26]. By the 1950s, freeze drying has established itself as a common process for drying pharmaceutical products. Toward the end of the twentieth century through to present day, the process has also gained attention for drying probiotics and nutraceutical products [21, 29, 31].

Despite being treated as a gold standard to which alternative drying methods must be compared, freeze drying suffers from a number of limitations, including the lengthy required drying time [31]. An array of alternative drying methods, ranging from bulk freeze drying and foam drying to rather different classes of drying techniques, have therefore been proposed and tested; some of them will be discussed in the latter chapters of the book.

2.3.2 Spray Drying

As mentioned earlier, it was Samuel Percy in 1872 who was credited for the invention of modern spray drying. He indeed described the spray-drying process as "The process of simultaneously atomizing and desiccating fluid and solid substances, and its application to the purpose of the exhaustion of moisture from such substances, and for the prevention of destructive chemical change" [5]. World War II was again the important driving force for the development and adoption of spray drying for continuous production of milk powder. The process has gone through a number of design modifications and is now widely used to convert an array of pumpable liquids into flowing powders of versatile applications [32].

Spray drying is probably the most mature alternative technology to freeze drying and can be applied to the production of many pharmaceutical products, especially when attributes such as particle size, morphology, and stability need to be accurately controlled [33]. Spray drying may be used to produce fine particles for pulmonary and nasal deliveries as well as large agglomerated powers for oral administration [34]; Exubera®, despite its failure, was indeed the first inhaled therapeutics that was manufactured by spray drying [31]. Spray drying owes its advantages to the ability to control the particle size, bulk density, degree of crystallinity, and residual solvent or moisture content of a final powdery product. Micro- and nanocapsules with therapeutic core and biocompatible coating material(s) can be well prepared by spray drying. The technique can also be used to enhance the solubility and dissolution rate of a poorly soluble drug, usually via the formation of inclusion complexes or via the development of solid dispersions.

The first use of spray drying in pharmaceutically related application was probably that of Robert Stauf in the early twentieth century for drying of blood [35]. A sterile version of spray dryer, which was used for drying plasma and serum, was, however, proposed by John F. Wilkinson, Kenneth Bullock, and William Cowen in the 1940s [36]. The technique has since been applied to manufacture infusions, extracts, inorganic medicinal salts, adrenaline, and some vitamins [31, 37–39]. Of particular use of this drying technique is the production of pharmaceutical excipients and active ingredients, which are difficult to crystallize [33].

It is interesting to note here a brief historical development of the three major components of a spray-drying system, namely, a liquid pump, nozzle (or atomizer), and powder collection unit. The first use of pump dated back to as long as 2000 BC in Egypt, and the progress has continued through the whole history, with the inventions of a piston vacuum pump by Otto von Guericke in 1650, packed plunger pump by Sir Samuel Morland in 1674, and screw pump by Revillion in 1830 [40]. However, it was the invention of a steam pump of Henry R. Worthington in 1840 that marked the beginning of a real progress in this area. Spray nozzle was indeed the invention of Stauf in 1901, while the powder collection was first patented in 1906 by Wilhelm F. L. Beth [7].

Spray drying nevertheless suffers some shortcomings. Aseptic processing is clearly more challenging in the case of spray drying when compared with freeze drying. There may also be some difficulties when hygroscopic powders need to be handled. As the material recovery can never reach 100%, high-cost pharmaceutical products may not be suitable to be processed via spray drying.

2.3.3 Fluidized-Bed Drying

The first application of a fluidized bed was probably that of Fritz Winkler in 1922 for coal gasification, while it was not until 1942 that the first production facility using the fluidized-bed concept for catalytic cracking of petroleum feedstock became operational [41]. Since then fluidized bed has found applications in such a wide array of industries as petrochemical, materials processing, food, and pharmaceuticals. Fluidized-bed dryer has become particularly popular in the food industry for drying a large number of particulate materials. Grain kernels such as rice [42] as well as potato granules, peas, and diced vegetables [43] are commonly dried in this type of dryer.

In the pharmaceutical industry, a fluidized bed is used not only for drying but also for blending, pelletizing, and coating [44–46]. Combined drying and granulation are among the common operations that have been conducted in this type of dryer to improve the flowability and compressibility of a pharmaceutical powder.

2.3.4 Supercritical Drying

Baron Charles Cagniard de la Tour was noted in 1822 to be the first person to observe the critical phenomena. By placing a flint ball in a digester that was partially filled with liquid, a splashing sound was generated as the ball penetrated the liquid–vapor interface. Upon heating, the splashing sound ceased above a certain temperature beyond the boiling temperature of the liquid. This marks the discovery of the supercritical fluid phase where the densities of the liquid and gas phases become equal and the distinction between them disappears, resulting in a single supercritical fluid phase. Cagniard de la Tour, however, did not use the term "critical point" to explain his observation. It was Thomas Andrews in 1869 who coined the term. Significant progress has been made since that time; the reader is referred to an excellent review by Berche et al. [47] for the summary of the first 150-year history of the field.

Supercritical drying works in a similar fashion to supercritical fluid extraction, with solvent to be removed as a solute and supercritical fluid as an extraction solvent. Supercritical drying using CO_2 (which is the most widely used supercritical solvent) has been applied to produce a number of products, including

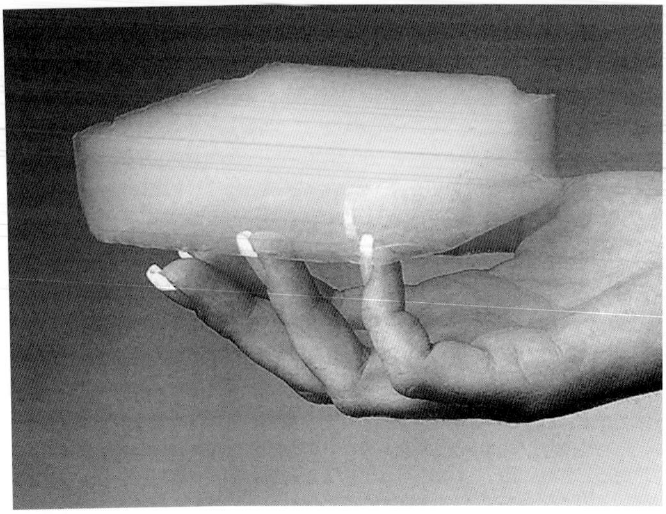

Figure 2.5 Aerogel block being held in a hand. Source: https://en.wikipedia.org/wiki/Aerogel#/media/File:Aerogel_hand.jpg (accessed 1 April 2018).

aerogels (Figure 2.5); high-value dried herbs and spices are also produced by this drying technique [48]. Among the noted advantages of supercritical drying, absence of the vapor–liquid interfaces is of particular interest. Such an absence leads to negligible surface tension and capillary-induced stress that may damage the microstructure of a material being dried [48, 49]. Samuel S. Kistler in the late 1920s was indeed the first who recognized such an advantage of a supercritical fluid when he tried to replace the liquid inside of a jelly without causing any shrinkage. In other words, he was trying to replace a liquid in a gel with a gas, thus creating a substance that was structurally a gel, but without the liquid [50].

Another important advantage of supercritical drying is its ability to operate at a lower temperature and hence the ability to dry highly heat-sensitive materials. In the pharmaceutical industry, supercritical fluid-assisted nebulization drying via the so-called Bubble Dryer® was used to prepare various dried powdery protein formulations and protein-loaded microparticles [51]. Supercritical solvents, e.g. supercritical CO_2, possess a number of unique properties, making them possible to process bioactive molecules and amorphous polymers without the use of toxic organic solvents. This type of solvent exhibits positive impacts on both micronization and encapsulation of microparticles [52]. Through the use of supercritical solvent for drying, microbial inactivation can also be achieved, thus alleviating concerns on aseptic processing as compared with the case of spray drying [31].

Other alternative technologies can also be applied to the drying of pharmaceutical products. Despite their ubiquity in other industries, namely, food and chemical industries, such technologies as vacuum drying and microwave drying still need to find more of their places in the pharmaceutical industry.

2.4 Concluding Remarks

In this chapter, a concise history of drying in general and pharmaceutical drying in particular is given. Brief histories of some major drying technologies that are in use in the pharmaceutical industry are also reviewed. Knowing the history, even in its brevity as is the case of this chapter, should give the reader a better appreciation (and more enjoyment!) of the exciting scientific and technological details of the various drying technologies applicable for an array of pharmaceutical products that will follow in the latter chapters of this book.

Acknowledgments

Financial support provided by the Thailand Research Fund (TRF) (grant number RTA 6180008), which allowed for the completion of the chapter, is greatly appreciated.

References

1 Hayashi, H. (1989). Drying technologies of foods: their history and future. *Drying Technology* 7: 315–369.
2 Borden, Jr., G. (1856). Improvement in concentration of milk. US Patent No. 15,553, issued 19 August 1856.
3 Valigra, L. (2013). Gail Borden Jr. 'Got Milk.' http://www.foodqualityandsafety.com/article/gail-borden-jr-got-milk (accessed 15 April 2017).
4 La Mont, C.A. (1865). Improvement in preserving eggs. US Patent No. 51,263, issued 28 November 1865.
5 Percy, S.R. (1872). Improvement in drying and concentrating liquid substances by atomizing. US Patent No. 125,406, issued 9 April 1872.
6 Filková, I., Huang, L., and Mujumdar, A.S. (2015). Industrial spray drying systems. In: *Handbook of Industrial Drying*, 4e (ed. A.S. Mujumdar), 191–226. Boca Raton: CRC Press.
7 Crew, M. (2015). The second quadrant – the birth of drug solubilization: 1840 through 1920. http://www.drug-dev.com/Main/Back-Issues/THE-SECOND-QUADRANT-The-Birth-of-Drug-Solubilizati-897.aspx (accessed 15 April 2017).
8 Lyophilization Technology, Inc. (2017). Freeze drying milestones. http://www.lyotechnology.com/fd-milestones.html (accessed 15 April 2017).
9 Couriel, B. (1980). Freeze drying: past, present, and future. *PDA Journal of Pharmaceutical Science and Technology* 34: 352–357.
10 Lewis, W.K. (1921). The rate of drying of solid materials. *The Journal of Industrial & Engineering Chemistry* 13: 427–432.
11 Sherwood, T.K. (1929a). The drying of solids-I. *Industrial & Engineering Chemistry* 21: 12–16.

12 Sherwood, T.K. (1929b). The drying of solids-II. *Industrial & Engineering Chemistry* 21: 976–980.

13 Lüllmann, H., Mohr, K., Ziegler, A., and Bieger, D. (2000). *Color Atlas of Pharmacology*, 2e. Stuttgart: Thieme.

14 Petrovska, B.B. (2012). Historical review of medicinal plants' usage. *Pharmacognosy Reviews* 6: 1–5.

15 Osler, W. (1896). *Thomas Dover (of Dover's powder): Physician and Buccaneer*. Baltimore: Friedenwald.

16 Timeline of Events in the History of Drugs (2018). https://inpud.wordpress.com/timeline-of-events-in-the-history-of-drugs (accessed 19 March 2018).

17 The History of Vaccines (2018). https://www.historyofvaccines.org/timeline#EVT_100874 (accessed 19 March 2018).

18 Chen, G. and Mujumdar, A.S. (2015). Drying of herbal medicines and tea. In: *Handbook of Industrial Drying*, 4e (ed. A.S. Mujumdar), 637–646. Boca Raton: CRC Press.

19 Pakowski, Z. and Mujumdar, A.S. (2015). Drying of pharmaceutical products. In: *Handbook of Industrial Drying*, 4e (ed. A.S. Mujumdar), 681–701. Boca Raton: CRC Press.

20 Chuño (2018). https://en.wikipedia.org/wiki/chuño (accessed 19 March 2018).

21 Franks, F. (2007). *Freeze-Drying of Pharmaceuticals and Biopharmaceuticals: Principles and Practice*. Cambridge: RSC Publishing.

22 de Haan, S., Burgos, G., Arcos, J. et al. (2010). Traditional processing of black and white chuño in the Peruvian Andes: regional variants and effect on the mineral content of native potato cultivars. *Economic Botany* 64: 217–234.

23 Peñarrieta, J.M., Alvarado, K.J.A., Bravo, J.A., and Bergenståhl, B. (2011). Chuño and tunta; the traditional Andean sun-dried potatoes. In: *Potatoes: Production, Consumption and Health Benefits* (ed. C. Caprara), 1–12. Hauppauge: Nova Science Publishers.

24 Dietrich, G. (2014). Fundamentals of pharmaceutical freeze drying. https://www.gea.com/en/stories/freeze-drying-fundamentals.jsp (accessed 19 March 2018).

25 Pirie, N.W. (1973). Freeze drying: a consequence of a cold Christmas. *New Scientist* 60: 833–834.

26 Freeze-drying (Inventions). (2018). http://what-when-how.com/inventions/freeze-drying-inventions (accessed 19 March 2018).

27 Strong, D.M. and MacKenzie, A.P. (1993). Freeze-drying of tissues. In: *Musculoskeletal Tissue Banking* (ed. W.W. Tomford), 181–208. New York: Raven Press.

28 Flosdorf, E.W. (1954). The development of freeze-drying. In: *Biological Applications of Freezing and Drying* (ed. R.J.C. Harris), 63–84. New York: Academic Press.

29 Hua, T.-C., Liu, B.-L., and Zhang, H. (2010). *Freeze-Drying of Pharmaceutical and Food Products*. Cambridge: Woodhead Publishing.

30 History of Freeze-drying. (2018). http://www.freeze-dry.com/2015/09/29/history-of-freeze-drying/ (accessed 19 March 2018).

31 Walters, R.H., Bhatnagar, B., Tchessalov, S. et al. (2014). Next generation drying technologies for pharmaceutical applications. *Journal of Pharmaceutical Sciences* 103: 2673–2695.

32 Anandharamakrishnan, C. and Ishwarya, S.P. (2015). *Spray Drying Techniques for Food Ingredient Encapsulation*. West Sussex: Wiley-Blackwell.

33 Gaspar, F. (2014). Spray drying in the pharmaceutical industry. *European Pharmaceutical Review* 19: 45–48.

34 Patil, J. (2016). Spray-drying: an emerging technique for pharmaceutical product development. *Journal of Pharmacovigilance* 4: e150.

35 Stauf, R. (1901). Process of desiccating blood, milk and the like. US Patent No. 666,711, issued 29 January 1901.

36 Wilkinson, J.F., Bullock, K., and Cowen, W. (1942). Continuous method of drying plasma and serum. *Lancet* 239: 281–284.

37 Arpagaus, C., Collenberg, A., Rütti, D. et al. (2018). Nano spray drying for encapsulation of pharmaceuticals. *International Journal of Pharmaceutics* 546: 194–214.

38 Woo, M.W. and Mujumdar, A.S. (2015). Product functionality-oriented drying process related to pharmaceutical particles engineering. In: *Handbook of Industrial Drying*, 4e (ed. A.S. Mujumdar), 985–998. Boca Raton: CRC Press.

39 Ziaee, A., Albadarin, A.B., Padrela, L. et al. (2019). Spray drying of pharmaceuticals and biopharmaceuticals: critical parameters and experimental process optimization approaches. *European Journal of Pharmaceutical Sciences* 127: 300–318.

40 World Pumps. (2009). A brief history of pumps. http://www.worldpumps.com/general-processing/features/a-brief-history-of-pumps (accessed 24 March 2018).

41 American Chemical Society (1998). *The Fluid Bed Reactor*. Washington, DC: American Chemical Society.

42 Prachayawarakorn, S., Taechapairoj, C., Nathakaranakule, A. et al. (2015). Drying of rice. In: *Handbook of Industrial Drying*, 4e (ed. A.S. Mujumdar), 595–609. Boca Raton: CRC Press.

43 Jayaraman, K.S. and Das Gupta, D.K. (2015). Drying of fruits and vegetables. In: *Handbook of Industrial Drying*, 4e (ed. A.S. Mujumdar), 611–635. Boca Raton: CRC Press.

44 Burggraeve, A., Monteyne, T., Vervaet, C. et al. (2013). Process analytical tools for monitoring, understanding, and control of pharmaceutical fluidized bed granulation: a review. *European Journal of Pharmaceutics and Biopharmaceutics* 83: 2–15.

45 Takasaki, H., Sakurai, A., Katayama, T. et al. (2019). Novel, lean and environment-friendly granulation method: green fluidized bed granulation (GFBG). *International Journal of Pharmaceutics* 557: 18–25.

46 Tardos, G.I. and Mort, P.R. (2003). Applications for coating and granulation. In: *Handbook of Fluidization and Fluid-Particle Systems* (ed. W.-C. Yang), 445–468. New York: Marcel Dekker.

47 Berche, B., Henkel, M., and Kenna, R. (2009). Critical phenomena: 150 years since Cagniard de la Tour. *Journal of Physical Studies* 13: 3201.

48 Brown, Z.K. (2010). The drying of foods using supercritical carbon dioxide. Ph.D. Thesis, Department of Chemical Engineering, The University of Birmingham, UK.

49 Supercritical Drying. (2018). http://www.aerogel.org/?p=345 (accessed 31 March 2018).

50 Kistler, S.S. (1931). Coherent expanded aerogels and jellies. *Nature* 127: 741.

51 Cape, S.P., Villa, J.A., Huang, E.T.S. et al. (2008). Preparation of active proteins, vaccines and pharmaceuticals as fine powders using supercritical or near-critical fluids. *Pharmaceutical Research* 25: 1967–1990.

52 Ginty, P.J., Whitaker, M.J., Shakesheff, K.M., and Howdle, S.M. (2005). Drug delivery goes supercritical. *Materials Today* 8: 42–48.

Part I

Drug Product Development

3

Importance of Drying in Small Molecule Drug Product Development

Paroma Chakravarty and Karthik Nagapudi

Genentech, Inc., 1 DNA Way, South San Francisco, CA 94080, USA

3.1 Introduction

Small molecule drug product development involves a number of pharmaceutical unit operations to manufacture the final dosage form, and drying is a critical unit operation involved in this process. Typically, drying operation involves the removal of small amounts of residual solvent (mostly water) from either the active pharmaceutical ingredient (API), the drug product intermediate (DPI), or the final drug product (DP) by using heat. This is a complex technology involving heat and mass transfer and is accompanied by physicochemical changes in the dried product, such as changes in particle size, morphology, chemical composition, and even solid-state phase transformations [1]. Moisture and/or other solvents may come in contact with pharmaceuticals (API or DP) at different stages of drug substance and drug product manufacturing, such as during chemical synthesis, crystallization, and unit operations such as lyophilization, spray drying, and wet granulation or upon handling and storage (US Pharmacopeia, Section 1241). Water may also migrate to active ingredients from the excipients used in the formulation, depending on the "state" of water (free or bound) associated with the formulation components [2–4]. Owing to such pernicious effects of water on a wide range of pharmaceutically relevant properties at different stages of development, it is therefore a quality and regulatory requirement that the water content be controlled both in the drug substance and dosage form to ensure the quality and performance of the final product.

Drying operations play an important role in controlling the moisture/solvent content in the final product, which is required to obtain and maintain desired product properties such as physical and chemical stability, powder flow and granule morphology, and tableting properties (compressibility, compactibility, tensile strength, hardness) and guarantee reliability and reproducibility in the final product performance such as disintegration and dissolution of tablets [5–10]. In addition, drying plays a vital role by removing moisture from pharmaceuticals to ensure adequate shelf life via prevention of moisture-induced chemical and microbial degradation [11]. Moreover, drying is also the most energy-intensive unit operation in drug product development and as such

Drying Technologies for Biotechnology and Pharmaceutical Applications, First Edition.
Edited by Satoshi Ohtake, Ken-ichi Izutsu, and David Lechuga-Ballesteros.

needs to be carefully monitored and controlled. The impact of drying on small molecules formulation development may be broadly classified into three categories: (a) effect on physical form of the API, (b) effect on powder flow and consequently formulation manufacture, and (c) as an aid in development of enabling formulations.

(a) *Effect on physical form*: For drug candidates, physical form selection and its maintenance through different stages of product development is critical and mandatory to ensure the efficacy and intended *in vivo* performance. Owing to its small size and ubiquitous nature, water is often absorbed in the lattice of crystalline solids, forming hydrates that may dehydrate to the anhydrous crystalline solid or an amorphous solid, depending on the location of water in the crystal lattice and the kinetics of moisture removal [4, 12]. For pharmaceuticals with a propensity to form hydrates, especially when the equilibrium water activity favoring hydrate formation is in the manufacturing relative humidity (RH) range (30–60%) or if the API has to undergo processing conditions involving water (such as wet granulation), the hydrate form may be obtained as an intermediate via process-related phase transformations. Formation of a hydrate during product development may not be desirable owing to the lower solubility of the hydrate in aqueous media compared to the anhydrate, which may affect *in vivo* exposure and bioavailability [13]. Debnath and Suryanarayanan have outlined this phenomenon for theophylline where formation of theophylline monohydrate upon storage led to dissolution failure of anhydrous theophylline tablets owing to lower dissolution rate of the hydrate. In situ hydrate formation in the tablets exposed to moisture also resulted in increased hardness [14]. Drying conditions (equipment and drying parameters) have to be chosen judiciously to ensure maintenance of the desired form in the final formulation.

Conversely, if the hydrate is the chosen form for development, drying conditions need to be optimized so as not to "over dry" the API and thus dehydrate the hydrate. Dehydration of a hydrate may lead to formation of dehydrated phases with varying degrees of crystallinity depending on the nature of the lattice water and the kinetics of water removal [15]. Such phase transition to either a crystalline anhydrate or anhydrous phases with partial to complete disorder (amorphous) may alter the pharmaceutically relevant properties of the drug product and affect its performance. For example, Phadnis and Suryanarayanan demonstrated formation of a metastable anhydrous phase obtained exclusively via the dehydration of theophylline monohydrate that was a highly reactive phase that converted to the stable anhydrous form in tablets upon exposure to moisture (33% or 52% RH, room temperature), leading to tablet dissolution failure. This metastable form also showed a more rapid conversion to the hydrate during dissolution from neat API compacts compared with those obtained from the stable form [16]. In order to prevent the formation of the undesired phase, a priori thorough understanding of thermodynamics of hydrate–anhydrate stability (i.e. water activity required for hydrate–anhydrate conversion at a

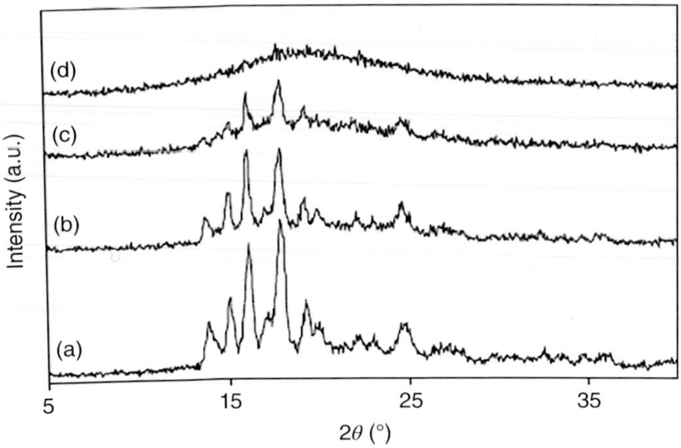

Figure 3.1 X-ray powder diffraction (XRPD) patterns of anhydrous trehalose obtained by isothermal dehydration of trehalose dihydrate at different drying temperatures: (a) 40 °C, (b) 60 °C, (c) 85 °C, and (d) 100 °C. Source: Rani et al. 2006 [17]. Reproduced with permission of Springer Nature.

particular temperature) along with an evaluation of the kinetics of drying (e.g. dryer type, airflow, temperature, use of reduced pressure, drying medium, duration) is required to determine the extent of drying related form changes and nature of the final dried product. There are several examples in literature on both theophylline and trehalose where dehydration of the respective hydrates leads to formation of different product phases with different physicochemical properties. Theophylline monohydrate, upon drying at 50 °C under ambient conditions, yielded an anhydrate that was 75% crystalline. Conversely, upon drying at 90 °C under reduced pressure, the anhydrate obtained did not have any detectable disorder [14]. Figure 3.1 shows the effect of drying on the solid-state form of the final product in trehalose dihydrate. The higher the drying temperature, the greater the lattice collapse, leading to the formation of a progressively more disordered anhydrous form [17].

Besides hydrate–anhydrate systems, the drying technique and conditions can also have a bearing on the different polymorphic forms of an active. Depending on the drying method and parameters chosen, the starting form may undergo a partial or a complete transformation to a different polymorphic form, especially in enantiotropic systems where the transition temperature resides below the melting points of the polymorphs [18]. Drying may also lead to the trapping and retention of a metastable polymorph if the rate of drying (such as that of wet-massed granules) is faster than the rate of solution mediated metastable-to-stable form conversion [19, 20]. For example, fluidized-bed drying of wet granulated glycine in the stable γ-form resulted in a mixture of the metastable α-form and stable γ-form in the dried granules. Faster drying at 80 °C resulted in an increased α-form content than that at 60 °C. Slower tray drying at 21 °C resulted in a much lower amount of the α-form in the dried granules compared with that obtained via fluidized-bed drying [19].

There are many scenarios where an amorphous active is preferred over its crystalline counterpart to exploit the apparent higher solubility of the amorphous form that may lead to greater *in vivo* bioavailability [21]. Such an approach comes with the caveat of reduced physical and chemical stability of the amorphous phase owing to its higher molecular mobility. Drying techniques such as spray drying and freeze drying (lyophilization) are often utilized to manufacture either the amorphous drug substance or the drug product, i.e. solid dispersion, in conjunction with one or more polymers or other carriers such as β-cyclodextrin or lipids [22–25]. In these cases where crystalline API is converted to its amorphous form, a thorough characterization of the "drying space" is required to ensure the formation of an amorphous drug substance or drug product that remains stable over the assigned shelf life. For both of these drying procedures, the feed material is typically a solution of the API alone or with a carrier such as a polymer or a lipid [11, 26]. Since the final product is a solid cake or a free-flowing powder, the process should be designed such that the maximum amount of solvent is removed in the most energy efficient way possible so that the final product has minimum residual moisture associated with it. This is important because water acts as a plasticizer and can lead to increased mobility and ultimately crystallization of the API [27]. Crystallization can also occur during the primary drying stage of the lyophilization process, where the frozen solution is exposed to reduced pressure wherein the amorphous solute (in the frozen solution) may crystallize out during heating and/or drying. For example, pH-dependent crystallization was observed in succinate and tartrate buffer systems when the rapidly frozen solutions of these salts were heated during primary drying [28]. Spray drying is the method of choice for bulk manufacturing of amorphous drug substance or product (solid dispersion) and the choice of drying parameters (feed concentration, inlet and outlet air temperature, pump rate, airflow), solvent used, and formulation composition can have a bearing on the solid-state form, particle size, and morphology of the API or drug product [29–31]. Roos has demonstrated the importance of determining the glass transition temperature to design the spray-drying process to obtain free-flowing, amorphous lactose particles and prevent crystallization as well as the formation of sticky agglomerates by maintaining product temperature at or below its glass transition [32]. Finally, while both of these drying techniques are used for vitrification of poorly soluble API, it has been well documented in the literature that the end product, although amorphous, may demonstrate differences in stability owing to their inherently different molecular mobility, which is sample history dependent. For example, Surana et al. have shown the effect of preparation method on the stability of amorphous trehalose, with the dehydrated samples (oven dried at 97 and 100 °C) being the least stable of all amorphous samples tested (Figure 3.2) [33]. A follow-up study by Bhardwaj et al., using dielectric spectroscopy, has demonstrated the differences in the relaxation profiles (α-relaxations) of amorphous trehalose,

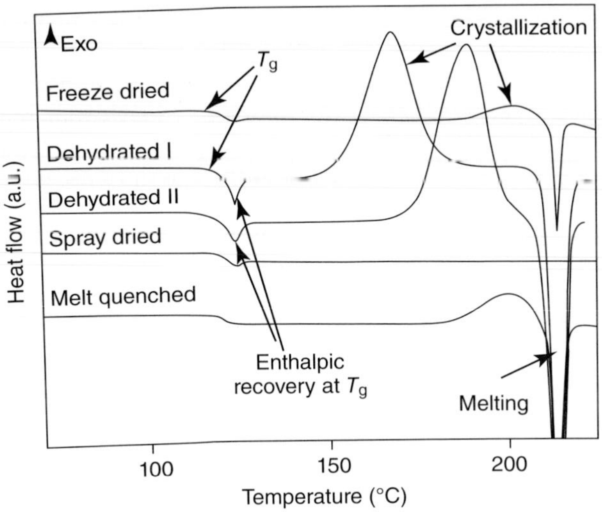

Figure 3.2 Differential scanning calorimetry (DSC) heating scans of amorphous trehalose prepared by different drying methods as compared to the melt-quenched sample. Post-drying at 60 °C to remove moisture, the samples were cooled to room temperature and heated to 230 °C at a heating rate of 10 °C/min. The dehydrated (dried at 97 and 100 °C) and freeze-dried samples crystallized out at temperatures >150 °C as evident from their enthalpy of crystallization shown in the figure. The spray-dried sample remained stable and did not show any crystallization post the glass transition temperature (T_g). Source: Surana et al. 2004 [33]. Reproduced with permission of Springer Nature.

obtained by different drying techniques, such as freeze drying, spray drying, and dehydration of trehalose dihydrate that explain the differences in the crystallization propensity of these samples [34].

(b) *Effect on powder and granule properties*: Most small molecule pharmaceuticals are administered as oral solid dosage forms, i.e. as tablets and capsules. Disintegration and dissolution are the two phenomena that need to occur prior to *in vivo* drug release and absorption, and these behaviors are strongly dependent on powder properties of API/excipient blend. Drying operation can impact a myriad of properties such as powder flow and compressibility, *in vivo* exposure, and kinetics of form change. Moisture may have a detrimental effect on powder flow as shown in a study by Schepky where granular flow was significantly inhibited upon exposure to moisture at ≥60% RH, 22 °C [8]. Powder flow, essential for tableting and capsule filling, is in turn affected by particle size and morphology, with smaller, needle-shaped particles often resulting in hopper clogging and poorer flow while larger, spherular particles being free flowing [35, 36]. Particle size and morphology also influence powder compactibility and tablet hardness, which in turn affect tablet integrity, disintegration, and dissolution times [37–39]. Additionally, particle size may also affect *in vivo* exposure, hygroscopicity, and kinetics of physical form change, through its relationship to surface area [40, 41].

In the wet granulation operation, the API/excipient blend is agglomerated via convective mixing using a binder solution (typically an aqueous polymer solution) for size enhancement. The wet mass that results is then further dried to obtain granules, which are usually free flowing (due to size enhancement) and are compressed into tablets. Much like primary particles of API, granule properties (surface area, size distribution, porosity) may influence tableting behavior and therefore the quality and performance of the final dosage form [35]. It has been well documented in literature that the structural and functional properties of granules are dependent on both drying technique and conditions employed [35, 42]. Tray dryers or fluidized-bed dryers are commonly used for drying of granules, with microwave drying being explored as another possible drying method. In a previous study, Bataille et al. have shown that granules obtained by microwave drying (30 minutes, 2450 MHz frequency, 12.24 cm wavelength) have greater porosity and lower fracture strength compared with those obtained by oven drying (12 hours, 40 °C) that produced less porous and harder, smaller-sized granules [43]. In both methods, granules were dried to a constant weight. Wlosnewski et al. have compared the physical properties and drug release behavior of formulated paracetamol pellets produced by extrusion that were dried using three different techniques: hot air drying, microwave drying, and freeze drying. The structural, mechanical, and functional properties of granules were found to vary considerably with the choice of drying method employed, with freeze drying producing weaker, larger, and more porous granules that showed a considerably faster drug release compared with the other two methods [44]. It has also been shown that static bed dryers such as oven or tray dryers yield granules with greater bulk density/strength and higher friability and exhibit faster drug dissolution compared with those obtained from fluidized-bed dryers [45, 46]. Intragranular porosity has been reported to be the most dominant factor dictating tablet strength, irrespective of tablet composition, in many studies. An increase in the intragranular porosity results in greater ability of the granules to fragment, leading to increased tablet strength. For granules less prone to fragmentation, intragranular porosity is critical for compressibility and the final tensile strength of the tablet [35, 36]. Johansson et al. have shown that greater intragranular porosity causes greater deformation, leading to a closed-knit intragranular pore structure and therefore stronger tablets [47]. Berggren has postulated that the drying rate affects the contraction and densification of granules and thus affects intragranular porosity, which influences granule tableting behavior [35]. Granule size and shape have shown to affect tablet strength with smaller granules producing tablets with greater strength and irregular-shaped granules facilitating increasing tablet strength compared with spherical granules of similar porosity [48, 49]. Finally, surface amorphization may occur during drying of granules owing to removal of water and formation of defects. Generation of disorder may be beneficial for powder compactibility by increasing surface reactivity and plastic deformation that causes a “sintering” effect and yields tablets with higher strength [50]. Hüttenrauch and Keiner have shown a linear correlation between extent of defect formation and loss of water upon drying, thereby conclusively proving that drying can generate a considerable amount of disorder in a material (Figure 3.3) [51]. This is

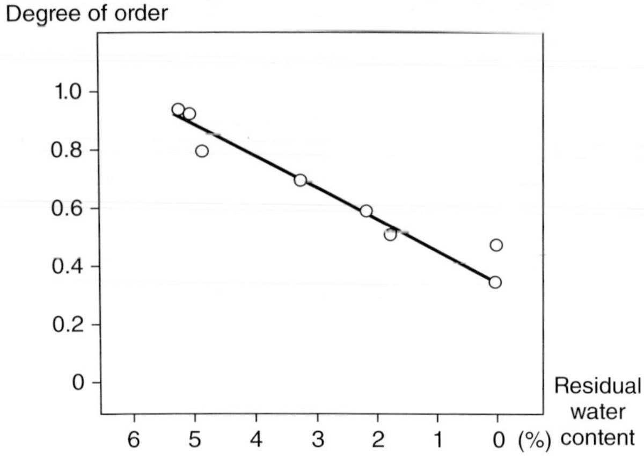

Figure 3.3 A plot showing a linear decrease in order with increase in drying time (decrease in residual water content) upon vacuum drying of α-lactose monohydrate. The degree of order was determined densimetically. Source: Hüttenrauch and Keiner 1979 [51]. Reproduced with permission of Elsevier.

definitely a cause for concern since the presence of small amount of surface disorder may result in localization of moisture in these surface defects, leading to chemical and physical instabilities. In order to prevent such undesirable phase transformations, the drying parameters should be optimized, and the solid-state properties of the dried granules should be monitored during the drying process as well as after completion of drying. Techniques such as water sorption, surface area analysis, inverse gas chromatography (to assess surface energy), X-ray powder diffractometry, and solid-state nuclear magnetic resonance (NMR) (to detect small amounts of disorder) may be used to evaluate changes in the solid-state properties of granule surfaces upon drying and detect formation or disorder [20].

Many studies have shown the effect of moisture on the mechanical properties and tableting behavior of excipients used for direct compression [5, 7, 48, 52–63]. Depending on the nature of water (surface adsorbed or tightly bound) and the extent of moisture sorption, the tensile strength and brittle fracture propensity of these excipients were found to be adversely affected at moisture content levels corresponding to twice that of tightly bound surface monolayer [53]. Studies with microcrystalline cellulose, the most widely used tablet diluent, have shown that increased moisture sorption first led to an increase in compactibility and volume followed by decrease in tablet tensile strength [5]. Similar results were observed for lactose, another tablet diluent, where it was recorded that increase in moisture content in anhydrous lactose (as little as 1–2% at 92% RH) resulted in decreased tablet hardness, and greater compression pressure was required to achieve target hardness values [9].

(c) *Development of enabling formulations and other specialized applications*: Drying techniques such as fluidized-bed drying, spray drying, and freeze drying are often utilized for formulating dosage forms for targeted drug delivery via other routes of administration (such as pulmonary and intravenous) and to obtain sufficient exposure in preclinical or clinical studies employing oral dosage forms. For heat-sensitive materials, freeze drying is an excellent route to obtain solid cakes that may be reconstituted into solution for intravenous delivery. This technique is almost exclusively used to manufacture parenteral drugs that are too unstable to remain in solution, such as antibiotics (e.g. cephalotin sodium, cefazolin sodium) [26]. Merck's Edecrin Sodium® is an example of a diuretic drug administered as an IV formulation manufactured by freeze drying to bring about rapid onset of diuresis and reduce edema. In recent years, freeze drying has been demonstrated to be a feasible method for ensuring long-term stability of colloidal nanoparticles by preventing aggregation and producing dried particles that can be reconstituted instantaneously into a colloidal suspension [64]. Freeze drying may also be employed for making amorphous solid dispersions (ASDs) for rapid release, but there are a few drawbacks to this procedure and therefore often not desirable for scale-up. Organic solvents often used for solubilizing the drug and carrier have low freezing points and may not exist in the frozen state upon ice sublimation, which is a requisite to obtain a dry, solid cake. Since the sample temperature has to be maintained below the glass transition of the frozen fraction for vitrification, lyophilization cycles can get prolonged with solvents having low freezing points. Finally, this method works best with solvents having high vapor pressure or else one may end up with cycle times of unacceptable duration [65].

Spray drying is the most widely used technique for manufacturing solid dispersions and a diverse range of formulations since it is a bulk manufacturing technique providing ease of scale-up and yields particles with a large surface area and narrow particle size distribution. Moreover, optimization of drying parameters can help tailor the flowability, size, morphology, and bulk density of the particles, thereby providing considerable flexibility in the formulation design space [35]. Due to this ability to engineer particle properties via adjustment of drying parameters, spray drying is used for manufacturing of different kinds of enabling formulations, such as (i) ASDs where the active is retained in an amorphous form in a carrier (polymer, β-cyclodextrin, lipid) to provide faster dissolution and increased solubility, (ii) controlled release solid dispersions where the release profile of the active is modulated by the use of water insoluble polymers, (iii) microspheres and nanoparticles, (iv) dry powder inhalation formulations, and (v) solid self-microemulsifying drug delivery system (SEDDS) (utilizing a solid carrier such as dextran) for poorly soluble drugs administered orally [23, 25, 66–78]

Fluidized-bed dryers are routinely used to dry wet masses obtained from wet granulation to generate free-flowing granules for tableting (batch process). They are also used for coating dry solid particles for various purposes in the food and pharmaceutical industries [79]. For example, there are studies demonstrating successful coating of bitter tasting drugs such as ibuprofen and indeloxazine hydrochloride using polymer and excipient solutions (coating material) for taste masking where the particles are encased in the coating solution that is subsequently dried off and a layer is deposited around the active, acting as a barrier to the undesirable taste [80, 81]. The Wurster fluidized-bed drying, which uses the bottom-spraying approach, is particularly popular for coating purposes for either taste masking or creating layers for the purpose of achieving controlled drug release. These coated particles are then compressed into tablets along with other suitable excipients [82]. In recent years fluidized-bed drying has also been utilized as a continuous granulation technique known as fluidized-bed granulation, which is a one-step enclosed process for particle agglomeration and drying. This involves fluidizing the particles, spraying a binder solution on them to create liquid bridges that aids agglomeration, and finally evaporation of the liquid to yield free-flowing granules with porous structures that enhance wettability [82, 83]. Masters has shown the use of a spray dryer in conjunction with a fluid-bed dryer to yield granules with good flowability. The outlet temperature of the spray dryer, linked externally to a fluidized bed, was lowered to allow for discharge of a moist product in the latter, where the particles underwent further agglomeration upon drying and were finally released as free-flowing granules [84].

The examples provided in these preceding sections showcase the importance of drying operation in pharmaceutical development. The drying step needs to be thoroughly studied and controlled since it influences critical properties of drug substance, drug product intermediates, and the performance of the final dosage form. The choice of dryers and drying method itself will depend on the nature of the material, i.e. its heat sensitivity, the solid-state of the drug substance, drying kinetics, ease of scale-up, cost and energy effectiveness, and the desired quality attributes of final drug product [11]. Figure 3.4 depicts a flowchart summarizing the effects of drying on the final solid in pharmaceutical drug product development and the corresponding physicochemical changes brought about by the removal of moisture.

3.2 Drying Materials and Dryer Types

A wide variety of pharmaceutical materials are subjected to drying, and they range from starting materials, the active itself (drug substance), drug product intermediates and the final drug product. Based on their physical form, these materials may be categorized as follows [11]:

(a) *Solids*: These are either wet cakes or granules obtained upon wet granulation to cause size enlargement via agglomeration.
(b) *Suspensions*: These include slurries or pastes. For example, the process of API crystallization often involves formation of crystal slurry with a given liquid to solid ratio that is filtered and finally dried to obtain crystallites of desired size.
(c) *Solutions*: These include clear solutions of either API or carrier (such as a polymer) or both that are commonly used to prepare ASDs by rapid removal of solvent either by sublimation or application of vacuum or heat that leads to formation of a solid cake or powder.

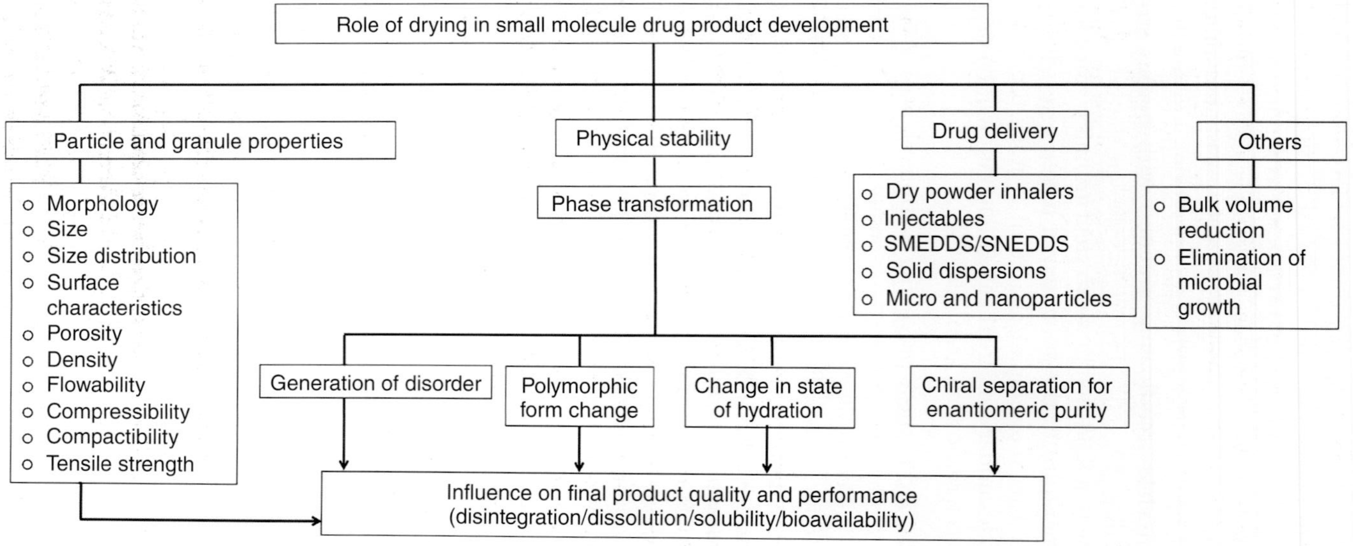

Figure 3.4 Schematic summarizing the importance of drying as a unit operation in pharmaceutical formulation development.

Table 3.1 Classification of dryers.

Criterion	Dryer type
Mode of operation	Batch, continuous
Heating principle/source	Conduction, convection, radiation, electromagnetic, combination of several modes, intermittent or continuous heating, direct or indirect
State of material in the dryer	Stationary, moving, agitated, dispersed
Operating pressure	Atmospheric or reduced (vacuum)
Drying medium (convection)	Air, superheated steam, supercritical fluid
Relative motion (between drying medium and solids)	Cocurrent or countercurrent or mixed flow
Residence time	Short (<1 min), medium (1–60 min), long (>60 min)
Number of stages	single step or multistage

Source: Adapted from Ref. [1].

Given the diversity of applications of drying processes to pharmaceutical materials, it is not surprising that there are a diverse range of dryers available. The dryers may be classified in several ways, based on either their mode of operation, operating pressure, heat input type, movement of feed material inside the dryer, drying temperature, drying time, drying medium, drying stages, or relative motion between drying medium and solids. These criteria are shown in Table 3.1 [1]. Pharmaceutical dryers are either batch or continuous and may be directly heated (adiabatic/convective type) or indirectly heated (nonadiabatic/conductive type). Directly heated dryers utilize the heat of the carrier gas in contact with the solid for evaporation of the liquid, whereas indirectly heated dryers do not require a carrier gas for liquid removal. Instead a heat transfer medium, usually separated from the solids by a metal wall, is used for evaporation of the liquid phase, and the heat is conducted via the wall and/or impellers. Although the majority of pharmaceutical dryers are convective, i.e. use a direct heat source, conductive/contact dryers are economically advantageous and environmentally friendly and provide greater thermal efficiency. Commonly used, directly heated batch dryers include tray dryers and fluidized-bed dryers, whereas the ones operating in continuous mode include turbo-tray dryers, pneumatic dryers, cyclone dryers, spouted bed dryers, vibrated bed dryers, fluidized-bed dryers, and spray dryers. Indirectly heated dryers include drum dryers, vacuum dryers, and freeze dryers. These dryers are capable of handling pharmaceutical materials of different kinds and consistencies such as wet solids, thermolabile materials, fibrous raw materials, granules, sludges or sticky materials, solutions, suspensions, thin slurries, and pastes [1, 11]. Some of these dryers and drying techniques will be discussed in detail in the following sections, with a brief overview of their drying principle, utility and challenges in pharmaceutical product development, and its effect on pharmaceutically relevant properties of the dried solids.

3.3 Directly Heated (Convective) Dryers

3.3.1 Tray Drying

3.3.1.1 Description

Tray dryers are enclosed systems, i.e. insulated chambers where trays are stacked on top of each other in trolleys and the solids (granules or wet cake) to be dried are placed on these trays. Moisture removal occurs by exposing the wet solids directly to circulating hot air (drying medium) by electric heaters or steam from radiator coils. Blower fans ensure uniform circulation of air to facilitate heat transfer, and the dryer is equipped with external control panel for temperature regulation. The rate of mass transfer is dependent on parameters such as drying temperature and airflow, both of which can be controlled. Drying end point is achieved when three subsequent losses on drying readings are identical for aliquots of the drying material that are removed periodically. Tray dryers can also be operated in the conductive mode (indirect heating) by heating the trays using underlying heating plates, wherein metal trays are employed to ensure good contact between the plates and the trays. For heat-sensitive materials, where direct contact with the heating medium may be detrimental, drying can be conducted at a lower temperature in conjunction with the use of vacuum, which also aids in solvent recovery. These are known as vacuum tray dryers and are some of the most commonly used batch dryers. Heat transfer to the feed occurs via conduction where the heating element (steam, water, hot oil) passes through heating plates, on which trays are mounted containing the feed material. Solvent vapors produced during drying are either removed directly or via a steam jet compressor to an external condenser. Non-condensable gases are extracted by the vacuum system. Unlike conventional tray dryers, turbo-tray dryers are operated in the continuous mode and are equipped for drying granular materials placed on rotating shelves with forced convective air above them that causes heat transfer and moisture removal. The feed material on the shelves is routinely perturbed by a series of stationary blades so that fresh layers of the drying material are periodically exposed to the drying medium, thereby facilitating uniform drying. After every rotation, the material is wiped off by the last blade, and it falls on to the lowermost shelf, thereby allowing fresh material to be introduced. These dryers are equipped with as many as 30 trays and provide large residence times. Turbo-tray dryers can also be hermetically sealed to facilitate solvent recovery [11, 85].

3.3.1.2 Utility

Owing to their relatively simple design, low cost, and ease of use, tray dryers are popular in the pharmaceutical industry, especially in places where manufacturing and drying need to occur in tandem. Such dryers are a good and economical option for drying of small batches, and the design, i.e. shelves loaded in an enclosed chamber, makes it portable enough for drying to occur during transportation as well [11]. Granular material, spread out on trays, have a larger surface area exposed to the drying medium, which facilitates moisture removal. Tray dryers are suitable for drying almost all kinds of materials, barring dusty solids/very fine particles [1]. The insulated design, sometimes equipped with a vacuum system, allows for recovery of expensive solvents. The use of heating plates placed below the trays (for indirect heating) and application of vacuum makes this method attractive for drying thermolabile materials [86]. In addition, this method also allows ease of sampling, i.e. removal of small aliquots of the drying material, for offline characterization.

Another added advantage of tray drying is that it allows for drying under humid conditions (humidity drying) wherein a specific headspace RH is generated by introducing a stream of dry and wet air (usually, nitrogen) and by regulating the airflow of the dry and wet streams. The RH is displayed using humidity sensors. Humidity drying is employed in the pharmaceutical industry for control of the solid-state form, especially for actives that are employed as hydrates. Maintenance of a headspace RH during the drying process, which corresponds to the equilibrium RH for hydrate stability, helps to ensure that the product is not overheated and the hydrate lattice water is not removed. Introduction of moisture in the headspace along with simultaneous heat transfer helps to maintain the desired state of hydration of the active and prevent undesirable phase transformations that may have deleterious effects downstream. This method of drying is even more pertinent for nonstoichiometric hydrates for which the lattice water content changes continually as a function of t water activity. Many nonstoichiometric hydrates dehydrate to their corresponding anhydrates where the lattice structure is retained when the water molecules are removed. Such isomorphic desolvates are high energy forms and may react with other formulation components that may alter the properties of the dosage form [87, 88]. For example, Bauer et al. have demonstrated that dehydration of erythromycin dihydrate into its corresponding isomorphic dehydrate led to dissolution failure in tablets due to binding of the anhydrate with magnesium hydroxide, a formulation excipient. This binding was found to be reversible upon exposure of the formulation to moisture, wherein the anhydrate reverted to the hydrate form, as illustrated in Figure 3.5 [89]. Owing to their ease of dehydration and rehydration, nonstoichiometric hydrates are typically not preferred for development, but in instances where such hydrate is the chosen solid-state form, humidity drying would be the preferred route to preserve the state of hydration and prevent inadvertent drying. Humidity drying may also be employed to bring about intentional phase transformation of the API, such as that shown by Chakravarty and Lubach, where a partially disordered active was converted to a completely amorphous form upon exposure to moisture at room temperature (RT) to provide a pathway to form control for regulatory purposes [90].

3.3.1.3 Drawbacks and Challenges

One of the main disadvantages of tray drying is the nonuniformity of the drying process itself. Nonuniformity of airflow distribution leads to nonuniform heat transfer to the feed material, which consequently results in long drying times (10–20 hours). Also, drying rates are typically the most inconsistent at the extremes, i.e. point of entry and exit of the circulating air [85]. Nonuniformity in drying results in inhomogeneity in moisture content in the sample bed, and this may have implications for physical and chemical stability and bulk properties of the granule. From a solid-state perspective, incomplete drying

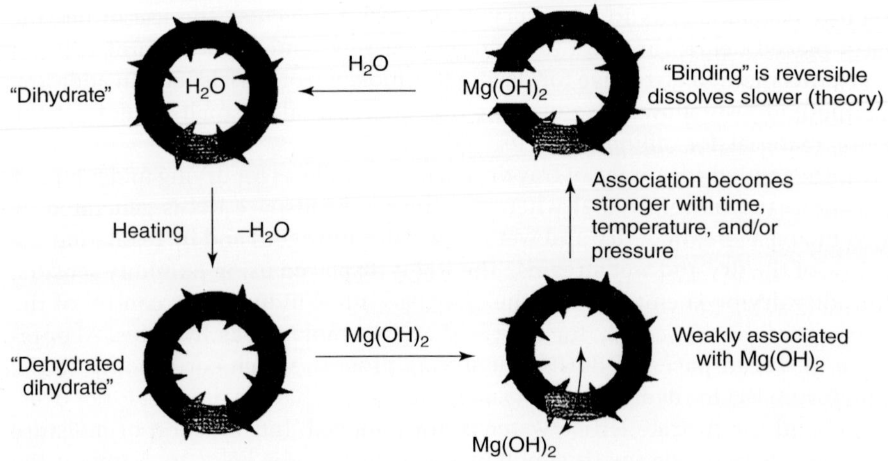

Figure 3.5 Schematic showing reversible binding in erythromycin dihydrate tablets. Drying leads to formation of isomorphic desolvate of the API that reversibly binds with the tablet excipient magnesium hydroxide, which leads to dissolution failure in tablets. Exposure to moisture causes competitive displacement of the excipient by water, and the hydrated form is restored. Source: Bauer et al. 1999 [89]. Reproduced with permission of John Wiley & Sons.

may lead to a series of phase transformations, resulting in a mixture of forms in the dried material, depending on the drying kinetics and the starting solid form. Depending on the extent and nature of the new phases so formed, the quality and performance of the drug product may be significantly altered. This is especially true for actives known to form hydrates where one of the following transitions may occur due to incomplete drying:

(A) *Anhydrate → hydrate → incomplete dehydration*: An anhydrous API may convert to the hydrate during wet-massing step of granulation, which may not completely revert back to the anhydrate if drying is inhomogeneous. The hydrate may persist along with the anhydrate, and the drug substance may exist as a mixture of these two forms in the final drug product. Since hydrates are typically less water soluble than their anhydrous counterparts, the dissolution and solubility of the drug product may be compromised. For example, the presence of the monohydrate form in anhydrous thiamine hydrochloride granules led to partial dehydration to the more stable hemihydrate that caused granule and, consequently, tablet hardening [91]. Anhydrate → hydrate → anhydrate transformations are common in carbamazepine, where wet massing of the different anhydrous polymorphic forms (I, II and III) results in different extents of conversion to the dihydrate (form IV), which exclusively dehydrates to the fine particles of form III upon drying [92].

(B) *Hydrate → anhydrate or dehydrated phase*: If the hydrate is the starting form and subjected to nonuniform drying, one or more products of dehydration may be generated in pockets of overdrying. The nature and degree of crystallinity of the dehydrated product and the extent of its formation will dictate the bulk properties of the granules (where the drug loading is high) and the quality of the final drug product, i.e. tablet. For example, the dehydrated phase may be completely disordered (amorphous), leading to potential moisture-induced chemical instability since amorphous forms possess high molecular mobility, are reactive, and easily interact with moisture. If the dehydrated phase is crystalline and anhydrous, it may possess different physicochemical properties compared with the hydrate that again may affect granule size, structure, and flow and other mechanical properties such compressibility, compactibility, and tablet tensile strength. Finally, if a metastable anhydrous form is obtained, such as an isomorphic anhydrate, it may interact unfavorably with other formulation components and affect drug product performance. Tantry et al. have shown that tray drying of theophylline monohydrate can lead to a mixture of metastable and stable anhydrous forms, the former converting to the stable anhydrate during storage, which leads to a lowering of the dissolution rate of tablets [93]. Poor control of drying process can lead to formation of such intermediate high energy forms that may compromise product performance either by having different physicochemical properties of their own or simply by reconverting to a more stable form that is undesirable.

3.3.2 Fluidized-Bed Drying

3.3.2.1 Description

Fluidized-bed drying is one of the most prevalent drying technologies used in small molecule formulation development and is the operation of choice for drying of granules obtained during wet granulation to be filled into capsules or compressed into tablets. In a fluidized-bed dryer, gas stream (heating medium) is passed from the bottom through a bed of particulate matter. At low air velocities, the bed remains static on a gas distributor plate. The fluidizing gas is uniformly distributed throughout the bed as it passes through the distributor. As the gas velocity is increased, the pressure gradually drops across the solid bed, and ultimately the entire bed is mobilized, i.e. fluidized in the gas stream, which supports the entire mass of the solid bed. This condition is known as the minimum fluidization condition, and the corresponding gas velocity is known as minimum fluidization velocity (u_{mf}). Typically fluidized-bed dryers are operated at 2–4 u_{mf}, with variations occurring according to the nature of the feed bed and the moisture content. After passing through the particulate bed, the gas stream enters the filter system to separate the fines from the exiting gas stream for external discharge. Sometimes, the exiting gas stream is partially recycled to save energy [11]. The kinetics of drying of pharmaceutical granules comprises of two stages: (i) stage 1 that is limited by heat transfer and involves the evaporation of surface or loosely bound water from the surface of granules and (ii) stage 2 that is diffusion limited and involves the diffusion of moisture from the granule core to its surface prior to evaporation. Each of these stages has a different time dependency and has been thoroughly modeled in previous studies [94]. Figure 3.6 shows a schematic of the fluidized-bed dryer consisting of a gas blower, heater, fluidization column, bag filters, precipitator, and scrubber. The dryer's body includes an

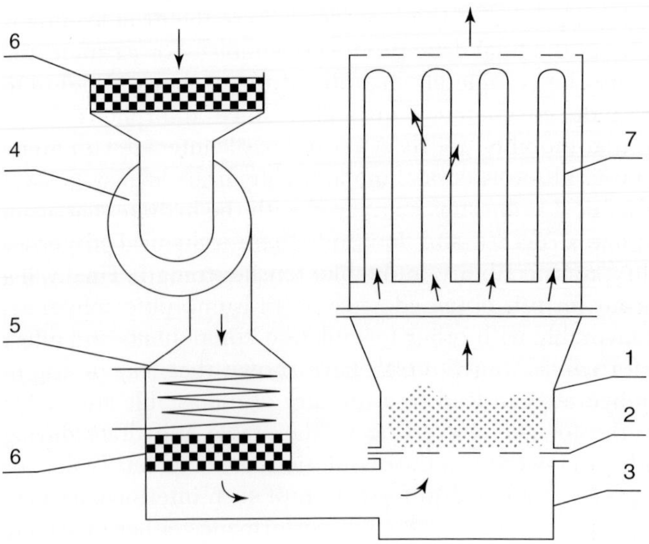

Figure 3.6 Schematic of a batch fluidized-bed dryer. (1) Fluidizing chamber. (2) Gas distributor. (3) Plenum chamber. (4) Blower. (5) Heater. (6) Filters. (7) Bag dust collector. Source: Mujumdar 2014 [11]. Reproduced with permission of Taylor & Francis.

air distribution chamber and an aerial exhaust air outlet opening to an emissions control system (cyclone or baghouse) for safe disposal of dust-laden air. There is a feed inlet for the bulk material and a regulated discharge outlet to obtain the dried solids. Fluidized-bed dryers can operate both in batch and continuous mode, the latter often being equipped with a vibrating base for the continuous movement of the solid bed [85].

Although a wide variety of materials are dried by fluidization, aeratable and sand-like particles are easier to fluidize when dry or partially dry, whereas fines (submicron range particles) and dense solids are difficult to fluidize due to strong cohesive forces in the former and bubbling of the bulk solid bed in the latter. The following are some characteristics of materials suitable for fluidized-bed drying [85]:

(1) Particles with size ranging from 20 μm to 10 mm are amenable to fluidized-bed drying. Submicron particles tend to clump together due to larger surface area, whereas larger particles may cause slugging when fluidization is applied.
(2) Particle size distribution needs to be sufficiently narrow to ensure that majority of the particles are fluidized and loss by entrainment is minimized.
(3) Larger spherical particles are preferred for efficient fluidization.
(4) Hard aggregates or lumps are undesirable since they may adversely affect the fluidity of the powder bed.
(5) Particles must have sufficient mechanical strength to tolerate the vigorous mixing action in the dryer.
(6) The final product should not be sticky at the outlet temperature for efficient discharge of the dried product.

3.3.2.2 Determination of End Point of Drying

The end point of drying is determined based on granule moisture content and size [95, 96]. Granules moisture content affects several bulk properties and performance such as granule breakage, flowability, friability, ease and speed of compaction, hardness, and ultimately disintegration of granules [96]. Granule size affects granule porosity and flowability. In addition, excess drying can cause generation of fines and subsequent product loss by entrainment in the airstream. As a result, these two parameters must be monitored and controlled effectively to ensure reliability of final dried solids. Unlike tray drying, where offline measurement, i.e. loss on drying, is conducted on aliquots removed periodically, fluidized-bed drying is an energy-intensive process, and therefore online measurement techniques are preferred to minimize energy usage by identifying optimal drying conditions [97]. Online monitoring also provides the added advantage of in-depth understanding of the process to improve standard operating procedures and to meet product quality specifications [96]. There are several studies in the literature exemplifying online monitoring of fluidized-bed drying by using process analytical techniques to monitor water content in the granule bed. For example, Buschmüller et al. developed microwave resonance sensors to reliably, accurately, and continuously monitor the water content in placebo granules dried in a GPCG-15 fluidized-bed dryer. This moisture measurement was conducted independently of product density, and the moisture content values so obtained during drying correlated well with those obtained using offline techniques such as loss on drying by infrared spectroscopy (LOD/IR) and Karl Fischer titration (Figure 3.7) [98]. Liu et al. employed near-infrared spectroscopy (NIR) for online determination of the residual moisture content of anhydrous dibasic calcium phosphate upon drying and found the data to agree well with offline LOD measurements [97]. Nieuwmeyer et al. used inline NIR measurements successfully to determine both moisture content and median granule size during drying by employing chemometrics. The NIR-based water model so developed was effective in distinguishing between different stages of drying, i.e. the constant rate period, the falling rate period, and the equilibrium

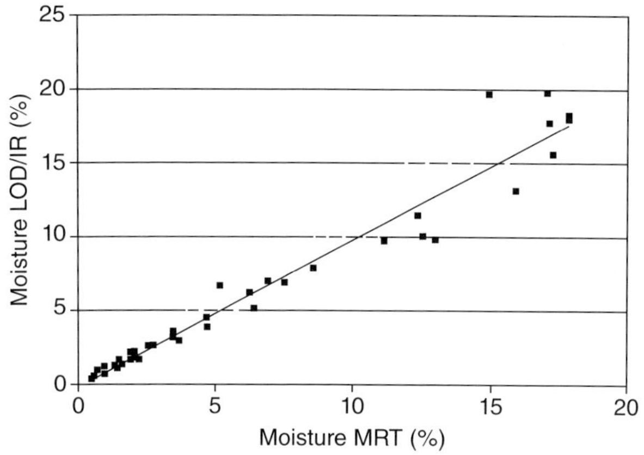

Figure 3.7 Correlation of moisture content as monitored in-line by microwave resonance technology (MRT) vs. that obtained by offline LOD/IR. Regression line $R^2 = 0.976$. Source: Buschmüller et al. 2008 [98]. Reproduced with permission of Elsevier.

period, and provided a reliable and faster determination of the drying end point compared with offline techniques [95].

3.3.2.3 Advantages, Utility, and Drawbacks

Owing to the fluidization principle, the solid particles are intimately mixed with the stream of air/gas, thereby allowing for efficient heat and mass transfer, which also leads to shorter drying time and a resultant solid bed homogeneous in temperature and moisture. Efficiency of heat and mass transfer enabled by fluidization also allows for drying of heat-sensitive materials at lower temperatures over relatively shorter periods of time compared with other adiabatic dryers. Additionally, due to the presence of fewer mechanical components, the maintenance cost is low. The ease and low cost of operation, ease of handling feed, flexibility of use in either batch or continuous mode, rapid heat transfer between gas and fluidized particles that minimizes overheating, and ease of material transport within the dryer make it an attractive choice for the industry [11, 85]. A fluidized-bed dryer can be modified in several ways to accommodate different kinds of solids for drying. Vibration may be applied for materials that are too wet to be fluidized, and a spouting mode (use of a high velocity gas jet to dislodge particles) may be added for larger particles that exhibit slugging under normal fluidization [11]. As mentioned before, fluidized-bed granulation and spray coating are the two other variants of this drying technique, both widely used in the pharmaceutical industry [82, 99, 100]. Fluidized-bed granulation is a "one-pot" enclosed process where a binder solution is sprayed from the top on particles that are fluidized to cause size enhancement via liquid bridging. Once the desired agglomerate size is reached, the drying process starts to evaporate solvent and produce granules. This method is highly favored in the pharmaceutical industry due to elimination of dust. Wurster fluidized-bed drying is another modification of this operation where a coating solution is bottom-sprayed on the fluidized bed for coating particles either to mask the bitter taste of the active or for layering purposes to create sustained release formulations [101–103]. The rapid mixing of solids in a fluidized-bed dryer can potentially be utilized for more intimate mixing of API and excipients in a formulation blend.

Disadvantages of fluidized-bed drying include the following: (i) energy-intensive process with high electricity consumption, (ii) unsuitability for very fine or large particles and sticky materials, and (iii) pulverization by attrition that may be caused by overheating. This causes generation of fines and subsequent entrainment of these fine particles by air, leading to substantial product loss [11, 85]. For small molecule pharmaceuticals, there is an additional challenge of changes in the solid-state form that may be brought about during moisture removal, which may have a bearing on product functionality. For example, fluid-bed drying of risedronate sodium hemipentahydrate (a mixed hydrate with both lattice and channel water) below a critical water activity value led to the complete removal of its channel water. When granules were made from the partially dehydrated hydrate compressed into tablets that were later exposed to humidity (60–70% RH), water was rapidly absorbed into the channels, resulting in noticeable swelling of the tablets and loss of tablet integrity in extreme cases (Figure 3.8). This was brought about by expansion of lattice parameters upon

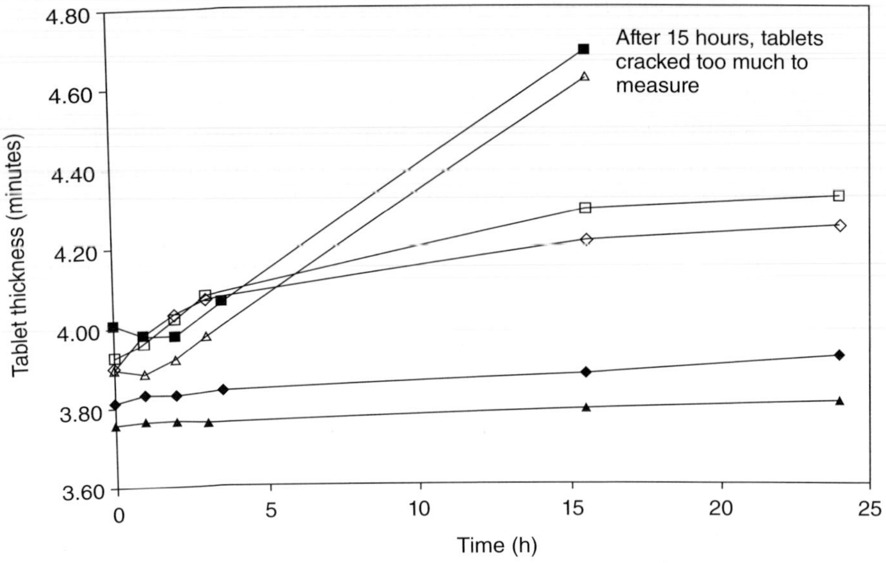

Figure 3.8 Effect of risedronate sodium rehydration on tablet thickness upon exposure to 60% RH (22 °C). The tablets showing marked increase in thickness and therefore cracking were the ones with the lowest granule water content of 1.13 (♦) and 1.46 (Δ) % w/w post fluid-bed drying. Source: Hausman et al. 2005 [104]. Reproduced with permission of Elsevier.

rehydration of the lattice channels, a phenomenon that is commonly observed in nonstoichiometric and/or channel hydrates [104–106]. In another study, the stable polymorphic form A of fosinopril sodium underwent a polymorphic transformation to the metastable form B upon rapid drying of a nonaqueous granulation mass since rapid drying kinetics often favors the trapping of a metastable phase [94]. As with other adiabatic or directly heated dryers where heat transfer occurs directly between the heating medium and the solid particles, it is necessary to construct a detailed phase diagram pertaining to polymorph stability (temperature vs. free energy or solubility) and hydrate–anhydrate stability (water activity vs. moisture content and form at a given temperature) to judiciously design the drying space. This will help to avoid any inadvertent phase transitions during the drying process.

3.3.3 Spray Drying

3.3.3.1 Description

Spray drying is a one-step continuous drying operation where a liquid or thin slurry feed is pumped into a hot chamber consisting of a gaseous drying medium and is converted into droplets via atomization when passed through an atomization device (single or dual fluid or rotating disk nozzles) located at the top of the air chamber [11]. Atomization converts the liquid to individual droplets that are then evaporated when they come in contact with the heating air. The resulting solids ultimately get collected using a cyclone separator or bag filter as dried powder. The airflow may be concurrent or countercurrent with respect to droplet movement. Owing to the intimate contact between droplets and the surrounding air, heat and mass transfer rates are high. Additionally, atomization brings about an increase in the interfacial surface area, resulting in high evaporation rates. These factors allow for a very short residence time of the droplets (5–30 seconds). Since the material is maintained at its wet bulb temperature for the majority of the drying period, higher heating temperatures can be used for thermolabile materials [1]. Short residence times lead to effective preservation of organoleptic properties of materials, and the end products, i.e. dried particles, are usually hollow or porous with low density, spherical in shape and with narrow particle size distribution [35]. For pharmaceuticals, spray drying leads to generation of fine particles that are then mixed with suitable excipients and compressed into tablets [11]. Advantages of this drying technique include continuous operation, complete automation of the operation, process flexibility, and short residence time enabling drying of heat-sensitive materials. Low thermal efficiency leading to high energy consumption, drying-induced solid-state phase transformation (changes in crystallinity, degree of solvation, and polymorphic form), low yield at laboratory scale (20–75%) owing to product deposition on drying chamber wall, high maintenance cost due to clogging of nozzles, and unsuitability of use for hygroscopic and thermoplastic materials are some of the drawbacks associated with this drying technique [107–109]. There are several spray-dryer designs available such as (i) open cycle, where drying medium is air and is discharged after use, and (ii) closed cycle, where organic solvents are used in the feed and therefore nitrogen is used as the drying medium that is recirculated and the solvents are recovered. Dryers may also be available where the drying air has reduced oxygen content to dry highly inflammable materials: (iii) semi-closed cycle and d) with or without aseptic control [29, 69]. A detailed description of the spray-drying operation has been provided chapter elsewhere in this book.

3.3.3.2 Role in Formulation Development

Spray drying is a versatile process and has been widely used to alter and control a range of properties such as particle size, shape, bulk density, porosity, moisture content, flowability, compression properties, physical form stability, and friability [110]. The following are some of the key aspects of small molecule drug product development impacted by this drying technique.

Impact on Physical Form For crystalline actives where the free form is poorly soluble and salts are not viable for manufacturing, an intentional change in the physical form, i.e. amorphization, is one of the routes employed to improve *in vivo* exposure owing to the apparent higher solubility of the amorphous state. Spray drying has been effectively utilized in this regard for scale-up and bulk conversion of crystalline to amorphous active. Essentially, the atomization and flash evaporation of the active in solution (typically organic solvents are used to dissolve API with poor aqueous solubility) leads to generation of the amorphous form, i.e. vitrification of the solid. Drying parameters such as feed concentration, inlet air temperature, and atomization conditions can influence the extent of amorphous formation. For example, Chidavaenzi et al. showed an increase in the feed concentration of an aqueous solution of lactose monohydrate to have an

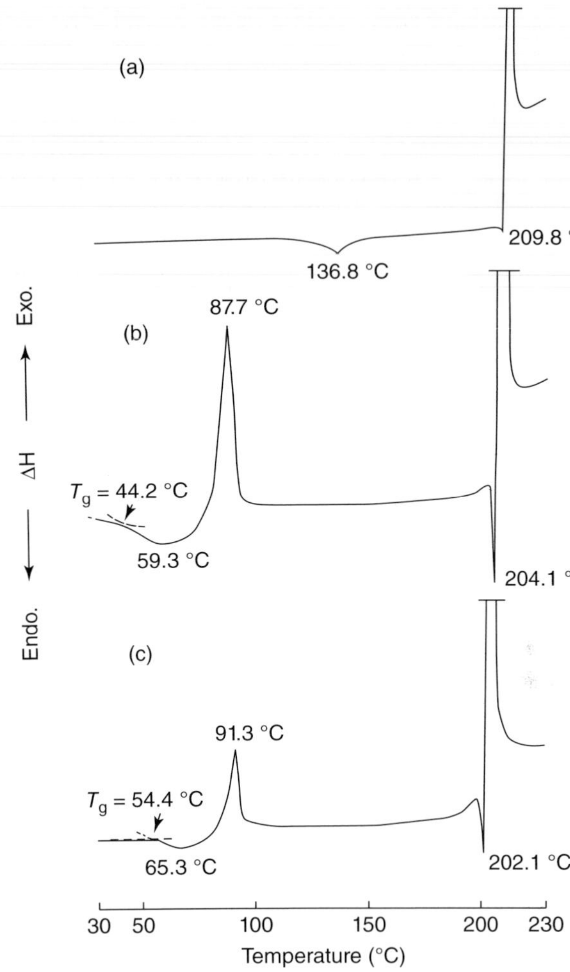

Figure 3.9 DSC traces of frusemide solid forms. (a) Crystalline form I. (b) Amorphous form A. (c) Amorphous form B. The two amorphous forms were obtained upon spray drying. Source: Matsuda et al. 1992 [112]. Reproduced with permission of John Wiley & Sons.

inverse effect on the amorphous content in the final dry powder [111]. Matsuda et al. showed that spray drying of frusemide at 50 or 150 °C resulted in two different amorphous forms A and B with different glass transition temperatures (44 °C for form A vs. 54 °C for form B) and activation energies for crystallization, as depicted in Figure 3.9 [112]. Spraying-drying of a dichloromethane solution of MAT [4″-0-(4-methoxyphenyl acetyltylosin] resulted in formation of amorphous phases with marked differences in crystallization propensity, i.e. different recrystallization temperatures (T_c) and heat of recrystallization (ΔH_c), depending on the inlet temperature ranging from 50 to 160 °C [113]. All of these forms had the same IR spectra and showed little scatter in their T_g values (102–103 °C). Both T_c and ΔH_c were found to be low when the inlet air temperature was greater or lesser than the T_g of the amorphous form. The most stable amorphous forms, with the highest T_c and ΔH_c values, were those obtained when the inlet air temperature was maintained between T_g and T_c. The most famous example of amorphization, albeit partial, via spray drying is possibly that of directly compressible, spray-dried lactose where change in physical form causes marked improvement in its compressibility. This directly compressible lactose is obtained by spray drying a suspension of α-lactose monohydrate crystals in a saturated lactose solution and then sieving the dried particles to obtain a size distribution for achieving the desired flow and tableting properties. Spray-dried lactose consists of predominantly crystalline lactose monohydrate (depending on the drying conditions) with the 9–12% w/w remaining being amorphous lactose [114]. This unique internal structure, wherein the crystals are embedded in an amorphous matrix, leads to improved plasticity and binding during tableting resulting in harder tablets with decreased friability and also disintegration times that are independent of the applied compression force [115]. Another example of a beneficial physical form change via spray drying was demonstrated by Martino et al. for the poorly compressible compound, acetaminophen. Spray drying of this active led to formation of a mixture of forms I and II, which showed a marked improvement in compressibility compared with the individual pure forms. The spherical shape and minor surface roughness of the spray-dried particles contributed to improved compressibility, whereas the intrinsic elasticity of the pure forms hindered compression [116].

However not all form changes are desirable or intentional, and spray drying has been shown to inadvertently alter the polymorphic form and/or state of solvation of a crystalline active [110]. Owing to the rapid drying of the atomized droplets, a metastable state, unobtainable by crystallization or other methods, may be formed in the dried solid. Therefore spray drying often emerges as a route for manufacturing of metastable or rare polymorphic forms. Since conversion of the metastable form to the stable form in the final drug product during storage may lead to changes in product properties and performance, continuous monitoring of the drying process and characterization of the final dry powder is required to assess the nature and extent of phase transformation, if any. There are several literature examples on spray drying-induced form changes. For example, in the case of phenylbutazone, spray drying from methylene chloride solution led to formation of different polymorphs (α, β and ε), depending on the drying temperature of the droplets. Of these, form ε was the rare polymorphic form that could not be obtained previously from any recrystallization method [117, 118]. Similarly, spray drying of an ethanolic solution of phenobarbitone (form II) resulted in the formation of polymorphic form III, irrespective of changes in the feed concentration, the spraying solvent composition, and inlet and outlet temperatures [119]. Likewise, griseofulvin, an antifungal agent, was found to form a solvate with chloroform when it was used as a spraying solvent [120]. Hulse et al. showed that spray drying of different commercial brands of D-mannitol (excipient used for tablet compression) existing either as the α-polymorph or a mixture of α and β resulted in complete conversion to the β-form upon drying [121]. Furthermore, Lee et al. showed that the polymorphic composition was particle size dependent when spray drying a 10% ethanol solution of mannitol. Fast evaporation of smaller droplets led to greater amount of metastable form α, while slow evaporation of larger droplets with enough moisture resulted in the stable β-form [41]. Yu and Ng have shown a strong dependence of the final solid form of glycine (salt and polymorphs) on pH of its aqueous spraying solution. At a pH of 6.2 (unadjusted solution pH), α-glycine was obtained, whereas γ-glycine, the

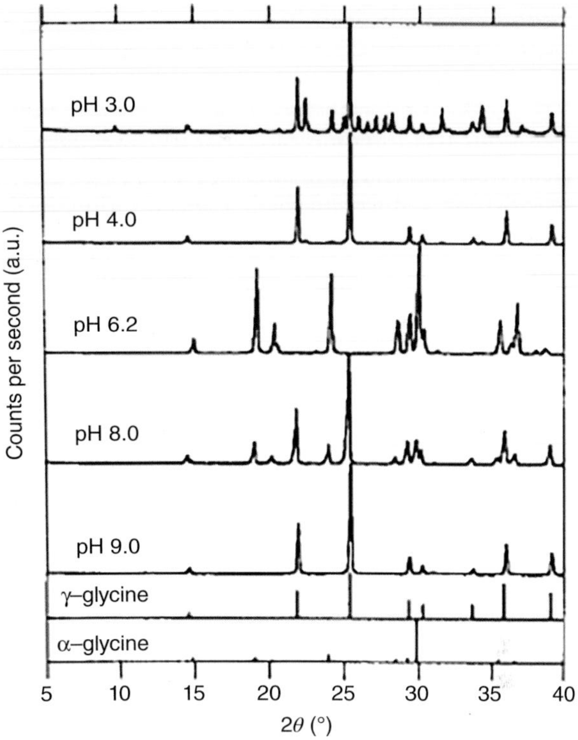

Figure 3.10 XRPD patterns depicting the effect of pH on the polymorphism of glycine free form. The patterns of α- and γ-glycine are included as reference. At the neutral pH of 6.2, α-glycine was obtained, whereas pH adjustment to 4 or 8 led to formation of the thermodynamically stable γ-form. Source: Yu and Ng 2002 [122]. Reproduced with permission of John Wiley & Sons.

thermodynamically most stable form, was obtained when the pH was adjusted to 4 or 8. This was a novel finding since β-glycine was always the preferred polymorph obtained upon lyophilization of a solution containing the neutral zwitterion. Since the γ-glycine form is the most stable of all three polymorphs, the authors proposed the use of spray drying using pH adjustment as a route to stabilize formulations containing glycine [122]. This dependence of polymorphic composition on pH is shown in Figure 3.10.

Particle Engineering One of the main advantages of spray drying lies in the ability to control a range of pharmaceutically relevant powder properties such as particle size and size distribution, morphology, surface roughness, texture, bulk density, porosity, flowability, moisture content, dispersibility, wettability, breaking strength, disintegration, dissolution, and compression properties [29]. Optimization of spray-drying process variables not only leads to design of a more efficient drying condition but also provides in-depth understanding of the process and effective particle engineering to meet the target product quality and performance attributes.

Spray drying has four distinct steps: atomization of the feed, sprayed droplet-air contact, drying of the atomized droplets, and finally the separation of the dried particles from the airstream. These steps are influenced by several process variables such as inlet air temperature, inlet air moisture content, feed concentration, feed rate, airflow rate, outlet temperature, and atomization pressure [111], all of which can have an impact on the final product properties and performance. For example, an increase in the atomization pressure at constant feed rate leads to generation of smaller, high density particles, whereas increasing the feed rate at constant operation conditions leads to formation of coarse particles with higher moisture content due to inefficient drying. Increase in the feed concentration leads to increase in feed viscosity that in turn leads to formation of a coarser spray and ultimately larger particles with greater bulk density. An increase in feed temperature may help to reduce the viscosity of a slurry or high concentration feed and may lead to formation of smaller droplets by atomization [123]. The type of atomizer used can also have an impact on particle size, such as plain-jet air-blast atomizers producing smaller droplets, and therefore finer particles in the respirable size range for dry powder inhalers compared with ultrasonic atomizers [124]. Variations in the feed solvent, feed composition, outlet drying temperature, and atomization rate can lead to tailoring of particle shape and surface properties [125–128]. Proper humidity control of the drying medium can lead to tailoring of the densities and aerodynamic properties of particles to be used for inhalation purposes, and drying conditions can also be maintained at dew point temperatures ranging from 0 to −40 °C [129]. Elversson et al. demonstrated the relationship between droplet and particle size for inhalable lactose by showing that atomization nozzle orifice size and airflow controlled droplet size. However, both droplet size and feed concentration influenced particle size, the latter having a nonlinear effect on the size of the dried particles. It was also shown that the shell thickness of the hollow spray-dried lactose particles increased with an increase in feed concentration [130]. In a separate study using several carbohydrates (lactose, mannitol, sucrose/dextran 4 : 1 mixture), it was shown that the particle size of these sugars increased with an increase in droplet size (with wider nozzle orifices) and feed concentration up to 5% w/w. Particles obtained from dilute feed solutions (1–5% w/w) were relatively more hygroscopic than those obtained from concentrated feeds. In terms of particle density, smaller droplet size led to finer particles with higher densities compared with larger particles. The solid state of the sugars influenced the particle surface roughness with amorphous lactose and sucrose/dextran particles having smooth surfaces while crystalline mannitol particles having substantial surface corrugations [131].

There are several studies in the literature demonstrating particle engineering via spray drying for the development of dry powder inhalers (DPI). The optimization of the drying parameters provides a means to tailor the particle size distribution, shape, and surface properties for carriers mixed with micronized active in DPI for their effective delivery to the deep lung. Although lactose monohydrate has been traditionally used as a carrier, it has some inherent drawbacks such as undesirable reaction (Maillard reaction) with primary amino group containing actives (e.g. budesonide) and variations in product quality during processing and storage. In addition lactose undergoes complete or partial amorphization during spray drying that may affect the adhesion between carrier and active particles. Therefore other sugars have been explored as carriers of choice, and spray drying has been utilized as viable technique to alter the properties of these carrier particles by optimizing the process variables [132]. For example, Littringer et al. have shown spray-dried mannitol to be an effective carrier for salbutamol sulfate in DPI by altering the surface properties of the carrier particles upon changing the outlet temperature in a pilot-scale spray dryer. Although spray drying generally produces spherical, hollow particles owing to high evaporation rates, it was seen that changes in the outlet temperature not only altered the surface roughness of the particles but also changed their shape. Lower outlet temperatures (67–80 °C) produce smooth, spherical particles, and higher temperatures (84–102 °C) produces partially collapsed raisin-like particles with increased surface roughness. Changes in particle shape and surface roughness were found to affect the fine particle fraction (FPF), i.e. the amount of active being delivered to the deep lung. The highest FPFs were obtained with rough, spherical particles, whereas decrease in surface roughness and/or irregular-shaped particles with cavities led to a decrease in the FPF [133]. Furthermore, Littringer et al. used a full factorial design to determine the effect of spray-drying process variables on the surface topography, size, breaking strength, and solid-state form of mannitol carrier particles to be used in dry powder inhalers. The factors examined were feed concentration, feed rate, heater temperature, and atomization rotation speed. The study revealed that surface roughness was affected by both outlet air temperatures (influenced by high heater temperature and feed rate) as well as feed concentration. High outlet air temperature and low feed rate produced smoother particles, whereas increase in feed concentration led to an increase in surface roughness (Figure 3.11). Median particle size was influenced by both atomizer rotation speed and feed concentration with higher speeds and lower concentration, resulting in smaller particle size. The breaking strength of particles (required to be a minimum to maintain particle stability during preparation, dosing, and administration of DPI) was found to increase with increase in heater temperature and was found to decrease with an increase in feed rate. Mannitol precipitated as crystalline form I under all conditions with changes in process variables having no impact on the form or crystallinity [133].

Spray drying is also frequently employed to manufacture co-processed excipients, used in direct compression of tablets, with superior compressibility and compactibility compared to the starting materials [134]. Here too, process parameters can be optimized to obtain particles with improved tableting properties. For example, Gonnissen et al. used a mixture of acetaminophen, a poorly compressible active, and several tableting excipients to obtain a "ready-to-compress" mixture for tableting by co-spraying a suspension of these ingredients. The impact of the feed concentration was assessed, and it was found that increasing the feed solids concentration increased the median particle size (by increasing feed viscosity and producing larger droplets), caused lowering of the particle moisture content and these two factors coupled to lower the bulk density. Larger particle size led to increased particle collision and agglomeration. Increase in feed solids concentration led to increased yield, reduced tensile tablet strength due to increased tablet porosity, and shortening of disintegration times. Finally, 27.2% w/w solids concentration was chosen for further optimization since it provided high process yield, short disintegration time, and excellent particle flowability. At this feed concentration, it was observed that the median particle size was affected by both inlet and outlet air temperatures, with a decrease in size observed with increasing outlet temperature (at constant inlet air temperature) and size enhancement observed upon increased inlet air temperature (with a constant outlet air temperature) [135]. Increased inlet air temperature also caused lowering of the bulk density of

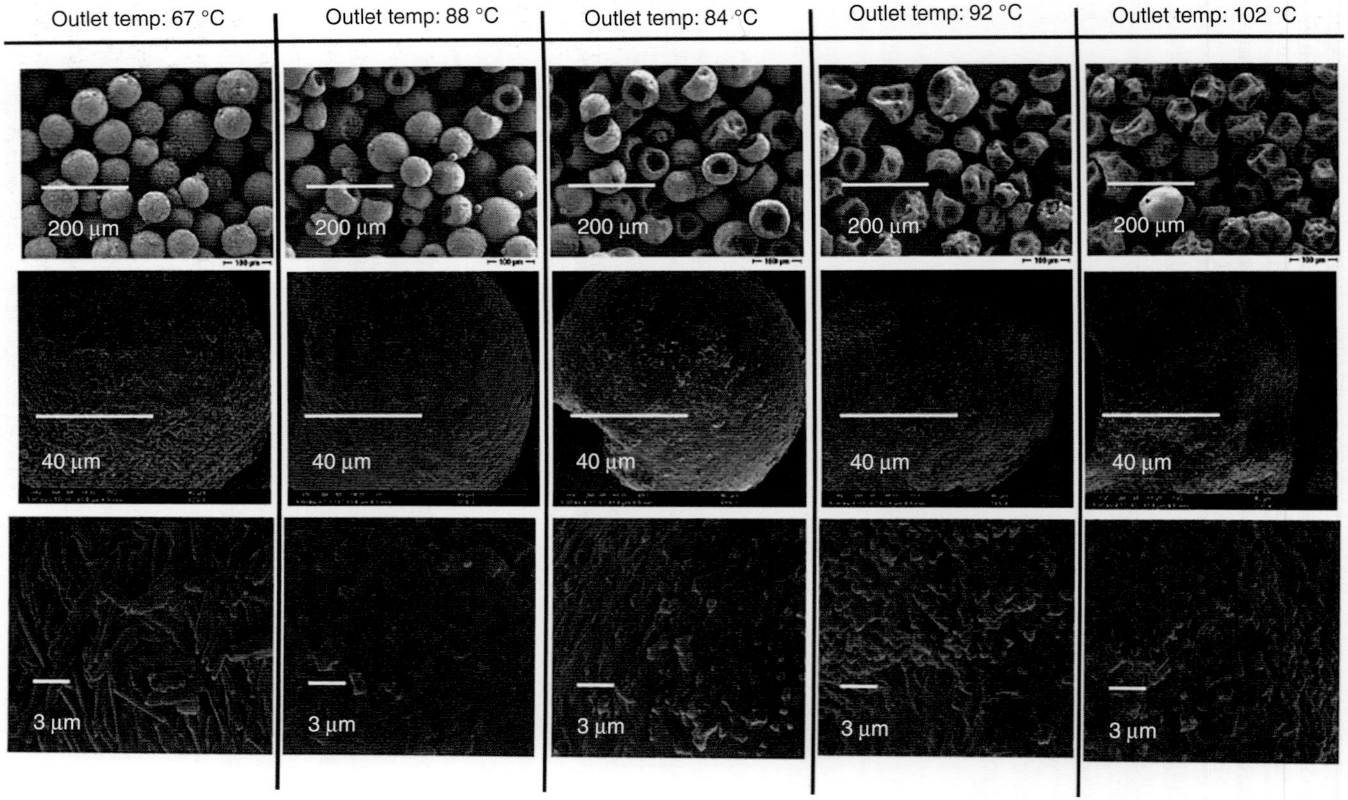

Figure 3.11 *Scanning electron microscopy (SEM) micrographs of mannitol spray-dried particles showing the effect of outlet temperature on particle morphology and surface roughness. Source: Littringer et al. 2012 [133]. Reproduced with permission of Elsevier.*

the particles attributed to case hardening of the droplets followed by expansion of the trapped air [136]. Low outlet air temperatures increased the moisture content of the granules but decreased the overall yield. Finally, a higher particle flowability index was obtained at lower drying temperatures (inlet, 170 °C; outlet, 60 °C) vs. higher drying temperatures (inlet, 230 °C; outlet, 90 °C). Based on these data, a numerical optimization was performed using statistical models to identify the parameters providing lowest residual moisture content and highest yield to further scale up the co-processed mixture [135]. A list of various spray-drying process parameters and their effect on particle properties is summarized in Table 3.2 to provide a comprehensive overview of "tunability" of particle properties by optimization of drying conditions [30].

Table 3.2 Spray-drying parameters and their importance.

Parameters	Importance in spray drying
Process	
Inlet air temperature	Increase in inlet temperature increases yield and produced less sticky particles with low moisture content
Outlet air temperature	Inversely affects final product moisture content
Humidity of drying gas	Impacts particle cohesion and moisture content; may reduce yield
Solution/suspension feed rate	Increase in feed rate forms coarser particles with higher moisture content due to inefficient drying
Drying gas flow	High gas flow decreases outlet temperature, produces smaller droplets, and therefore lowers particle size
Actuator design	Regulates airflow into the spray chamber to enhance drying precision and regulate particle size
Atomization pressure (commonly used fluid nozzles)	Increase in atomization pressure at constant feed rate results in formation of smaller, high density particles
Formulation	
Feed composition (API/excipients/solvents)	Affects particle size, morphology, cohesive properties, and solid-state form
Solvent type (organic/hydroalcoholic/aqueous)	Affects particle rheology, porosity, density, morphology, crystallinity, solid-state form, atomization conditions, and therefore size
% w/w solid content in spray solution	Affects crystallinity of the final product
Feed viscosity	Affects rate of evaporation and particle size
Surface tension of spray solution	Lower surface tension leads to generation of smaller particles

Source: Patel et al. 2015 [30]. Reproduced with emission of Elsevier.

Drug Delivery via Enabling Formulations Spray drying has been successfully used as a manufacturing technique for several targeted drug delivery systems and formulation-mediated solubility enhancement approaches. Some of these approaches are discussed in this section.

(A) *Solubility enhancement*: For oral solid drug product development, ASDs offer a viable path to administer BCS class II drugs (high permeability and low solubility) when salt formation is not viable. The poorly soluble active is molecularly dispersed in the amorphous form in a carrier matrix, which can be a polymer or a lipid or other carriers such as β-cyclodextrin or carbohydrates or silica particles. The high energy of the amorphous state leads to increased solubility and therefore increased bioavailability. Judicious choice of the carrier is required to maintain sufficient supersaturation and stabilization of the amorphous API via inhibition of crystallization. In recent years, spray drying has evolved to be the preferred solvent-based technique to manufacture ASDs owing to its continuous operation, relative ease of scale-up, and cost-effectiveness [137]. Arias et al. have shown that a spray-dried dispersion of triamterene (active) and D-mannitol (carrier) showed faster dissolution compared with the dispersion obtained by melting the carrier owing to amorphization of the active and strong drug–carrier interaction [138]. In spray drying, the active is co-sprayed with a suitable carrier, and rapid evaporation of the atomized feed causes the API to precipitate in the amorphous form and be kinetically trapped in the polymer matrix. This method often results in the formation of a supersaturated molecular dispersion with the carrier acting as the crystallization inhibitor/stabilizer [137, 139]. The spray-dried particles are then further co-processed in various ways for inclusion in either immediate or controlled release tablets or capsules. Being a solvent-based method, spray drying allows for the use of polymers with high glass transition temperatures (such as polyvinyl pyrrolidone), which could not have otherwise been employed in manufacturing ASD by the conventional melting technique without the use of a plasticizer [140]. A comprehensive list of examples from the literature for spray-dried dispersions with the API, carriers (such as vinyl polymers, cellulosic polymers, polyethylene oxide and derivatives, lipidic carriers, and acrylate polymers), molecular weights of the carriers, the solvent system used, solubility parameters, ASD hygroscopicity (75% RH, RT), and their glass transitions/melting temperatures has been provided by Paudel et al. [137].

Co-carriers comprising of a polymer blend are sometimes employed for preparing solid dispersions. Here, the different polymers adopt different stabilization roles and must be chosen based on their solubility in organic solvents and binary or ternary interactions in the feed solution. Al-Obaidi et al. prepared solid dispersions of proton acceptors such as griseofulvin, progesterone, or phenindione with polyvinylpyrrolidone (PVP), another proton-accepting polymer, and an additional polymer, poly(*N*-(2-hydroxypropyl)methacrylamide) (PHPMA), which acted as both hydrogen bond acceptor and donor. Inclusion of this second polymer resulted in marked improvement in the physical stability of these immiscible ASDs by promoting miscibility [141, 142]. PHPMA was also found to cooperatively strengthen the H-bonding between griseofulvin and hydroxypropyl methylcellulose acetate succinate (HPMC-AS), a proton-donating polymer, thereby increasing physical stability with minimum impact on dissolution [143]. Ternary ASDs were also prepared by spray drying using components other than stabilizers to facilitate downstream manufacturing. These are surfactants, glidants, pH modifiers, or disintegrants and are being included to improve post-processability by modifying the particulate and bulk properties of the ASD such as wettability and flowability. Inclusion of functional excipients in the preparation of ASD can affect solubility, drug-stabilizer interaction in solution, and mode of particle formation owing to changes in the solvent evaporation rate during drying. The latter can have significant impact on particle properties such as size, morphology, texture, and surface energetics and therefore on final crystallinity, miscibility, and the physical stability of the ternary dispersions compared with their binary counterparts [137]. Janssens et al. have reported increased dissolution in ternary dispersions of itraconazole with PVP-VA64 and polymeric surfactant such as Inutec® SP1 compared with the binary ASD without the surfactant. This increased dissolution was attributed to increase in solubilization via the surfactant's ability to promote wettability of the active [144–147]. In another example, addition of adsorbent such as Aerosil® 200 (fumed silica) as a drying aid helped to improve the flowability of spray-dried dispersion of simvastatin (a low T_g drug) with PVP [22].

Owing to feasibility of particle engineering via spray drying, this technique has been used for other solubility enhancement approaches, such as drying of nanosuspensions to yield nanoparticles or nanocrystalline dispersions of poorly soluble API [148–150]. Hecq et al. utilized spray drying to obtain dry powder nanoparticles from a nanosuspension of the poorly soluble API nifedipine. Mannitol was used as a carrier to prevent particle agglomeration and facilitate wettability and redispersion of the nanoparticles. Nifedipine nanoparticles were found to show a significant improvement in dissolution rate over unmilled commercial API with 95% of the nanoparticles being dissolved within 60 minutes compared with only 5% of the unmilled API (Figure 3.12) [71]. Other solubility enhancement approaches such as formation of co-crystals or SEDDS can also be pursued via spray drying. Co-crystals, which are a molecular complex comprising stoichiometric ratios of two molecular or ionic compounds exhibiting non-covalent interactions, have been shown to demonstrate improved *in vivo* performance either via faster dissolution or greater solubility [151]. Owing to some of their purported advantages, co-crystals are now increasingly being pursued as an alternate solid form for drug product development. Alhalaweh and Velaga demonstrated spray drying as a feasible method of co-crystal formation by spraying stoichiometric ratios of carbamazepine and glutaric acid. In contrast to the conventional solvent evaporation method where a mixture of phases of co-crystal and pure components were obtained, spray drying produced pure co-crystals. The authors

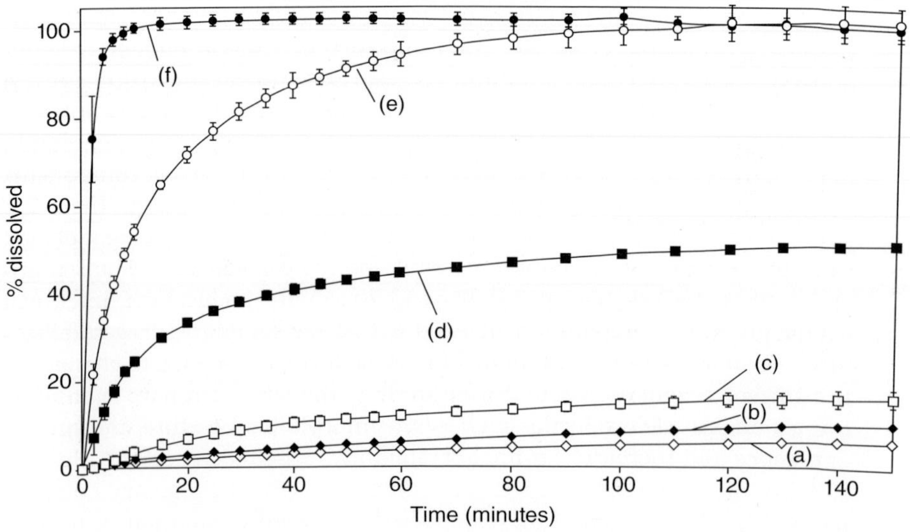

Figure 3.12 Dissolution profiles of different nifedipine formulations in deionized water (pH 7, 37 °C). The profiles shown are that of (a) unmilled commercial nifedipine, (b) nifedipine–HPMC physical mixture, (c) spray-dried mannitol-less nanoparticles with no milling, (d) spray-dried mannitol-less nanoparticles with Turrax® milling, (e) spray-dried mannitol-less nanoparticles with high pressure homogenizer milling, and (f): spray-dried mannitol-containing nanoparticles with high pressure homogenizer milling. Mannitol prevents particle agglomeration and promotes faster dissolution. Source: Hecq et al. 2005 [71]. Reproduced with permission of Elsevier.

postulated the formation of pure co-crystals could either be a kinetically controlled phenomenon or driven by the intermediate glassy state [66]. SEDDS is another solubility enhancement approach via solubilization of a poorly water-soluble API. Here the API is dissolved in a blend of a lipidic component such as triglycerides or partial glycerides, and a surfactant or cosurfactant, which when it comes in contact with the gastrointestinal fluids, causes the API to be dispersed into fine particles to aid absorption [152]. SEDDS have been primarily used as liquids or in capsules, but these approaches have several drawbacks such as high manufacturing cost, patient compliance issues, storage stability (precipitation of API or excipients at lower temperatures), and incompatibility with soft gelatin capsules [78, 153]. An alternate approach is to use solid SNEDDS/SMEDDS (self-nanoemulsifying drug delivery systems or self-microemulsifying drug delivery systems) by removal of water from liquid SNEDDS formulation. For example, Kang et al. have shown that spray drying of a liquid SNEDDS formulation of flurbiprofen in polyvinyl acetate (PVA), Na-CMC, and HP-β-CD resulted in the formation of a solid dispersion [72]. Similarly, Yi et al. obtained a solid SMEDDS by spray drying a liquid formulation ethyl oleate, Labrasol®, Cremophor® RH 40, and the active nimodipine using dextran 40 as a carrier [78]. Comparison of the droplet size of the microemulsions formed by solid and liquid SMEDDS revealed no difference when examined by transmission electron microscope and photo correlation spectrometer. The efficacy of a solid SEDDS is measured by its reconstitution efficiency and bioavailability compared with the liquid SEDDS. Thus a judicious choice of a suitable spray-drying carrier/bulking agent is required since it affects the crystallinity, dissolution, and therefore bioavailability of the solid SEDDS. A carrier able to maintain the desired API particle size and minimize particle agglomeration is preferred [72].

(B) *Sustained release*: Besides immediate release formulations, spray drying can be effectively harnessed to prepare sustained release products where the API release is modulated to prolong its effect. Bhalekar et al. formulated glipizide (used orally for the treatment of type II diabetes and administered either as BID or TID) as microspheres by spray-drying since they are suitable as oral sustained release formulation with minimized risk of dose dumping. The active was spray-dried using xyloglucan. Process and formulation variables such as carrier concentration in the feed, feed rate, and amount of cross-linking agent were optimized using a statistical design to obtain the desired time for 80% drug release and percent drug entrapped in the microspheres. The microspheres so obtained had particle size in the 3–6 μm range, with nearly 99% active loading (present in the amorphous form), and showed controlled release, sustaining beyond seven hours [154]. A combination product for sustained release from dry powder inhaler was obtained by spray drying a 70% v/v ethanolic solution of the two micronized actives salmeterol xinafoate and fluticasone propionate along with a surfactant (leucine) and a polymer as drug release modifier (HPMC). The dry powder so obtained was characterized to be an amorphous coprecipitate with optimal particle size (1.2–1.5 μm) and narrow size distribution owing to the leucine–HPMC combination. The particles also showed a sustained release profile in *in vitro* dissolution studies with 30–64% of the actives being released within 45 minutes. The drug release duration was found to increase with increased concentration of HPMC [155]. Chen et al. obtained a solid dispersion of acetaminophen via spray drying and using chitosan as a carrier wherein the active was entrapped in the amorphous form. Furthermore, infrared and solid-state NMR spectroscopy confirmed hydrogen bond formation between the hydroxyl group of acetaminophen and the amino group in chitosan in these solid dispersions. Dispersions obtained in the 1 : 5 mixing ratio of API/polymer showed a sustained release drug profile in dissolution studies at both pH 1.2 and 6.8 (37 °C) [68].

(C) *Targeted drug delivery*: As has been discussed in detail in the previous section, owing to the feasibility of particle engineering, spray drying has emerged as the method of choice to manufacture dry powder inhalers for pulmonary delivery of actives. The effectiveness of pulmonary delivery relies on the extent of drug deposition in the deep lung and reproducibility in dosing. To satisfy the former criterion, the active particle size is required to be in the 1–5 μm range, which leads to extremely high degree of cohesion, leading to agglomeration, poor flow, and therefore problems in manufacturability. Thus it is customary to mix the micronized active particles with larger carrier particles 50–100 μm in size and typically consisting of a sugar such as α-lactose monohydrate or mannitol. Spray drying is routinely used to prepare these carrier particles owing to the narrow size distribution and spherical particle shape obtained from this technique that produces uniform adhesion with the active particles, promotes flowability, and facilitates filling of the inhalation device. In addition, the carrier particles should have surface properties conducive for adhesion high enough to ensure homogeneous mixing with the active and low enough to ensure detachment of active particles and their release into the deep lung tissues [132]. Spray drying is advantageous in this aspect as well, since surface roughness that influences contact area and therefore adhesion can be altered by varying the outlet temperature [156]. Surface roughness also depends on the droplet size and particle size distribution that can be altered by changing the atomization nozzle type [132, 156]. A detailed discussion on the effect of drying parameters on carrier particle properties has been discussed in the previous Section 3.3.3.2.2. An interesting example of directly producing low density API containing particles with good flowability for pulmonary drug delivery can be found in the study conducted by Steckel and Brandes. The authors spray-dried a suspension consisting of the active salbutamol sulfate, surfactant (poloxamer or phosphatidylcholine), a bulking agent (lactose or a cyclodextrin derivative), and a lipid phase comprising a liquefied propellant. Spray drying resulted in formation of hollow, irregular-shaped particles with a geometric mean size of <5 μm, low density of 0.02 g/cc, and a drug load of 40% w/w. The particle size and dispersibility could be altered by changing the composition of the aqueous phase and the poloxamer concentration in the feed, respectively. The agglomeration tendency of the irregular particles was further reduced by addition of dichloromethane in the propellant phase [157].

3.4 Indirectly Heated (Conductive) Dryers

3.4.1 Rotary Drying

3.4.1.1 Description

Rotary dryers are also commonly used in the drying operation in the pharmaceutical industry owing to their ability to handle large amounts of feed. The dryer consists of a cylindrical shell rotated on ball bearings, with a slight slope in the horizontal plane [11]. The wet feed is introduced from the top from where it makes its way to the bottom via tumbling action and rotation, wherein it is finally collected as free-flowing dry powder. Rotary dryers can be directly or indirectly heated and can operate in batch or continuous mode. In directly heated rotary dryers, hot air is passed through either concurrently or countercurrent to the direction of the feed, depending on the properties of the feed material. These dryers are also equipped with paddles to facilitate constant movement and cascading of the feed so as to enhance heat exchange between the drying materials and the hot air. For more heat-sensitive materials where direct contact with the heating medium may not be desirable, the shell is equipped with a heating jacket through which the heating medium (steam or hot air) can be circulated. Although directly heated rotary dryers have the lion's share of drying applications, indirectly heated ones offer the advantages of tight process control and drying of fine materials without having the issue of losing the dried particles by entrainment in the airstream. Owing to their design where the furnace exhaust is kept separate from the process gas, less treatment of the exit gas is required. Indirectly heated rotary dryers are therefore helpful for drying thermolabile, highly combustible, and fine materials [11, 158].

3.4.1.2 Advantages and Drawbacks

Rotary dryers are often considered the "workhorse" in an industrial setting owing to their ability to accept various kinds of feed in substantially greater loads. The drying operation can be continuous, requires little supervision, and is a robust method to withstand inconsistencies in the feedstock as well as changes in the process parameters. Owing to the cascading action of the feed, there is good contact between the particles and drying air, allowing for effective heat and mass transfer. Although thermal efficiency is less than fluid-bed drying, the energy consumption may be lowered by operating at decreased capacities. Due to their availability in different designs (direct and indirect heating), rotary dryers can be used to dry a range of materials. Disadvantages include greater maintenance due to the presence of more moving parts, generation of fines, and product degradation due to attrition caused by the "lifting and dropping" action inside the dryer [158].

3.4.2 Freeze Drying

3.4.2.1 Description

Freeze drying or lyophilization is a drying process commonly employed for thermolabile materials where a solution of the labile active along with excipients is converted to a stable solid cake for storage, distribution, and dosing upon aqueous reconstitution. Typically, industrial freeze dryers consist of a drying chamber with temperature-controlled shelves that is connected to a condenser chamber via a valve. This condenser chamber comprises plates or coils that can be maintained at very low temperatures (<−50 °C). The condenser chamber is also connected to one or more vacuum pumps to achieve operating pressures in the range of 0.03–0.3 Torr. The drying operation consists of three stages: (i) freezing stage where the shelf temperature is brought down to as low as −40 °C to convert most of the water to ice followed by (ii) primary drying stage where the pressure is lowered and the shelf temperature is increased in a controlled manner to remove the ice directly by sublimation and finally (iii) secondary drying stage where any remaining unfrozen water is removed via desorption by further increasing the shelf temperature in the range of 25–50 °C. Of these three stages, the primary drying process is the longest and may take days and sometimes even weeks, if the process design and formulation are not adequately optimized. Since a large amount of heat is required for sublimation, the product temperature is well below the shelf temperature during primary drying. Secondary drying is much shorter in duration and occurs over several hours, and the product and shelf temperature are nearly identical in this stage. The water removed from the product is converted to ice by the condenser. The final solid cake, obtained upon drying, is typically an amorphous, porous non-shrunken mass that is dispersed or dissolved in a suitable vehicle before administration [11, 26]. Cake elegance, stability (physical and chemical), and reconstitution time are some of the product properties that are of importance for the freeze-dried product. Further details on freeze drying can be found in Chapter 6.

3.4.2.2 Advantages and Drawbacks

Freeze drying is a low-temperature drying operation and therefore suitable for labile materials since the risk of thermal degradation is low. Besides aqueous solutions, freeze drying can also be conducted using organic solvents, provided the solvents have a high enough vapor pressure so as not to prolong the drying cycle. The removal of water, i.e. desiccation, leads to better preservation and longer shelf life of pharmaceutical products such as biologics, injectables, tablets, and wafers [26, 159, 160]. Water removal leads to formation of a porous, dry cake that can be easily reconstituted in the appropriate vehicle for administration. Using this technique, sterile and particulate-free environment can be maintained for parenterals, rapidly dissolving sublingual tablets can be manufactured, and adequate protection can be provided to oxygen-sensitive formulations by stoppering of vials within the drying chamber [161]. However, freeze dryers are expensive equipment, and drying cycles can be long and time consuming [26]. Additionally, this drying technique is unsuitable for low-temperature/freeze-sensitive compounds.

3.4.2.3 Role in Small Molecule Formulation Development

Although freeze drying is primarily used for the development of protein formulations, it is included in small molecule drug product development as well and has been used to prepare injectables for antibiotics, fast-dissolving tablets, and lyophilized polymer wafers for buccal drug delivery. Though the risk of thermal degradation is low in this drying technology, stresses imparted by freezing and application of vacuum may lead to unwanted phase transformations in either the active or the stabilizing excipients or both [20, 26]. The following sections include detailed discussion and case studies on the effect of freeze drying on physical stability of formulation components as well as its varied role in drug delivery.

Phase Transformation in Formulation Components Solutions subjected to freeze drying contain both the active and formulation aids, i.e. excipients that stabilize the active during drying and in the final lyophilized cake. During freezing, the ice crystals start separating out, and the solution, being maximally concentrated, is also known as the freeze concentrate [162]. In this stage, primary stabilizers such as trehalose and sucrose are rendered amorphous, whereas solutes like mannitol and glycine tend to crystallize in the freeze concentrate. The crystallization behavior of these components is influenced by both process and formulation variables [20]. The former, i.e. process parameters, will be discussed further in context of the effect of drying operation on solid-state form change. In a previous study, the cooling rate of the starting solution was found to have an influence on the polymorphic composition in the final cake for mannitol. The δ-form was the major polymorph observed in the final lyophilized cake upon slow cooling, while uncontrolled, rapid cooling caused the α-polymorph to crystallize out as the dominant solid phase [163]. The effect of cooling rate on the polymorphism in glycine was reported by Pyne and Suryanarayanan where rapid or slow (20 or 2 °C/min) cooling of an aqueous solution of glycine (15% v/v) resulted in the formation of the β-polymorph. Quench cooling of the solution by immersion in liquid nitrogen rendered mannitol amorphous in the freeze concentrate, but upon further heating, β-glycine reappeared only to convert to the more stable γ-form upon annealing. The extent of this conversion depended on the annealing temperature [164]. It is desirable to have the bulking agents, such as glycine and mannitol that impart structural integrity to the dried cake, to remain crystalline in the final product. This can be facilitated by annealing the frozen solutions as it increases the molecular mobility in the freeze concentrate and causes crystallization of these solutes [165–168]. The temperature during solute crystallization was also shown to have an effect on the physical form. Using mannitol as a model compound, Mehta et al. showed that mannitol hemihydrate (MHH) was formed at solute crystallization temperatures ≤−20 °C, whereas anhydrous mannitol was obtained at temperatures ≥−10 °C (Figure 3.13) [169]. There are several literature reports of hydrate formation during the freezing step, such as in the case of cefazolin sodium, nafcillin sodium, dibasic sodium phosphate, and mannitol, where cooling of an aqueous solution led to crystallization of these solutes as hydrates [170–173]. Hydrates so formed during freezing may undergo further solid-state transformation during the subsequent steps of primary and secondary drying where a combination of increased temperature and reduced pressure is

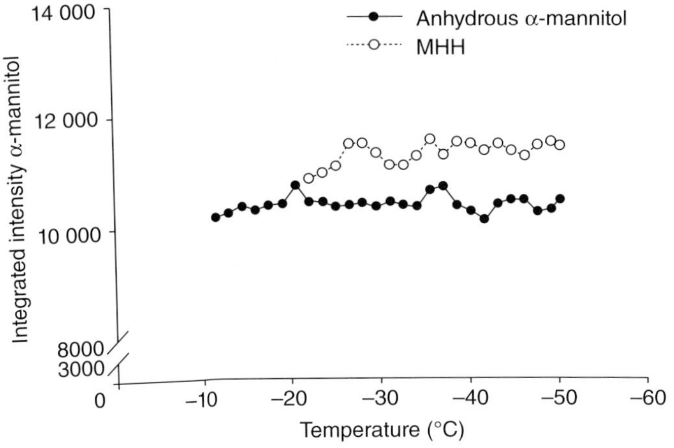

Figure 3.13 Intensity of the characteristic peaks of anhydrous α-mannitol and mannitol hemihydrate (MHH) as a function of temperature in annealed solutions, as monitored by synchrotron XRPD. Solutions cooled from 0 to −10 °C and annealed for 16 hours contained anhydrous α-mannitol, whereas those annealed at −20 °C showed hemihydrate crystallization. Source: Mehta et al. 2013 [169]. Reproduced with permission of Elsevier.

applied to remove the ice and unfrozen water by sublimation and desorption, respectively. For example, Cavatur and Suryanarayanan monitored in situ phase transformations in freeze drying using X-ray powder diffractometry and showed that sodium nafcillin hydrate, which crystallized out in the frozen solution at −4 °C, underwent partial dehydration during primary drying at −10 °C to form a poorly crystalline hemihydrate [170]. Pyne et al. showed that disodium hydrogen phosphate, which formed a dodecahydrate during freezing, underwent dehydration during primary drying to an amorphous anhydrate [171]. Hydrate formation during freeze drying is of concern since the removal of the hydrate may require aggressive secondary drying conditions that may lead to thermal degradation or collapse of the lyophilized cake. Furthermore, the hydrate so formed may release water upon storage and compromise the stability of the formulation [169]. Since there may be multiple phase transformations during freeze drying, it is advisable to do an in situ monitoring of the freeze concentrate at different stages of drying rather than simply characterizing the final, dry cake so as to assess the nature and extent of the product phases formed at each step and their impact on cake quality and performance [170]. The final form of the solutes present in the dried cake may not be the same as the starting form and does not provide any indication of the series of form changes that may occur during the drying operation. Therefore, monitoring the in situ phase transformation via X-ray diffractometry or spectroscopy is an effective way to detect these solid form changes and evaluate their influence on final product properties [168, 170, 172, 174].

Drug Product Development Freeze drying is the preferred operation for manufacturing of products intended for parenteral use. Sterilization and particulate-free environment are the two essential requirements for parenteral products. In the case of freeze drying, the sterile filtration of the fill solution before it is aseptically filled in vials followed by the drying process in an enclosed chamber unperturbed by human contact allows for a sterile and particulate-free environment to be maintained as compared with other dry powder handling methods [26]. The application in small molecules includes manufacturing of parenteral formulations of β-lactam antibiotics (cephalosporins) that are too unstable to withstand terminal sterilization in solution. In addition, freeze drying has found much success in the manufacturing of fast-dissolving oral or sublingual tablets. A commercially viable example is the Zydis® (Catalent) orally dissolving tablet. It is a freeze-dried oral solid dosage form that disperses almost instantly in the mouth without any need for water, thereby providing rapid drug release and enhancing patient compliance. These are laminar tablets with a "spongy" internal structure and are prepared by freeze drying tablet molds into which the formulation solution is poured [175]. The Lyopan® fast-dissolve technology is another patented technique by Catalent Pharma to produce rapidly dissolving lyophilized tablets. In other examples of rapidly disintegrating oral tablets, Ahmed et al. prepared tablets of griseofulvin, an antifungal agent, by freeze drying an oil in water emulsion of the active with a 2% w/v gelatin solution as the water phase and a medium chain triglyceride such as Miglyol 812 N® or sesame oil as the oil phase along with emulsifiers such as hydroxypropyl methylcellulose or a 4 : 1 Tween 80/Span 80 blend. The lyophilized dry emulsion tablets were found to enhance both *in vitro* dissolution and *in vivo* absorption of griseofulvin compared with the neat drug and the commercially available immediate release tablet, respectively. The authors attributed this rapid drug release to the large surface area provided by the lipid droplets upon tableting and/or the solubilization effect of the API by the oily components [176]. Besides fast-dissolving tablets, freeze drying has also been extensively used for development of polymer wafers as a potential drug delivery system via the buccal mucosa and for wound treatment. For wafers and films to act as effective wound dressing materials, efficient drug release, ease of hydration, and suitable mechanical strength are requisite properties for targeted drug delivery and to provide necessary muco-adhesion to moist surfaces. In a previous study employing freeze-dried wafers of the active paracetamol in polymer gels such as sodium alginate or carboxymethylcellulose for wound treatment, it was shown that lyophilization produced highly porous structures in wafers with higher drug loading and water absorption capacity compared with solvent-cast films of carboxymethylcellulose (Figure 3.14). The wafers also showed more rapid *in vitro* drug release than the films, and this was attributed to their internal porous network [159, 177]. Patel and Amiji explored freeze-dried hydrogels comprising chitosan and polyethylene oxide as a means of localized drug delivery of antibiotics in the stomach. Owing to the highly porous semi-penetrating matrix created by cross-linking the polymers, these freeze-dried hydrogels showed a very high swelling index (16.1) after one hour in simulated gastric fluid and released >65% of amoxicillin and 59% metronidazole after two hours in the same medium. Thus by employing cationic hydrogels with pH swelling properties and creating a highly porous internal structure feasible for rapid hydration and swelling, targeted drug delivery of antibiotics was possible in the acidic stomach pH where they are typically unstable [178]. Freeze drying is also used as an effective means

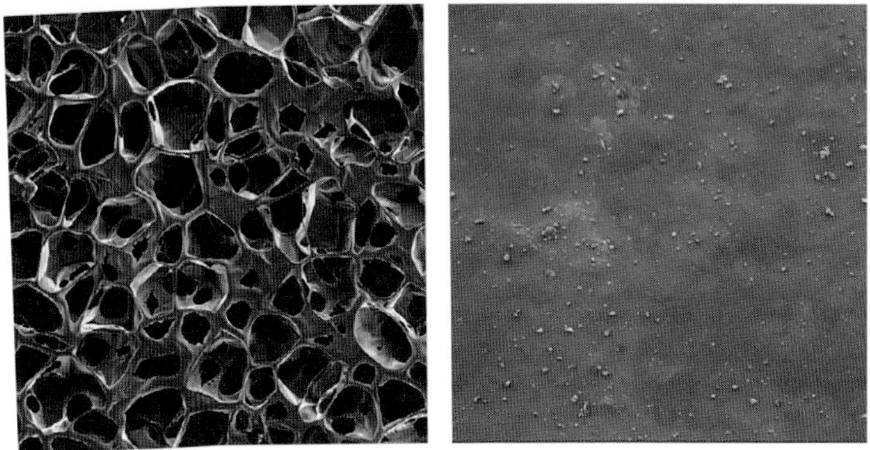

(a) (b)

Figure 3.14 SEM micrographs of paracetamol-containing freeze-dried wafers (a) vs. solvent-cast films (b) obtained from 2% w/w CMC solution. Difference in the physical structure between the porous wafers and the nonporous films is evident from these images. Source: Boateng et al. 2009 [177]. Reproduced with permission of Elsevier.

to remove water and therefore stabilize colloidal nanoparticles, microparticles, and lyospheres [64, 161].

3.5 Emerging Drying Technologies

Drying is an extremely energy-intensive process, and often stresses of temperature and reduced pressure may lead to irreversible changes in material properties, thereby affecting final product quality and performance. Therefore, new drying techniques are being explored for pharmaceutical R&D and manufacturing for further improvement of existing technology. Improvements have been sought in the following areas: energy efficiency and therefore lower energy costs, enhanced drying capacity, improved quality control, use of renewable energy for reduced environmental impact, shorter processing times without compromising product quality, and lower operational and maintenance costs [86]. Of the several emerging techniques, supercritical fluid (SCF) drying and microwave drying are gaining popularity in small molecule drug development and will be discussed further.

3.5.1 Supercritical Fluid (SCF) Drying

3.5.1.1 Description

SCF-drying technology utilizes an SCF as a drying medium instead of air, the supercritical state being achieved by a substance when its temperature and pressure exceed their respective critical values [179, 180]. The phase diagram pertaining to the supercritical state of carbon dioxide is shown in Figure 3.15. In this state, the distinction between the liquid and gas phase disappears, and neither increase in pressure nor temperature can liquefy or vaporize the fluid. SCF physicochemical properties such as density, diffusivity, viscosity, and dielectric constant can be readily altered by changing temperature and pressure without any corresponding phase change [180]. SCF have densities and solubilities comparable with a liquid, and their compressibility, viscosity, and diffusivity resembles that of a gas. SCF density, which can be readily regulated by changing the pressure, dictates its solvation power, whereas its gas-like properties facilitate mass transfer [181]. Carbon dioxide is the most widely used SCF for pharmaceutical applications as it is nonflammable and nontoxic, provides for easy removal from the final product, is inexpensive, and has a low critical temperature of 31.2 °C and pressure of 7.4 MPa, both of which are easily attainable [182].

3.5.1.2 Advantages and Drawbacks

There are several advantages of SCF drying over conventional drying operations prevalent in the pharmaceutical industry. One of the biggest advantages of SCF-drying technology is that there are no surface tension effects and no occurrence of liquid–gas phase change during drying. As a result, highly porous materials can be dried effectively without collapse that occurs upon the removal of water achieved through conventional drying. The solvent-like properties aid in

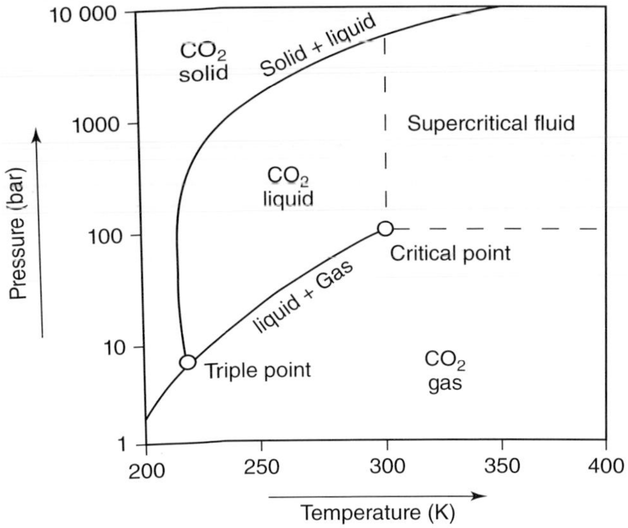

Figure 3.15 Phase diagram of carbon dioxide. Source: Benali and Boumghar 2014 [179]. Reproduced with permission of Taylor & Francis.

drug solubilization, plasticization of polymers, and solvent/impurity extraction, while the gas-like properties of lower viscosity and higher diffusivity facilitate more efficient mass transfer [180, 181]. Owing to its low critical temperature and pressure values, the use of carbon dioxide as an SCF is beneficial for drying thermolabile materials to eliminate the risk of thermal degradation. SCF properties can be easily regulated by changes in temperature and pressure, and this in turn helps to establish a high degree of control over the dried product properties, thereby enabling particle engineering [182]. Finally, SCF drying is a single-step, solvent-free, "green" technology with provision of recovering and recycling the drying medium [182]. A potential drawback is the use of a nonpolar compound like carbon dioxide that excludes the solubilization of polar compounds. This can be addressed by adding small amounts of polar cosolvents such as ethanol to the fluid. Although this may decrease processing times and increase yield, this introduces complications in the thermodynamics of drying along with a substantial increase in operational cost [180]. Being a high pressure application, safety aspects encountered during scale-up procedures also require careful consideration [183].

3.5.1.3 Pharmaceutical Applications

In recent years, the utilization of SCF drying for a wide variety of pharmaceutical applications has increased tremendously owing to the versatility of this drying technology. The applications include crystallization, solvent/impurity extraction and separation, particle size control for enhancement in dissolution rate via size reduction (micro and nanoparticle formation), particle engineering for inhalation therapy, and formation of solid dispersions and complexes [184, 185]. These different applications are enabled by the role of SCF as solvent, cosolvent, solute, or cosolute [179]. Each of these methodologies offer different mechanisms of nucleation and growth and are selected depending on the target product properties [186]. Some of the important pharmaceutical applications are discussed in detail in the following sections.

(A) *Form control and polymorphism*: The rapid expansion supercritical solution (RESS) technology is utilized where the SCF acts as a solvent during crystallization, provided the solute shows appreciable solubility in the fluid. Typically, the solute is first dissolved in carbon dioxide (SCF), followed by passing the solution through a heated nozzle at supersonic speed that leads to rapid expansion and a dramatic decrease in density and solubilizing power of the SCF solution. As a result, supersaturation occurs and solid solute particles are precipitated [186]. This technique was employed to obtain fine particles (mean particle size of 1.59 μm) of the metastable β-polymorph of phenylbutazone from the stable δ-form [187]. Micronization-aided wettability and dispersibility along with the greater solubility of the metastable form was postulated to enhance the bioavailability of phenylbutazone upon oral administration. In the case of tolbutamide, a hypoglycemic agent, and barbital, a sedative, the effect on SCF operating conditions (extraction pressure of 18–26 MPa and temperature of 32–80 °C) was found to play a role in the polymorphic form obtained. The extent of solute supersaturation in the SCF during expansion was found to affect both particle size and polymorphic form obtained. For tolbutamide, the metastable form II or mixtures of metastable forms II and IV dominated at higher pressures (26 MPa), whereas a lower extraction pressure (18 MPa) favored the stable form I. For barbital, the starting form was found to be a mixture of stable form I and metastable form II that converted to stable form I using SCF RESS process at 26 MPa and 60 °C for three hours. All high pressure and temperature combinations produced metastable form II [188]. Precise control of RESS parameters can not only enable precipitation of desired polymorphs with high purity but also offer a route to obtain new polymorphic forms that cannot be crystallized otherwise using conventional methods. Carbamazepine, existing as four anhydrous polymorphs and one dihydrate form, was used as the model compound to demonstrate formation of pure polymorphic forms by changing the SCF processing conditions. By using SCF, complete conversion to the stable polymorphic form III was obtained from a starting mixture of forms, thereby demonstrating that SCF can be used to obtain pure phases from a mixture of polymorphs without the use of any organic solvent [189]. A new polymorphic form was obtained for the excipient deoxycholate when treated under carbon dioxide purge in a pressure vessel for one hour at 12 MPa and 60 °C [190].

SCF technology where the fluid is used as an anti-solvent is known as solution-enhanced dispersion (SEDS) and is applicable in scenarios where the solute is not soluble in SCF but the base solvent is compatible or miscible with the SCF. The principle is based on the bidirectional mass transfer of the solvent to SCF and vice versa. Dissolution of the solvent in the SCF causes supersaturation that is also brought about by dilution of the SCF in the solvent, leading to density lowering and lesser solubilization.

This supersaturation, augmented by solvent–SCF miscibility causes direct precipitation of the solid as dry, fine particles due to high mass transfer rates [179, 184, 191]. For compounds with poor solubility in SCF, SEDS provides a pathway for form control as well. All three sulfathiazole polymorphs could be obtained by using methanol as a solvent, whereas acetone produced only form I. The operational temperature also had a bearing on the polymorph obtained, with lower temperatures favoring forms III and IV, while higher temperature produced form I [192]. By this process, flunisolide (used in nasal spray to treat allergic rhinitis) produced a new polymorphic form III with acetone at 100 bar pressure and 60 or 40 °C and form IV with methanol at 80 °C [191]. Finally, the use of SEDS has been shown to be a promising approach for controlling enantiomeric purity, such as in the case of ephedrine racemates, via a diastereomeric salt formation with mandelic acid. The resolution achieved, as determined by capillary electrophoresis, appeared to vary as a function of SCF temperature and density (Figure 3.16). The racemate was used as a starting material, and crystals of >90% diastereomeric excess were obtained via a single crystallization step. These crystals showed greater purity and smoother morphology compared with those obtained by conventional crystallization techniques [193]. Oakes et al. reported exclusive pressure-optimized diastereoselectivity achieved via the use of SCF drying at ~110 bar of carbon dioxide in the asymmetric catalytic sulfoxidation of cysteine and methionine. A diastereomeric purity of ~95% was obtained by this method, which could not be achieved by using conventional solvents [194].

(B) *Particle engineering and micronization*: Conventional techniques for micronization produce particles with high surface energy that tend to show static charging, undergo agglomeration, and thus have poor flow [182, 195].

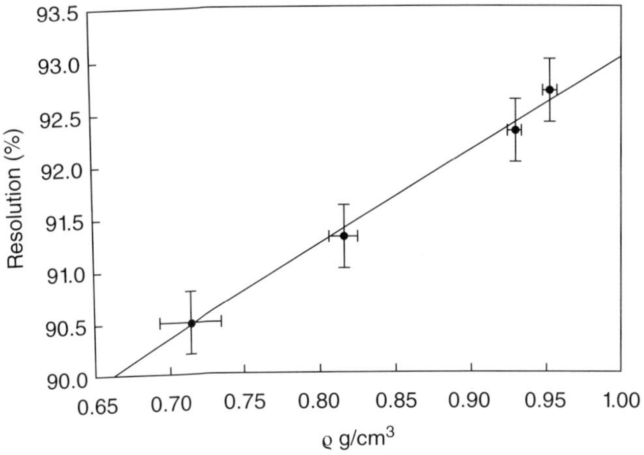

Figure 3.16 Diastereomeric resolution of SEDS-crystallized ephedrine mandalate as a function of carbon dioxide density. The resolution increases with increasing density at constant temperature. Source: Kordikowski et al. 1999 [193]. Reproduced with permission of John Wiley & Sons.

In addition, shear stresses experienced during conventional micronization may lead to generation of disorder that may jeopardize the physical and chemical stability of the material during further processing or storage. Therefore particle design technologies offering size reduction with minimal stress and low surface energy micronized particles are highly desirable. SCF drying has been identified to be extremely promising with regard to both particle micronization and engineering of particle properties. Unlike conventional micronization techniques with poor control of particle size distribution, propensity of attrition, and thermal degradation, SCF drying has been shown to successfully obtain micro- and nano-sized particles with a narrow size distribution [182]. This one-step approach toward controlled micronization has found utilization in pulmonary delivery wherein a tight particle size distribution is desired (particle size of 1–5 μm) for delivery to the bronchial and alveolar tissues in the lung [196–198]. SCF drying has been shown to be an effective technique to produce free-flowing micronized powders with reduced adhesion and cohesion [199]. Moreover, the low-temperature operating conditions make this process ideal for micronization of thermolabile materials. For example, Bettini et al. utilized the SCF RESS technology to obtain micronized particles of acetylsalicylic acid (ASA). Not only was the particle size reduced effectively, but the study also showed a linear correlation between particle size and the operating pressure. There was no alteration in the solid-state form of the micronized particles [200]. Türk et al. used carbon dioxide as an SCF solvent for micronization and obtained a very narrow size distribution for naphthalene (1.5–3 μm), benzoic acid (0.8–1.2 μm), and cholesterol (<0.35 μm) [201]. The RESS process was similarly used to increase dissolution rate and therefore improve bioavailability for griseofulvin and β-sitosterol by size reduction of particles to a diameter of 200 nm [202]. Unlike other size reduction techniques, SCF drying can be equally effective in micronizing poorly soluble compounds by using SCF as an anti-solvent where the solubilizing power of the primary solvent (where the compound of interest remains dissolved) is drastically reduced by introducing SCF, which leads to solvent depletion, supersaturation, nucleation, and ultimately particle growth [184, 203]. Factors such as temperature, pressure, solvent to SCF ratio, rate of SCF addition, and solvent miscibility in SCF dictate the particle size distribution [204]. By utilizing the SEDS process, where the drug dissolved solvent and SCF were simultaneously introduced and mixed into a reaction vessel using a coaxial nozzle, droplets and consequently particles of very small size were produced due to increased mass transfer rate and intimate mixing between the solvent and SCF [205]. High mass transfer rates of SCF into the base solvent was attributed to be the driver for rapid nucleation and formation of smaller particles showing less agglomeration propensity [206]. Yeo and Lee demonstrated that the injection rate of supercritical carbon dioxide may have a bearing on particle morphology, as seen during recrystallization of sulfamethizole solutions in acetone. Low injection rates produced large, tabular crystals, while higher injection rates led to formation of small particles that were thin and plate-like. The choice of solvent also led to changes in particle size and shape, with large platy crystals being obtained from dimethyl formamide (DMF) irrespective of injection rate [207]. SCF as anti-solvent and SC carbon dioxide-aided atomization have been successfully used to produce micron and submicron particles of several actives such as tartaric acid, cefonicid, tetracycline, terbutaline, and rifampicin with controlled particle size distribution [208–212]. Many of these micronization studies also explored the operation variables such as rate of carbon dioxide injection, temperature of crystallization, nozzle geometry, solute concentration, solvent to anti-solvent ratio, application of sonication to atomization, and solvent choice, all of which were shown to influence the shape, size, and physical form of the dried particles [207, 213]. These examples amply demonstrate the ability of SCF drying in manipulating particle properties for different drug delivery applications.

(C) *Drug delivery systems*: SCF-drying technology is being explored to prepare inclusion complexes or solid dispersion without the use of organic solvents, which is a common practice in other dispersion preparation techniques. For example, owing to the high solubility of ibuprofen in SC carbon dioxide, an attempt was made to form inclusion complexes using three different types of β-cyclodextrin (substituted or unsubstituted) via SCF. A physical mixture, an amorphous dried product, and a new crystalline single phase were obtained for the three different cyclodextrins used, with the single crystalline form being a true inclusion complex as determined by calorimetric and spectroscopic analyses [214–218]. Moribe et al. postulated that the high solubility of the substituted β-cyclodextrin in SC carbon dioxide was the driver for inclusion complex formation [184]. The particles from gas saturated solution (PGSS) technique in SCF drying, where the SCF is dissolved in a melted substrate or a solution or suspension of the substrate, followed by rapid expansion of the saturated solution or slurry through a nozzle, has been successfully utilized for drug encapsulation [219]. For example, using the SEDS process, a suspension of hydrocortisone particles in a poly(d,l-lactide-co-glycolide) (PLG) solution in dimethazone was sprayed into SC carbon dioxide to obtain sustained drug-releasing microparticles where the active was successfully coated by PLG. Higher polymer to drug ratios was found to increase the encapsulation efficiency. Rodriguez et al. also demonstrated a proof-of-concept study to outline the use of SCF in preparing microcomposites of theophylline with hydrogenated palm oil (HPO) for controlled drug release. Higher expansion pressures led to spherical particles (mean particle size range of 2.5–3.0 μm) with theophylline encapsulated in the HPO matrix [219]. Dissolution studies showed that theophylline released from the HPO matrix follows Higuchi's model for simple diffusional processes after an initial burst of API in the dissolution medium [220, 221].

3.5.2 Microwave Drying

Microwave drying utilizes high frequency radio waves ranging from 300 MHz to 300 GHz, which upon interaction with the substrate lead to the removal of moisture via energy conversion to heat [1, 11]. A high frequency generator is used to guide the waves into an oven, which prevents them from leaving the chamber. The depth of penetration, required for effective and uniform drying, and the extent of dehydration are determined by the choice of the appropriate wavelength and material properties [85]. The advantages of microwave drying include high process speed, reduction in drying time, efficiency of energy conversion leading to significant energy savings, improved and rapid process control, less floor space requirement, selective heating, and increase in efficiency since the electromagnetic radiation couples with the solvent, leading to exclusive heating of the moisture and its removal while the solid is heated by conduction. This can lead to an improvement of product quality and elimination of case hardening due to overdrying since the solid surface is not typically overheated. Caution must be exercised while using microwave drying since this is a rapid drying technique and uncontrolled heating rates may lead to substantial product burns and degradation. Besides, uniformity of heating may be a problem if the appropriate wavelength is not selected for adequate depth of penetration to occur. In recent years microwave drying has been combined with other drying techniques such as freeze drying, vacuum drying, and convective drying to overcome problems of uneven heating due to focusing, corner and edge heating, inhomogeneity of electromagnetic field, and irregular substrates with nonuniform composition [86, 222–232]. A detailed discussion on microwave drying and its modifications may be found in Chapter 10.

3.5.2.1 Pharmaceutical Applications

Microwave drying enjoyed a revival in the 1980s when ICI introduced a production-scale, batch microwave-drying system with a capacity of up to 100 kg, into operations for drying of potent, granular pharmaceuticals. As a result, less dusty tablets were produced as compared with conventional drying techniques in significantly less time [233–235]. Current applications include integration of a microwave source with granulation techniques to enhance drying efficiency and the use of continuous microwave-drying system for larger production capacity. The primary pharmaceutical use of microwave drying lies in drying of granules because microwave energy can efficiently dry large quantities of binder solutions in aqueous granulations. Microwave drying may also allow mixing, granulation, lubrication, and dry sizing in a single step and provide advantages of operator safety, equipment cleaning, energy savings, and greater environmental control during scale-up, as compared with other conventional drying techniques [11]. There are several examples in literature demonstrating the use of single-pot microwave-assisted drying in granulation operations. For example, Loh et al. employed microwave-assisted drying in a one-pot high shear granulation process for ASA granules, which were dried in situ. Formulation variables such as powder load and granule shape and size appeared to have an effect on drying rate. Owing to the volumetric heating provided by microwave drying, larger granules showed faster drying rates than the finer particles. Finally, drying time was found to correlate negatively with API stability [236].

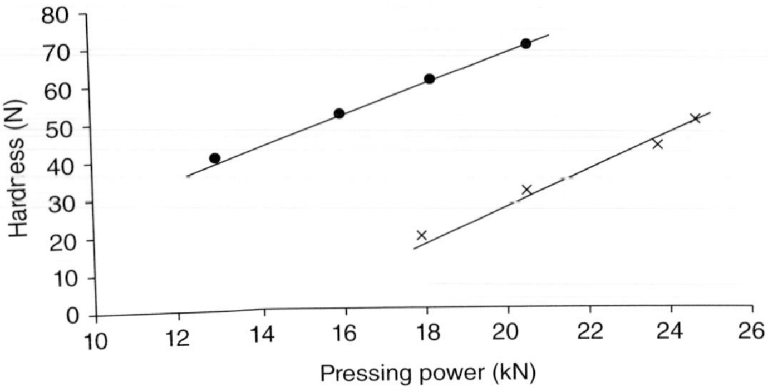

Figure 3.17 Tablet hardness vs. pressing power (compression force) for granules obtained via microwave drying (×) vs. granules obtained by fluidized-bed drying (•). The former produced granules with low porosity, high bulk, and tap densities that required greater compression force to produce tablets of equal hardness as compared with fluidized-bed-dried granules. Source: Hegedűs and Pintye-Hódi 2007 [238]. Reproduced with permission of Elsevier.

In another study, Chee et al. showed microwave drying to be a superior drying method compared with hot air oven and fluid-bed drying while determining the stability of moisture-sensitive active ASA in dried granules obtained from high shear granulation. Granules dried with a dynamic bed microwave dryer showed the lowest percentage of ASA degradation compared with other drying methods. This was attributed to improved dissipation of heat and moisture by mixing that led to enhanced drying capability and therefore stability of ASA [237]. Hegedus and Pintye-Hodi conducted a study to compare the properties of granules dried either by fluid-bed drying or microwave vacuum drying after granulation in a high shear granulator. Granules obtained via microwave vacuum drying were spherical and showed lower porosity and higher bulk and tap densities compared with those obtained by fluid-bed drying. These granules were also readily compressible to produce thinner tablets compared with the fluidized-bed-dried granules owing to differences in granule structure. However, greater compression force had to be applied for microwave-vacuum-dried granules compared with fluidized-bed-dried granules to obtain tablets of comparable hardness (Figure 3.17). The difference in compression force did not affect the disintegration time of the tablets. Ultimately, the observed differences in granule shape, porosity, and density were attributed to the specialized drying characteristics intrinsic to microwave vacuum drying, such as volumetric heating and slow, gentle, and more uniform expulsion of moisture. As a result, granule primary physical structure and shape remains more intact. In contrast, the impact and rapid moisture removal experienced during fluid-bed drying leads to particulate erosion and substantial damage to particle physical structure [86, 238].

Table 3.3 captures a summary of all the drying techniques discussed in this chapter detailing their advantages, drawbacks, pharmaceutical applications, and influence on solid-state properties of small molecules.

Table 3.3 Overview of the advantages, drawbacks, pharmaceutical applications, and influence on solid-state/physical properties of different drying techniques.

Drying technique	Advantages	Challenges	Applications	Effect on physical form
Directly heated dryers				
Tray drying	(a) Simplicity of design (b) Low cost and ease of use (c) Portability (d) Rapid moisture removal due to increased surface area (e) Suitable for drying thermolabile materials (f) Provision for solvent recovery (g) Humidity drying possible (h) Sampling and offline characterization possible	(a) Nonuniformity in drying leads to inhomogeneous moisture content and longer drying times (b) Drying rates are typically inconsistent at sample extremities	Small batch drying of pharmaceuticals [85, 86]	Change in the state of hydration of drug substance [89, 91, 93]
Fluidized-bed drying	(a) Efficient heat and mass transfer leading to shorter drying times (b) Homogeneity in temperature and moisture across product bed (c) Good for drying heat-sensitive materials (d) Low cost of maintenance, ease of operation and feed handling, ease of material transport (e) Operable in batch or continuous mode (f) Overheating is minimized due to rapid heat transfer (g) Several modifications possible to dry different kinds of solids	(a) Energy-intensive process with high electricity consumption (b) Unsuitable for very fine or large particles and sticky materials (c) Pulverization by attrition causes generation of fines and subsequent entrainment of these fine particles by air may lead to substantial product loss	(a) Generation of free-flowing granules for compression into tablets or capsule filling (b) Coating of solid particles, such as taste masking of bitter actives or for layering in sustained release formulations (c) Facilitates intimate mixing of API and excipients [79–84, 99–103]	(a) Change in the state of hydration of the active (b) Polymorphic form change [94, 104–106, 215]

Spray drying	(a) Bulk manufacturing technique providing ease of scale-up (b) Continuous drying operation with process flexibility and complete automation (c) Yields particles with large surface area and narrow size distribution (d) Particle properties (flow, texture, size, bulk density, morphology) can be altered by adjusting drying parameters (e) High heat and mass transfer as well as evaporation rates achievable (f) Drying occurs mostly at wet bulb temperatures thus enabling use of higher heating rate for thermolabile materials (g) Short residence time enables preservation of organoleptic properties	(a) Low thermal efficiency leading to high energy consumption (b) Low yield at laboratory scale (20–75%) (c) High maintenance cost due to clogging of nozzles (d) Unsuitable for hygroscopic and thermoplastic materials	(a) Used for bulk conversion of crystalline active into amorphous form to improve solubility and potentially bioavailability (b) Suitable for manufacturing of different kinds of enabling formulations, such as amorphous solid dispersions (to enhance solubility), controlled release solid dispersions, microspheres, nanoparticles, dry powder inhalation formulations, and solid self-microemulsifying drug delivery Manufacturing method for spray-dried lactose, a directly compressible tableting excipient and other co-processed excipients [22, 23, 25, 66, 67, 69–78, 132–134, 137–143, 147–150, 154, 156, 157]	(a) Change in degree of crystallinity of active (partial or complete amorphization) (b) Change in the state of solvation of drug substance (c) Polymorphic form change: may lead to formation of rare, metastable form [41, 110–122]
Indirectly heated dryers				
Rotary drying	(a) Can handle large quantities of feed (b) The drying operation can be continuous, requires little supervision, and is a robust method to withstand inconsistencies in the feedstock as well as changes in the process parameters (c) Owing to the cascading action of the feed, there is good contact between the particles and drying air, allowing for effective heat and mass transfer (d) Indirectly heated rotary dryers are more suitable for drying thermolabile substances, highly combustible, and fine materials (e) Can operate in batch or continuous mode (f) Less treatment of exit gas needed due to design	(a) Higher maintenance required due to the presence of more moving parts (b) Leads to generation of fines and product degradation due to attrition caused by the "lifting and dropping" action inside the dryer (c) Thermal efficiency is less compared with fluidized-bed dryer		

(*continued*)

Table 3.3 (Continued)

Drying technique	Advantages	Challenges	Applications	Effect on physical form
Freeze drying	(a) Low temperature drying operation and therefore suitable for labile materials (b) Can also be conducted using organic solvents, provided the solvents have a high enough vapor pressure (c) Desiccation leads to better preservation and longer shelf life of pharmaceutical products (d) Used for obtaining sterile and particulate-free environment for parenterals	(a) Expensive equipment (b) Drying cycles are long and time consuming (c) Not suitable for freeze-sensitive compounds	(a) Used for manufacturing of parenterals (proteins and small molecules such as injectable antibiotics), fast-dissolving tablets, freeze-dried hydrogels for targeted drug delivery, and lyophilized polymer wafers for buccal drug delivery	Solid-state phase transformation can occur in both active and excipients, such as polymorphic form change or change in the state of hydration during freezing and subsequent drying steps [163–174]
Emerging drying technologies				
Supercritical fluid drying	(a) No surface tension effects enables drying of highly porous materials without collapse (b) Solvent-like drying properties aid in drug solubilization, plasticization of polymers, and solvent/impurity extraction, while the gas-like properties facilitate more efficient mass transfer (c) Carbon dioxide as SCF is beneficial for drying thermolabile materials (d) SCF properties can be easily regulated by changes in temperature and pressure that helps to establish control over the dried product properties, thereby enabling particle engineering (e) This is a single-step, solvent-free, "green" technology with provision of recovering and recycling the drying medium	Use of a nonpolar compound like carbon dioxide as SCF excludes the solubilization of polar compounds	(a) Crystallization: form control and obtaining desired polymorphic form of high purity (b) Solvent/impurity extraction and separation (c) Particle size control for enhancement in dissolution rate via size reduction (micro- and nanoparticle formation) (d) Particle engineering for inhalation therapy (e) Micronization to produce free-flowing powders with reduced adhesion and cohesion (f) Formation of solid dispersions and complexes [179, 181, 182, 184–193, 196–200, 206–216, 218, 219]	New or metastable polymorphic forms may be obtained by this specialized drying technique [184, 188–190, 192]

Microwave drying	(a) High process speed (b) Reduction in drying time (c) Efficiency of energy conversion leading to significant energy savings (d) Improved and rapid process control (e) Less floor space requirement (f) Selective heating and increase in efficiency since the electromagnetic radiation couples with the solvent, leading to exclusive heating of the moisture and its removal while the solid is heated by conduction. This can lead to an improvement of product quality and elimination of case hardening due to overdrying (g) Suitable for drying moisture-sensitive materials	(a) This is a rapid drying technique, and uncontrolled heating rates may lead to substantial product burns and degradation (b) Uniformity of heating may be a problem if the appropriate wavelength is not selected for adequate depth of penetration to occur	(a) Integration of a microwave source with granulation techniques to enhance drying efficiency (b) Continuous microwave-drying system may be employed for larger production capacity (c) Provides efficient drying of tablet granules and helps to preserve granule primary structure and shape as compared with fluidized-bed drying (d) Allows mixing, granulation, lubrication, and dry sizing in a single step (microwave-assisted drying has been used in single-pot granulation operations) [233–238]

Numbers in parentheses indicate the relevant references for pharmaceutical applications and solid-state changes encountered upon drying.

3.6 Summary

Drying is an extremely energy-intensive unit operation that is integral to small molecule formulation development. Moisture removal serves manifold purposes of reducing product bulk to facilitating transportation, enhancing product stability by eliminating microbial growth, and altering the physicochemical properties of the feed to make them conducive for more downstream processing, such as tablet compression and capsule filling. However, drying is a complex operation involving several rate processes such as heat and mass transfer that may bring about a series of physical and chemical transformations in the solids, which in turn may affect the final product quality and performance. Therefore, judicious selection of a dryer, optimization of drying conditions, and continuous monitoring of the process are imperative for a thorough understanding of the drying process and to achieve tight control on product properties and quality.

References

1 Parikh, D.M. (2014). Solids drying: basics and applications. *Chemical Engineering* 121 (4): 42–45.
2 Carstensen, J. (1988). Effect of moisture on the stability of solid dosage forms. *Drug Development and Industrial Pharmacy* 14 (14): 1927–1969.
3 Du, J. and Hoag, S.W. (2001). The influence of excipients on the stability of the moisture sensitive drugs aspirin and niacinamide: comparison of tablets containing lactose monohydrate with tablets containing anhydrous lactose. *Pharmaceutical Development and Technology* 6 (2): 159–166.
4 Khankari, R.K. and Grant, D.J. (1995). Pharmaceutical hydrates. *Thermochimica Acta* 248: 61–79.
5 Khan, F., Pilpel, N., and Ingham, S. (1988). The effect of moisture on the density, compaction and tensile strength of microcrystalline cellulose. *Powder Technology* 54 (3): 161–164.
6 Kontny, M.J. and Zografi, G. (1995). Sorption of water by solids. *Drugs and the Pharmaceutical Sciences* 70: 387.
7 Nokhodchi, A. (2005). Effect of moisture on compaction and compression. *Pharmaceutical Technology* 6: 46–66.
8 Schepky, G. (1989). Preformulation the role of moisture in solid dosage forms. *Drug Development and Industrial Pharmacy* 15 (10): 1715–1741.
9 Shukla, A.J. and Price, J.C. (1991). Effect of moisture content on compression properties of directly compressible high beta-content anhydrous lactose. *Drug Development and Industrial Pharmacy* 17 (15): 2067–2081.
10 Stubberud, L., Arwidsson, H.G., and Graffner, C. (1995). Water-solid interactions: I. A technique for studying moisture sorption/desorption. *International Journal of Pharmaceutics* 114 (1): 55–64.
11 Mujumdar, A.S. (2014). *Handbook of Industrial Drying*. Boca Raton, FL: CRC Press.

12 Gillon, A.L., Feeder, N., Davey, R.J., and Storey, R. (2003). Hydration in molecular crystals a Cambridge Structural Database analysis. *Crystal Growth & Design* 3 (5): 663–673.

13 Shefter, E. and Higuchi, T. (1963). Dissolution behavior of crystalline solvated and nonsolvated forms of some pharmaceuticals. *Journal of Pharmaceutical Sciences* 52 (8): 781–791.

14 Debnath, S. and Suryanarayanan, R. (2004). Influence of processing-induced phase transformations on the dissolution of theophylline tablets. *AAPS PharmSciTech* 5 (1): 39–49.

15 Giron, D., Goldbronn, C., Mutz, M. et al. (2002). Solid state characterizations of pharmaceutical hydrates. *Journal of Thermal Analysis and Calorimetry* 68 (2): 453–465.

16 Phadnis, N.V. and Suryanarayanan, R. (1997). Polymorphism in anhydrous theophylline—implications on the dissolution rate of theophylline tablets. *Journal of Pharmaceutical Sciences* 86 (11): 1256–1263.

17 Rani, M., Govindarajan, R., Surana, R., and Suryanarayanan, R. (2006). Structure in dehydrated trehalose dihydrate—evaluation of the concept of partial crystallinity. *Pharmaceutical Research* 23 (10): 2356–2367.

18 Lohani, S. and Grant, D.J. (2006). Thermodynamics of polymorphs. In: *Polymorphism: In the Pharmaceutical Industry* (ed. R. Hilfiker). Weinheim: Wiley.

19 Davis, T.D., Peck, G.E., Stowell, J.G. et al. (2004). Modeling and monitoring of polymorphic transformations during the drying phase of wet granulation. *Pharmaceutical Research* 21 (5): 860–866.

20 Govindarajan, R. and Suryanarayanan, R. (2006). Processing-induced phase transformations and their implications on pharmaceutical product quality. In: *Polymorphism: In the Pharmaceutical Industry* (ed. R. Hilfiker), 333–364. Germany: Wiley-VCH Verlag GmbH & Co. KGaA.

21 Yu, L. (2001). Amorphous pharmaceutical solids: preparation, characterization and stabilization. *Advanced Drug Delivery Reviews* 48 (1): 27–42.

22 Ambike, A.A., Mahadik, K., and Paradkar, A. (2005). Spray-dried amorphous solid dispersions of simvastatin, a low Tg drug: in vitro and in vivo evaluations. *Pharmaceutical Research* 22 (6): 990–998.

23 Chauhan, B., Shimpi, S., and Paradkar, A. (2005). Preparation and characterization of etoricoxib solid dispersions using lipid carriers by spray drying technique. *AAPS PharmSciTech* 6 (3): E405–E412.

24 Chen, J., Ormes, J.D., Higgins, J.D., and Taylor, L.S. (2015). Impact of surfactants on the crystallization of aqueous suspensions of celecoxib amorphous solid dispersion spray dried particles. *Molecular Pharmaceutics* 12 (2): 533–541.

25 Chhaprel, P., Talesara, A., and Jain, A.K. (2012). Solubility enhancement of poorly water soluble drug using spray drying technique. *International Journal of Pharmaceutical Studies and Research* 3 (2): 1–5.

26 Pikal, M.J. (2006). Freeze drying. *Encyclopedia of Pharmaceutical Technology* 1 (1): 1807–1833.

27 Hancock, B.C. and Zografi, G. (1994). The relationship between the glass transition temperature and the water content of amorphous pharmaceutical solids. *Pharmaceutical Research* 11 (4): 471–477.

28 Shalaev, E.Y., Johnson-Elton, T.D., Chang, L., and Pikal, M.J. (2002). Thermophysical properties of pharmaceutically compatible buffers at sub-zero temperatures: implications for freeze-drying. *Pharmaceutical Research* 19 (2): 195–201.

29 Re, M.-I. (2006). Formulating drug delivery systems by spray drying. *Drying Technology* 24 (4): 433–446.

30 Patel, B.B., Patel, J.K., Chakraborty, S., and Shukla, D. (2015). Revealing facts behind spray dried solid dispersion technology used for solubility enhancement. *Saudi Pharmaceutical Journal* 23 (4): 352–365.

31 Patel, R., Patel, M., and Suthar, A. (2009). Spray drying technology: an overview. *Indian Journal of Science and Technology* 2 (10): 44–47.

32 Roos, Y.H. (2002). Importance of glass transition and water activity to spray drying and stability of dairy powders. *Le Lait* 82 (4): 475–484.

33 Surana, R., Pyne, A., and Suryanarayanan, R. (2004). Effect of preparation method on physical properties of amorphous trehalose. *Pharmaceutical Research* 21 (7): 1167–1176.

34 Bhardwaj, S.P. and Suryanarayanan, R. (2012). Molecular mobility as an effective predictor of the physical stability of amorphous trehalose. *Molecular Pharmaceutics* 9 (11): 3209–3217.

35 Berggren, J. (2003). Engineering of pharmaceutical particles: modulation of particle structural properties, solid-state stability and tabletting behaviour by the drying process. Doctoral Thesis. Uppsala: Acta Universitatis Upsaliensis, Uppsala University.

36 Berggren, J. and Alderborn, G. (2001). Effect of drying rate on porosity and tabletting behaviour of cellulose pellets. *International Journal of Pharmaceutics* 227 (1): 81–96.

37 Alderborn, G., Borjesson, E., Glazer, M., and Nystrom, C. (1988). Studies on direct compression of tablets. XIX: the effect of particle size and shape on the mechanical strength of sodium bicarbonate tablets. *Acta Pharmaceutica Suecica* 25 (1): 31–40.

38 Alderborn, G. and Nyström, C. (1982). Studies on direct compression of tablets. III. The effect on tablet strength of changes in particle shape and texture obtained by milling. *Acta Pharmaceutica Suecica* 19 (2): 147.

39 Alderborn, G. and Nyström, C. (1982). Studies on direct compression of tablets. IV. The effect of particle size on the mechanical strength of tablets. *Acta Pharmaceutica Suecica* 19 (5): 381.

40 Hintz, R.J. and Johnson, K.C. (1989). The effect of particle size distribution on dissolution rate and oral absorption. *International Journal of Pharmaceutics* 51 (1): 9–17.

41 Lee, Y.-Y., Wu, J.X., Yang, M. et al. (2011). Particle size dependence of polymorphism in spray-dried mannitol. *European Journal of Pharmaceutical Sciences* 44 (1): 41–48.

42 Chatrath, M. and Staniforth, J.N. (1990). The relative influence of dielectric and other drying techniques on the physico-mechanical properties of a

pharmaceutical tablet excipient. Part I: compaction characteristics. *Drying Technology* 8 (5): 1089–1109.

43 Bataille, B., Ligarski, K., Jacob, N. et al. (1993). Study of the influence of spheronization and drying conditions on the physico-mechanical properties of neutral spheroids containing Avicel PH 101 and lactose. *Drug Development and Industrial Pharmacy* 19 (6): 653–671.

44 Wlosnewski, J.C., Kumpugdee-Vollrath, M., and Sriamornsak, P. (2010). Effect of drying technique and disintegrant on physical properties and drug release behavior of microcrystalline cellulose-based pellets prepared by extrusion/spheronization. *Chemical Engineering Research and Design* 88 (1): 100–108.

45 Dyer, A., Khan, K., and Aulton, M. (1994). Effect of the drying method on the mechanical and drug release properties of pellets prepared by extrusion-spheronization. *Drug Development and Industrial Pharmacy* 20 (20): 3045–3068.

46 Remon, J. and Schwartz, J. (1987). Effect of raw materials and processing on the quality of granules prepared from microcrystalline cellulose-lactose mixtures. *Drug Development and Industrial Pharmacy* 13 (1): 1–14.

47 Johansson, B., Wikberg, M., Ek, R., and Alderborn, G. (1995). Compression behaviour and compatibility of microcrystalline cellulose pellets in relationship to their pore structure and mechanical properties. *International Journal of Pharmaceutics* 117 (1): 57–73.

48 Li, L. and Peck, G. (1990). The effect of moisture content on the compression properties of maltodextrins. *Journal of Pharmacy and Pharmacology* 42 (4): 272–275.

49 Riepma, K., Vromans, H., Zuurman, K., and Lerk, C. (1993). The effect of dry granulation on the consolidation and compaction of crystalline lactose. *International Journal of Pharmaceutics* 97 (1–3): 29–38.

50 Huttenrauch, R. (1983). Modification of starting materials to improve tabletting properties. *Pharmazeutische Industrie* 45 (4): 435–440.

51 Hüttenrauch, R. and Keiner, I. (1979). Producing lattice defects by drying processes. *International Journal of Pharmaceutics* 2 (1): 59–60.

52 Khan, K., Musikabhumma, P., and Warr, J. (1981). The effect of moisture content of microcrystalline cellulose on the compressional properties of some formulations. *Drug Development and Industrial Pharmacy* 7 (5): 525–538.

53 Malamataris, S., Goidas, P., and Dimitriou, A. (1991). Moisture sorption and tensile strength of some tableted direct compression excipients. *International Journal of Pharmaceutics* 68 (1): 51–60.

54 Amidon, G.E. and Houghton, M.E. (1995). The effect of moisture on the mechanical and powder flow properties of microcrystalline cellulose. *Pharmaceutical Research* 12 (6): 923–929.

55 Armstrong, N.A., Patel, A., and Jones, T.M. (1986). The compressional properties of dextrose monohydrate and anhydrous dextrose of varying water contents. *Drug Development and Industrial Pharmacy* 12 (11–13): 1885–1901.

56 Craik, D. (1958). The flow properties of starch powders and mixtures. *Journal of Pharmacy and Pharmacology* 10 (1): 73–79.

57 Craik, D. and Miller, B. (1958). The flow properties of powders under humid conditions. *Journal of Pharmacy and Pharmacology* 10 (S1): 136T–144T.

58 Dawoodbhai, S. and Rhodes, C.T. (1989). The effect of moisture on powder flow and on compaction and physical stability of tablets. *Drug Development and Industrial Pharmacy* 15 (10): 1577–1600.

59 Jaffe, J. and Foss, N.E. (1959). Compression of crystalline substances. *Journal of the American Pharmaceutical Association (Scientific ed)* 48 (1): 26–29.

60 Lerk, C., Andreae, A., Boer, A. et al. (1983). Increased binding capacity and flowability of α-lactose monohydrate after dehydration. *Journal of Pharmacy and Pharmacology* 35 (11): 747–748.

61 Pande, G.S. and Shangraw, R.F. (1995). Characterization of β-cyclodextrin for direct compression tableting: II. The role of moisture in the compactibility of β-cyclodextrin. *International Journal of Pharmaceutics* 124 (2): 231–239.

62 Shotton, E. and Harb, N. (1966). The effect of humidity and temperature on the cohesion of powders. *Journal of Pharmacy and Pharmacology* 18 (3): 175–178.

63 Train, D. (1956). An investigation into the compaction of powders. *Journal of Pharmacy and Pharmacology* 8 (1): 745–761.

64 Abdelwahed, W., Degobert, G., Stainmesse, S., and Fessi, H. (2006). Freeze-drying of nanoparticles: formulation, process and storage considerations. *Advanced Drug Delivery Reviews* 58 (15): 1688–1713.

65 Vo, C.L.-N., Park, C., and Lee, B.-J. (2013). Current trends and future perspectives of solid dispersions containing poorly water-soluble drugs. *European Journal of Pharmaceutics and Biopharmaceutics* 85 (3): 799–813.

66 Alhalaweh, A. and Velaga, S.P. (2010). Formation of cocrystals from stoichiometric solutions of incongruently saturating systems by spray drying. *Crystal Growth & Design* 10 (8): 3302–3305.

67 Chauhan, B., Shimpi, S., and Paradkar, A. (2005). Preparation and evaluation of glibenclamide-polyglycolized glycerides solid dispersions with silicon dioxide by spray drying technique. *European Journal of Pharmaceutical Sciences* 26 (2): 219–230.

68 Chen, R., Okamoto, H., and Danjo, K. (2006). Particle design using a 4-fluid-nozzle spray-drying technique for sustained release of acetaminophen. *Chemical and Pharmaceutical Bulletin* 54 (7): 948–953.

69 Chow, A.H., Tong, H.H., Chattopadhyay, P., and Shekunov, B.Y. (2007). Particle engineering for pulmonary drug delivery. *Pharmaceutical Research* 24 (3): 411–437.

70 Giri, T.K., Kumar, K., Alexander, A. et al. (2012). A novel and alternative approach to controlled release drug delivery system based on solid dispersion technique. *Bulletin of Faculty of Pharmacy, Cairo University* 50 (2): 147–159.

71 Hecq, J., Deleers, M., Fanara, D. et al. (2005). Preparation and characterization of nanocrystals for solubility and dissolution rate enhancement of nifedipine. *International Journal of Pharmaceutics* 299 (1): 167–177.

72 Kang, J.H., Oh, D.H., Oh, Y.-K. et al. (2012). Effects of solid carriers on the crystalline properties, dissolution and bioavailability of flurbiprofen in solid self-nanoemulsifying drug delivery system (solid SNEDDS). *European Journal of Pharmaceutics and Biopharmaceutics* 80 (2): 289–297.

73 Jain, A., Teja, M.R., Pariyani, L. et al. (2013). Formulation and evaluation of spray-dried esomeprazole magnesium microspheres. *Tropical Journal of Pharmaceutical Research* 12 (3): 299 304.

74 Shan-Yang, L. and Yuh-Horng, K. (1989). Solid particulates of drug-β-cyclodextrin inclusion complexes directly prepared by a spray-drying technique. *International Journal of Pharmaceutics* 56 (3): 249–259.

75 Palmeri, G.F., Wehrlé, P., and Stamm, A. (1994). Evaluation of spray-drying as a method to prepare microparticles for controlled drug release. *Drug Development and Industrial Pharmacy* 20 (18): 2859–2879.

76 Fernandes, C.M., Vieira, M.T., and Veiga, F.J.B. (2002). Physicochemical characterization and in vitro dissolution behavior of nicardipine–cyclodextrins inclusion compounds. *European Journal of Pharmaceutical Sciences* 15 (1): 79–88.

77 Cabral-Marques, H. and Almeida, R. (2009). Optimisation of spray-drying process variables for dry powder inhalation (DPI) formulations of corticosteroid/cyclodextrin inclusion complexes. *European Journal of Pharmaceutics and Biopharmaceutics* 73 (1): 121–129.

78 Yi, T., Wan, J., Xu, H., and Yang, X. (2008). A new solid self-microemulsifying formulation prepared by spray-drying to improve the oral bioavailability of poorly water soluble drugs. *European Journal of Pharmaceutics and Biopharmaceutics* 70 (2): 439–444.

79 Sohi, H., Sultana, Y., and Khar, R.K. (2004). Taste masking technologies in oral pharmaceuticals: recent developments and approaches. *Drug Development and Industrial Pharmacy* 30 (5): 429–448.

80 Shen, R.W. (1996). Taste masking of ibuprofen by fluid bed coating. Google Patents, EP0524180B1, filed 26 Febraury 1991.

81 Lunstroth, D., Schill, D., and Siegrist, M. (1999). Improving the taste of gut lavage with lemon flavor. *Krankenhauspharmazie* 20: 126–128.

82 Srivastava, S. and Mishra, G. (2010). Fluid bed technology: overview and parameters for process selection. *International Journal of Pharmaceutical Sciences and Drug Research* 2 (4): 236–246.

83 Vervaet, C. and Remon, J.P. (2005). Continuous granulation in the pharmaceutical industry. *Chemical Engineering Science* 60 (14): 3949–3957.

84 Masters, K. (2002, 2002). *Process Stages and Spray Drying Systems in Spray Drying in Practice*, 1–35. Charlottenlund, Denmark: SprayDryConsult International.

85 United Nations Industrial Development Organization. (2010). Classification of dryers. [Internet]. www.unido.org (accessed 5 September 2016).

86 Mujumdar, A.S. and Law, C.L. (2010). Drying technology: trends and applications in postharvest processing. *Food and Bioprocess Technology* 3 (6): 843–852.

87 Chakravarty, P., Berendt, R.T., Munson, E.J. et al. (2010). Insights into the dehydration behavior of thiamine hydrochloride (vitamin B1) hydrates: part II. *Journal of Pharmaceutical Sciences* 99 (2): 816–827.

88 Stephenson, G.A., Groleau, E.G., Kleemann, R.L. et al. (1998). Formation of isomorphic desolvates: creating a molecular vacuum. *Journal of Pharmaceutical Sciences* 87 (5): 536–542.

89 Bauer, J.F., Dziki, W., and Quick, J.E. (1999). Role of an isomorphic desolvate in dissolution failures of an erythromycin tablet formulation. *Journal of Pharmaceutical Sciences* 88 (11): 1222–1227.

90 Chakravarty, P. and Lubach, J.W. (2013). Characterization of a water–solid interaction in a partially ordered system. *Molecular Pharmaceutics* 10 (11): 4294–4300.

91 Wöstheinrich, K. and Schmidt, P. (2001). Polymorphic changes of thiamine hydrochloride during granulation and tableting. *Drug Development and Industrial Pharmacy* 27 (6): 481–489.

92 Otsuka, M., Hasegawa, H., and Matsuda, Y. (1999). Effect of polymorphic forms of bulk powders on pharmaceutical properties of carbamazepine granules. *Chemical and Pharmaceutical Bulletin* 47 (6): 852–856.

93 Tantry, J.S., Tank, J., and Suryanarayanan, R. (2007). Processing-induced phase transitions of theophylline—implications on the dissolution of theophylline tablets. *Journal of Pharmaceutical Sciences* 96 (5): 1434–1444.

94 Morris, K.R., Griesser, U.J., Eckhardt, C.J., and Stowell, J.G. (2001). Theoretical approaches to physical transformations of active pharmaceutical ingredients during manufacturing processes. *Advanced Drug Delivery Reviews* 48 (1): 91–114.

95 Nieuwmeyer, F.J., Damen, M., Gerich, A. et al. (2007). Granule characterization during fluid bed drying by development of a near infrared method to determine water content and median granule size. *Pharmaceutical Research* 24 (10): 1854–1861.

96 Portoghese, F., Berruti, F., and Briens, C. (2008). Continuous on-line measurement of solid moisture content during fluidized bed drying using triboelectric probes. *Powder Technology* 181 (2): 169–177.

97 Liu, X., Muzzio, F.J., Khinast, J.G., and Glasser, B.J. (2013). Fluidized bed drying of pharmaceutical materials:moisture measurement and effects of particle size. *American Pharmaceutical Review.*

98 Buschmüller, C., Wiedey, W., Döscher, C. et al. (2008). In-line monitoring of granule moisture in fluidized-bed dryers using microwave resonance technology. *European Journal of Pharmaceutics and Biopharmaceutics* 69 (1): 380–387.

99 Faure, A., York, P., and Rowe, R. (2001). Process control and scale-up of pharmaceutical wet granulation processes: a review. *European Journal of Pharmaceutics and Biopharmaceutics* 52 (3): 269–277.

100 Teunou, E. and Poncelet, D. (2002). Batch and continuous fluid bed coating–review and state of the art. *Journal of Food Engineering* 53 (4): 325–340.

101 Saleh, K., Cherif, R., and Hemati, M. (1999). An experimental study of fluidized-bed coating: influence of operating conditions on growth rate and mechanism. *Advanced Powder Technology* 10 (3): 255–277.

102 Wurster, D.E. (1959). Air-Suspension technique of coating drug particles: a preliminary report. *Journal of the American Pharmaceutical Association (Scientific ed)* 48 (8): 451–454.

103 Iida, K., Todo, H., Okamoto, H. et al. (2005). Preparation of dry powder inhalation with lactose carrier particles surface-coated using a Wurster fluidized bed. *Chemical and Pharmaceutical Bulletin* 53 (4): 431–434.

104 Hausman, D.S., Cambron, R.T., and Sakr, A. (2005). Application of on-line Raman spectroscopy for characterizing relationships between drug hydration state and tablet physical stability. *International Journal of Pharmaceutics* 299 (1): 19–33.

105 Lester, C., Lubey, G., Dicks, M. et al. (2006). Dehydration of risedronate hemi-pentahydrate: analytical and physical characterization. *Journal of Pharmaceutical Sciences* 95 (12): 2631–2644.

106 Redman-Furey, N., Dicks, M., Bigalow-Kern, A. et al. (2005). Structural and analytical characterization of three hydrates and an anhydrate form of risedronate. *Journal of Pharmaceutical Sciences* 94 (4): 893–911.

107 Sosnik, A. and Seremeta, K.P. (2015). Advantages and challenges of the spray-drying technology for the production of pure drug particles and drug-loaded polymeric carriers. *Advances in Colloid and Interface Science* 223: 40–54.

108 Ozioko, C. (n.d.). Spray dryer. https://www.pharmapproach.com/spray-dryer (accessed October 2016).

109 Schwartzbach, H. (2010). The possibilities and challenges of spray drying. http://www.pharmtech.com/possibilities-and-challenges-spray-drying (accessed October 2016).

110 Corrigan, O. (1995). Thermal analysis of spray dried products. *Thermochimica Acta* 248: 245–258.

111 Chidavaenzi, O.C., Buckton, G., Koosha, F., and Pathak, R. (1997). The use of thermal techniques to assess the impact of feed concentration on the amorphous content and polymorphic forms present in spray dried lactose. *International Journal of Pharmaceutics* 159 (1): 67–74.

112 Matsuda, Y., Otsuka, M., Onoe, M., and Tatsumi, E. (1992). Amorphism and physicochemical stability of spray-dried frusemide. *Journal of Pharmacy and Pharmacology* 44 (8): 627–633.

113 Yamaguchi, T., Nishimura, M., Okamoto, R. et al. (1992). Glass formation of 4″-O-(4-methoxyphenyl) acetyltylosin and physicochemical stability of the amorphous solid. *International Journal of Pharmaceutics* 85 (1–3): 87–96.

114 Bolhuls, G., Kussendrager, K., and Langridge, J. (2004). New developments in spray-dried lactose. *Pharmaceutical Technology* 22: 26–31.

115 Sollohub, K. and Cal, K. (2010). Spray drying technique: II. Current applications in pharmaceutical technology. *Journal of Pharmaceutical Sciences* 99 (2): 587–597.

116 Di Martino, P., Scoppa, M., Joiris, E. et al. (2001). The spray drying of acetazolamide as method to modify crystal properties and to improve compression behaviour. *International Journal of Pharmaceutics* 213 (1): 209–221.

117 Matsuda, Y., Kawaguchi, S., Kobayashi, H., and Nishijo, J. (1980). Polymorphism of phenylbutazone by a spray drying method. *Journal of Pharmacy and Pharmacology* 32 (1): 579–580.

118 Matsuda, Y., Kawaguchi, S., Kobayashi, H., and Nishijo, J. (1984). Physicochemical characterization of spray-dried phenylbutazone polymorphs. *Journal of Pharmaceutical Sciences* 73 (2): 173–179.

119 Corrigan, O., Sabra, K., and Holohan, E. (1983). Physicochemical properties of spray dried drugs: phenobarbitone and hydroflumethiazide. *Drug Development and Industrial Pharmacy* 9: 1–2):1–20.

120 Tusda, Y., Ishida, M., Suzuki, E., and Sekiguchi, K. (1988). Spray drying of griseofulvin solution forming its solvate. *Chemical and Pharmaceutical Bulletin* 36 (6): 2193–2196.

121 Hulse, W.L., Forbes, R.T., Bonner, M.C., and Getrost, M. (2009). The characterization and comparison of spray-dried mannitol samples. *Drug Development and Industrial Pharmacy* 35 (6): 712–718.

122 Yu, L. and Ng, K. (2002). Glycine crystallization during spray drying: the pH effect on salt and polymorphic forms. *Journal of Pharmaceutical Sciences* 91 (11): 2367–2375.

123 Masters, K. (1991). *Handbook of Spray Drying*, 5e. London: Longman.

124 Dunbar, C.A., Concessio, N.M., and Hickey, A.J. (1998). Evaluation of atomizer performance in production of respirable spray-dried particles. *Pharmaceutical Development and Technology* 3 (4): 433–441.

125 Chew, N.Y. and Chan, H.-K. (2001). Use of solid corrugated particles to enhance powder aerosol performance. *Pharmaceutical Research* 18 (11): 1570–1577.

126 Chew, N.Y., Tang, P., Chan, H.-K., and Raper, J.A. (2005). How much particle surface corrugation is sufficient to improve aerosol performance of powders? *Pharmaceutical Research* 22 (1): 148–152.

127 Gilani, K., Najafabadi, A.R., Barghi, M., and Rafiee-Tehrani, M. (2005). The effect of water to ethanol feed ratio on physical properties and aerosolization behavior of spray dried cromolyn sodium particles. *Journal of Pharmaceutical Sciences* 94 (5): 1048–1059.

128 Maa, Y.-F., Costantino, H.R., Nguyen, P.-A., and Hsu, C.C. (1997). The effect of operating and formulation variables on the morphology of spray-dried protein particles. *Pharmaceutical Development and Technology* 2 (3): 213–223.

129 Chen, D., Batycky, R.P., Johnston, L., and Mintzes, J. (2005). Control of process humidity to produce large, porous particles. Google Patents, US7469488B2, filed 29 October 2004.

130 Elversson, J., Millqvist-Fureby, A., Alderborn, G., and Elofsson, U. (2003). Droplet and particle size relationship and shell thickness of inhalable lactose particles during spray drying. *Journal of Pharmaceutical Sciences* 92 (4): 900–910.

131 Elversson, J. and Millqvist-Fureby, A. (2005). Particle size and density in spray drying—effects of carbohydrate properties. *Journal of Pharmaceutical Sciences* 94 (9): 2049–2060.

132 Littringer, E.M., Mescher, A., Eckhard, S. et al. (2012). Spray drying of mannitol as a drug carrier—the impact of process parameters on product properties. *Drying Technology* 30 (1): 114–124.

133 Littringer, E.M., Mescher, A., Schroettner, H. et al. (2012). Spray dried mannitol carrier particles with tailored surface properties–the influence of carrier surface roughness and shape. *European Journal of Pharmaceutics and Biopharmaceutics* 82 (1): 194–204.

134 Gonnissen, Y., Remon, J.P., and Vervaet, C. (2007). Development of directly compressible powders via co-spray drying. *European Journal of Pharmaceutics and Biopharmaceutics* 67 (1): 220–226.

135 Gonnissen, Y., Goncalves, S., De Geest, B. et al. (2008). Process design applied to optimise a directly compressible powder produced via a continuous manufacturing process. *European Journal of Pharmaceutics and Biopharmaceutics* 68 (3): 760–770.

136 Wallman, H. and Blyth, H. (1951). Pilot plants. Product control in Bowen-type spray dryer. *Industrial & Engineering Chemistry* 43 (6): 1480–1486.

137 Paudel, A., Worku, Z.A., Meeus, J. et al. (2013). Manufacturing of solid dispersions of poorly water soluble drugs by spray drying: formulation and process considerations. *International Journal of Pharmaceutics* 453 (1): 253–284.

138 Arias, M., Gines, J., Moyano, J. et al. (1995). Influence of the preparation method of solid dispersions on their dissolution rate: study of triamterene-D-mannitol system. *International Journal of Pharmaceutics* 123 (1): 25–31.

139 Miller, D.A. and Gil, M. (2012). Spray-drying technology. *Formulating Poorly Water Soluble Drugs* 32: 363–442.

140 Leuner, C. and Dressman, J. (2000). Improving drug solubility for oral delivery using solid dispersions. *European Journal of Pharmaceutics and Biopharmaceutics* 50 (1): 47–60.

141 Al-Obaidi, H., Brocchini, S., and Buckton, G. (2009). Anomalous properties of spray dried solid dispersions. *Journal of Pharmaceutical Sciences* 98 (12): 4724–4737.

142 Al-Obaidi, H., Ke, P., Brocchini, S., and Buckton, G. (2011). Characterization and stability of ternary solid dispersions with PVP and PHPMA. *International Journal of Pharmaceutics* 419 (1): 20–27.

143 Al-Obaidi, H. and Buckton, G. (2009). Evaluation of griseofulvin binary and ternary solid dispersions with HPMCAS. *AAPS PharmSciTech* 10 (4): 1172–1177.

144 Janssens, S., De Armas, H.N., Roberts, C.J., and Van den Mooter, G. (2008). Characterization of ternary solid dispersions of itraconazole, PEG 6000, and HPMC 2910 E5. *Journal of Pharmaceutical Sciences* 97 (6): 2110–2120.

145 Janssens, S., Denivelle, S., Rombaut, P., and Van den Mooter, G. (2008). Influence of polyethylene glycol chain length on compatibility and release characteristics of ternary solid dispersions of itraconazole in polyethylene glycol/hydroxypropylmethylcellulose 2910 E5 blends. *European Journal of Pharmaceutical Sciences* 35 (3): 203–210.

146 Janssens, S., Nagels, S., De Armas, H.N. et al. (2008). Formulation and characterization of ternary solid dispersions made up of Itraconazole and two excipients, TPGS 1000 and PVPVA 64, that were selected based on a

supersaturation screening study. *European Journal of Pharmaceutics and Biopharmaceutics* 69 (1): 158–166.

147 Janssens, S., Van Humbeeck, J., and Van den Mooter, G. (2008). Evaluation of the formulation of solid dispersions by co-spray drying itraconazole with Inutec SP1, a polymeric surfactant, in combination with PVPVA 64. *European Journal of Pharmaceutics and Biopharmaceutics* 70 (2): 500–505.

148 Heng, D., Lee, S.H., Ng, W.K., and Tan, R.B. (2011). The nano spray dryer B-90. *Expert Opinion on Drug Delivery* 8 (7): 965–972.

149 Peltonen, L., Valo, H., Kolakovic, R. et al. (2010). Electrospraying, spray drying and related techniques for production and formulation of drug nanoparticles. *Expert Opinion on Drug Delivery* 7 (6): 705–719.

150 Vehring, R. (2008). Pharmaceutical particle engineering via spray drying. *Pharmaceutical Research* 25 (5): 999–1022.

151 Schultheiss, N. and Newman, A. (2009). Pharmaceutical cocrystals and their physicochemical properties. *Crystal Growth and Design* 9 (6): 2950–2967.

152 Mistry, R.B. and Sheth, N.S. (2011). A review: self-emulsifying drug delivery system. *International Journal of Pharmacy and Pharmaceutical Sciences* 3 (2): 23–28.

153 Balakrishnan, P., Lee, B.-J., Oh, D.H. et al. (2009). Enhanced oral bioavailability of dexibuprofen by a novel solid self-emulsifying drug delivery system (SEDDS). *European Journal of Pharmaceutics and Biopharmaceutics* 72 (3): 539–545.

154 Bhalekar, M., Madgulkar, A., Gunjal, S., and Bagal, A. (2013). Formulation and optimisation of sustained release spray-dried microspheres of glipizide using natural polysaccharide. *PDA Journal of Pharmaceutical Science and Technology* 67 (2): 146–154.

155 Shah, N., Kondawar, M., Shah, R., and Shah, V. (2011). Sustained release of spray-dried combination dry powder inhaler formulation for pulmonary delivery. *Asian Journal of Pharmaceutical and Clinical Research.* 4 (4): 112–118.

156 Maas, S.G., Schaldach, G., Littringer, E.M. et al. (2011). The impact of spray drying outlet temperature on the particle morphology of mannitol. *Powder Technology* 213 (1): 27–35.

157 Steckel, H. and Brandes, H.G. (2004). A novel spray-drying technique to produce low density particles for pulmonary delivery. *International Journal of Pharmaceutics* 278 (1): 187–195.

158 Capitaine, S.L. and Peppin, C. (2012) Rotary dryer or fluid bed dryer. http://feeco.com/rotary-dryer-or-fluid-bed-dryer (accessed October 2016).

159 Boateng, J.S., Auffret, A.D., Matthews, K.H. et al. (2010). Characterisation of freeze-dried wafers and solvent evaporated films as potential drug delivery systems to mucosal surfaces. *International Journal of Pharmaceutics* 389 (1): 24–31.

160 Corveleyn, S. and Remon, J.P. (1999). Stability of freeze-dried tablets at different relative humidities. *Drug Development and Industrial Pharmacy* 25 (9): 1005–1013.

161 Kumar, G., Prashanth, N., and Kumari, B. (2011). Fundamentals and applications of lyophilization. *Journal of Advanced Pharmaceutical Technology & Research* 2: 157–169.

162 Baheti, A., Kumar, L., and Bansal, A.K. (2010). Excipients used in lyophilization of small molecules. *Journal of Excipients and Food Chemicals* 1 (1): 41–54.

163 Cannon, A.J. and Trappler, E.H. (1999). The influence of lyophilization on the polymorphic behavior of mannitol. *PDA Journal of Pharmaceutical Science and Technology* 54 (1): 13–22.

164 Pyne, A. and Suryanarayanan, R. (2001). Phase transitions of glycine in frozen aqueous solutions and during freeze-drying. *Pharmaceutical Research* 18 (10): 1448–1454.

165 Carpenter, J.F., Pikal, M.J., and Chang, B.S. (1997). Randolph TW. Rational design of stable lyophilized protein formulations: some practical advice. *Pharmaceutical Research* 14 (8): 969–975.

166 Liao, X., Krishnamurthy, R., and Suryanarayanan, R. (2007). Influence of processing conditions on the physical state of mannitol—implications in freeze-drying. *Pharmaceutical Research* 24 (2): 370–376.

167 Milton, N., Nail, S.L., and Akers, M.J. (1997). The crystallization kinetics of glycine hydrochloride from 'frozen' solution. *Cryo-letters* 18 (6): 335–342.

168 Pyne, A., Surana, R., and Suryanarayanan, R. (2002). Crystallization of mannitol below Tg′ during freeze-drying in binary and ternary aqueous systems. *Pharmaceutical Research* 19 (6): 901–908.

169 Mehta, M., Bhardwaj, S.P., and Suryanarayanan, R. (2013). Controlling the physical form of mannitol in freeze-dried systems. *European Journal of Pharmaceutics and Biopharmaceutics* 85 (2): 207–213.

170 Cavatur, R.K. and Suryanarayanan, R. (1998). Characterization of phase transitions during freeze-drying by in situ X-ray powder diffractometry. *Pharmaceutical Development and Technology* 3 (4): 579–586.

171 Pyne, A., Chatterjee, K., and Suryanarayanan, R. (2003). Crystalline to amorphous transition of disodium hydrogen phosphate during primary drying. *Pharmaceutical Research* 20 (5): 802–803.

172 Pyne, A. and Suryanarayanan, R. (2003). The effect of additives on the crystallization of cefazolin sodium during freeze-drying. *Pharmaceutical Research* 20 (2): 283–291.

173 Yu, L., Milton, N., Groleau, E.G. et al. (1999). Existence of a mannitol hydrate during freeze-drying and practical implications. *Journal of Pharmaceutical Sciences* 88 (2): 196–198.

174 De Beer, T., Vercruysse, P., Burggraeve, A. et al. (2009). In-line and real-time process monitoring of a freeze drying process using Raman and NIR spectroscopy as complementary process analytical technology (PAT) tools. *Journal of Pharmaceutical Sciences* 98 (9): 3430–3446.

175 Bauer, K.H. (2007). A partially freeze-dried lyophilization technology for producing fast-melting tablets. *Pharmaceutical Technology Europe* 19 (9) www.PharmTech.com (accessed October 2016).

176 Ahmed, I.S. and Aboul-Einien, M.H. (2007). In vitro and in vivo evaluation of a fast-disintegrating lyophilized dry emulsion tablet containing griseofulvin. *European Journal of Pharmaceutical Sciences* 32 (1): 58–68.
177 Boateng, J.S., Matthews, K.H., Auffret, A.D. et al. (2009). In vitro drug release studies of polymeric freeze-dried wafers and solvent-cast films using paracetamol as a model soluble drug. *International Journal of Pharmaceutics* 378 (1): 66–72.
178 Patel, V.R. and Amiji, M.M. (1996). Preparation and characterization of freeze-dried chitosan-poly (ethylene oxide) hydrogels for site-specific antibiotic delivery in the stomach. *Pharmaceutical Research* 13 (4): 588–593.
179 Benali, M. and Boumghar, Y. (2014). Supercritical fluid-assisted drying. In: *Handbook of Industrial Drying*, 4e (ed. A.S. Mujumdar), 1261–1269. Boca Raton, FL: CRC Press.
180 Sihvonen, M., Järvenpää, E., Hietaniemi, V., and Huopalahti, R. (1999). Advances in supercritical carbon dioxide technologies. *Trends in Food Science & Technology* 10 (6): 217–222.
181 Pasquali, I., Bettini, R., and Giordano, F. (2008). Supercritical fluid technologies: an innovative approach for manipulating the solid-state of pharmaceuticals. *Advanced Drug Delivery Reviews* 60 (3): 399–410.
182 Pasquali, I., Bettini, R., and Giordano, F. (2006). Solid-state chemistry and particle engineering with supercritical fluids in pharmaceutics. *European Journal of Pharmaceutical Sciences* 27 (4): 299–310.
183 Munshi, P. and Bhaduri, S. (2009). Supercritical CO_2: a twenty-first century solvent for the chemical industry. *Current Science* 97 (1): 63–72.
184 Moribe, K., Tozuka, Y., and Yamamoto, K. (2008). Supercritical carbon dioxide processing of active pharmaceutical ingredients for polymorphic control and for complex formation. *Advanced Drug Delivery Reviews* 60 (3): 328–338.
185 Phillips, E.M. and Stella, V.J. (1993). Rapid expansion from supercritical solutions: application to pharmaceutical processes. *International Journal of Pharmaceutics* 94 (1): 1–10.
186 Yeo, S.-D. and Kiran, E. (2005). Formation of polymer particles with supercritical fluids: a review. *The Journal of Supercritical Fluids* 34 (3): 287–308.
187 Moribe, K., Tsutsumi, S.-i., Morishita, S. et al. (2005). Micronization of phenylbutazone by rapid expansion of supercritical CO_2 solution. *Chemical and Pharmaceutical Bulletin* 53 (8): 1025–1028.
188 Shinozaki, H., Oguchi, T., Suzuki, S. et al. (2006). Micronization and polymorphic conversion of tolbutamide and barbital by rapid expansion of supercritical solutions. *Drug Development and Industrial Pharmacy* 32 (7): 877–891.
189 Bettini, R., Bonassi, L., Castoro, V. et al. (2001). Solubility and conversion of carbamazepine polymorphs in supercritical carbon dioxide. *European Journal of Pharmaceutical Sciences* 13 (3): 281–286.
190 Tozuka, Y., Kawada, D., Oguchi, T., and Yamamoto, K. (2003). Supercritical carbon dioxide treatment as a method for polymorph preparation of deoxycholic acid. *International Journal of Pharmaceutics* 263 (1): 45–50.

191 Velaga, S.P., Berger, R., and Carlfors, J. (2002). Supercritical fluids crystallization of budesonide and flunisolide. *Pharmaceutical Research* 19 (10): 1564–1571.

192 Kordikowski, A., Shekunov, T., and York, P. (2001). Polymorph control of sulfathiazole in supercritical CO_2. *Pharmaceutical Research* 18 (5): 682–688.

193 Kordikowski, A., York, P., and Latham, D. (1999). Resolution of ephedrine in supercritical CO_2: a novel technique for the separation of chiral drugs. *Journal of Pharmaceutical Sciences* 88 (8): 786–791.

194 Oakes, R.S., Clifford, A.A., Bartle, K.D. et al. (1999). Sulfur oxidation in supercritical carbon dioxide: dramatic pressure dependant enhancement of diastereoselectivity for sulfoxidation of cysteine derivatives. *Chemical Communications* (3): 247–248.

195 Rehman, M., York, P., and Kippax, P. (2003). Particle engineering for improved dispersion in dry powder inhalers. *Pharmaceutical Technology Europe* 15: 34–39.

196 Bustami, R., Chan, H., and Foster, N. (eds.) (2000). Aerosol delivery of protein powders processed by supercritical fluid technology. In: *Proceedings of the Conference on Respiratory Drug Delivery*. Tarpon Springs, Florida: Palm Harbor (14–18 May 2000).

197 Bustami, R.T., Chan, H.-K., Dehghani, F., and Foster, N.R. (2000). Generation of micro-particles of proteins for aerosol delivery using high pressure modified carbon dioxide. *Pharmaceutical Research* 17 (11): 1360–1366.

198 Shekunov, B.Y., Feeley, J.C., Chow, A.H. et al. (2003). Aerosolisation behaviour of micronised and supercritically-processed powders. *Journal of Aerosol Science* 34 (5): 553–568.

199 Rehman, M., Shekunov, B.Y., York, P. et al. (2004). Optimisation of powders for pulmonary delivery using supercritical fluid technology. *European Journal of Pharmaceutical Sciences* 22 (1): 1–17.

200 Bettini, R., Rossi, A., Lavezzini, E. et al. (2003). Thermal and morphological characterization of micronized acetylsalicylic acid powders prepared by rapid expansion of a supercritical solution. *Journal of Thermal Analysis and Calorimetry* 73 (2): 487–497.

201 Türk, M. (1999). Formation of small organic particles by RESS: experimental and theoretical investigations. *The Journal of Supercritical Fluids* 15 (1): 79–89.

202 Türk, M., Hils, P., Helfgen, B. et al. (2002). Micronization of pharmaceutical substances by the rapid expansion of supercritical solutions (RESS): a promising method to improve bioavailability of poorly soluble pharmaceutical agents. *The Journal of Supercritical Fluids* 22 (1): 75–84.

203 Bristow, S., Shekunov, T., Shekunov, B.Y., and York, P. (2001). Analysis of the supersaturation and precipitation process with supercritical CO_2. *The Journal of Supercritical Fluids* 21 (3): 257–271.

204 Werling, J.O. and Debenedetti, P.G. (1999). Numerical modeling of mass transfer in the supercritical antisolvent process. *The Journal of Supercritical Fluids* 16 (2): 167–181.

205 Hanna, M. and York, P. (1998). Method and apparatus for the formation of particles. UK patent 5,851,453. (Inventors) University of Bradford, West Yorkshire, England, assignee.
206 Palakodaty, S. and York, P. (1999). Phase behavioral effects on particle formation processes using supercritical fluids. *Pharmaceutical Research* 16 (7): 976–985.
207 Yeo, S.-D. and Lee, J.-C. (2004). Crystallization of sulfamethizole using the supercritical and liquid antisolvent processes. *The Journal of Supercritical Fluids* 30 (3): 315–323.
208 Reverchon, E. and De Marco, I. (2004). Supercritical antisolvent micronization of Cefonicid: thermodynamic interpretation of results. *The Journal of Supercritical Fluids* 31 (2): 207–215.
209 Reverchon, E., De Marco, I., and Della Porta, G. (2002). Rifampicin microparticles production by supercritical antisolvent precipitation. *International Journal of Pharmaceutics* 243 (1): 83–91.
210 Reverchon, E. and Della Porta, G. (2003). Micronization of antibiotics by supercritical assisted atomization. *The Journal of Supercritical Fluids* 26 (3): 243–252.
211 Reverchon, E. and Della, P.G. (2003). Terbutaline microparticles suitable for aerosol delivery produced by supercritical assisted atomization. *International Journal of Pharmaceutics* 258 (1): 1–9.
212 Reverchon, E. and Spada, A. (2004). Erythromycin micro-particles produced by supercritical fluid atomization. *Powder Technology* 141 (1): 100–108.
213 Kröber, H. and Teipel, U. (2002). Materials processing with supercritical antisolvent precipitation: process parameters and morphology of tartaric acid. *The Journal of Supercritical Fluids* 22 (3): 229–235.
214 Blatchford, M.A., Raveendran, P., and Wallen, S.L. (2003). Spectroscopic studies of model carbonyl compounds in CO_2: Evidence for cooperative C-H-O interactions. *The Journal of Physical Chemistry A* 107 (48): 10311–10323.
215 Hirunsit, P., Huang, Z., Srinophakun, T. et al. (2005). Particle formation of ibuprofen–supercritical CO_2 system from rapid expansion of supercritical solutions (RESS): A mathematical model. *Powder Technology* 154 (2): 83–94.
216 Mura, P., Bettinetti, G., Manderioli, A. et al. (1998). Interactions of ketoprofen and ibuprofen with β-cyclodextrins in solution and in the solid state. *International Journal of Pharmaceutics* 166 (2): 189–203.
217 Shankland, N., Florence, A.J., Cox, P.J. et al. (1996). Crystal morphology of ibuprofen predicted from single-crystal pulsed neutron diffraction data. *Chemical Communications* (7): 855–856.
218 Tozuka, Y., Fujito, T., Moribe, K., and Yamamoto, K. (2006). Ibuprofen-cyclodextrin inclusion complex formation using supercritical carbon dioxide. *Journal of Inclusion Phenomena and Macrocyclic Chemistry* 56 (1–2): 33–37.
219 Rodrigues, M., Peiriço, N., Matos, H. et al. (2004). Microcomposites theophylline/hydrogenated palm oil from a PGSS process for controlled drug delivery systems. *The Journal of Supercritical Fluids* 29 (1): 175–184.

220 Higuchi, T. (1961). Rate of release of medicaments from ointment bases containing drugs in suspension. *Journal of Pharmaceutical Sciences* 50 (10): 874–875.

221 Higuchi, T. (1963). Mechanism of sustained-action medication. Theoretical analysis of rate of release of solid drugs dispersed in solid matrices. *Journal of Pharmaceutical Sciences* 52 (12): 1145–1149.

222 Askari, G., Emam-Djomeh, Z., and Mousavi, S. (2009). An investigation of the effects of drying methods and conditions on drying characteristics and quality attributes of agricultural products during hot air and hot air/microwave-assisted dehydration. *Drying Technology* 27 (7–8): 831–841.

223 Cui, Z.-W., Li, C.-Y., Song, C.-F., and Song, Y. (2008). Combined microwave-vacuum and freeze drying of carrot and apple chips. *Drying Technology* 26 (12): 1517–1523.

224 Duan, X., Zhang, M., and Mujumdar, A.S. (2007). Studies on the microwave freeze drying technique and sterilization characteristics of cabbage. *Drying Technology* 25 (10): 1725–1731.

225 Huang, L.-l., Zhang, M., Mujumdar, A.S. et al. (2009). Studies on decreasing energy consumption for a freeze-drying process of apple slices. *Drying Technology* 27 (9): 938–946.

226 Reyes, A., Ceron, S., Zuniga, R., and Moyano, P. (2007). A comparative study of microwave-assisted air drying of potato slices. *Biosystems Engineering* 98 (3): 310–318.

227 Scaman, C. and Durance, T. (2005). Combined microwave vacuum drying. In: *Emerging Technologies for Food Processing* (ed. D. Sun), 507–534. Waltham: Elsevier Academic.

228 Setiady, D., Tang, J., Younce, F. et al. (2009). Porosity, color, texture, and microscopic structure of russet potatoes dried using microwave vacuum, heated air, and freeze drying. *Applied Engineering in Agriculture* 25 (5): 719–724.

229 Stępień, B. (2008). Effect of vacuum-microwave drying on selected mechanical and rheological properties of carrot. *Biosystems Engineering* 99 (2): 234–238.

230 Wang, R., Zhang, M., Mujumdar, A.S., and Sun, J.-C. (2009). Microwave freeze–drying characteristics and sensory quality of instant vegetable soup. *Drying Technology* 27 (9): 962–968.

231 Wang, W. and Chen, G. (2005). Theoretical study on microwave freeze drying of an aqueous pharmaceutical excipient with the aid of dielectric material. *Drying Technology* 23 (9–11): 2147–2168.

232 Witrowa-Rajchert, D. and Rząca, M. (2009). Effect of drying method on the microstructure and physical properties of dried apples. *Drying Technology* 27 (7–8): 903–909.

233 Cliff, M. (1986). Applications of microwaves in the pharmaceutical industry. *IChemE North Western Branch Papers* 3: 4.1–4.12.

234 Cliff, M. (ed.). (1986) Use of microwaves to dry pharmaceutical granules. *Proceedings of IEE Colloquium – Electricity in Pharmaceuticals and Specialised Organics*, pp 1–4.

235 McLoughlin, C., McMinn, W., and Magee, T. (2003). Microwave drying of multi-component powder systems. *Drying Technology* 21 (2): 293–309.
236 Loh, Z., Liew, C., Lee, C., and Heng, P. (2008). Microwave-assisted drying of pharmaceutical granules and its impact on drug stability. *International Journal of Pharmaceutics* 359 (1): 53–62.
237 Chee, S.N., Johansen, A.L., Gu, L. et al. (2005). Microwave drying of granules containing a moisture-sensitive drug: a promising alternative to fluid bed and hot air oven drying. *Chemical and Pharmaceutical Bulletin* 53 (7): 770–775.
238 Hegedűs, Á. and Pintye-Hódi, K. (2007). Comparison of the effects of different drying techniques on properties of granules and tablets made on a production scale. *International Journal of Pharmaceutics* 330 (1): 99–104.

4

Drying for Stabilization of Protein Formulations

Jacqueline Horn[2], Hanns-Christian Mahler[1], and Wolfgang Friess[2]

[1] *Lonza AG, Drug Product Services, Hochbergerstrasse 60A, Basel 4057, Switzerland*
[2] *Ludwig-Maximilians-Universität, Muenchen, Department of Pharmacy, Pharmaceutical Technology and Biopharmaceutics, Butenandtstrasse 5, Muenchen 81377, Germany*

Between 2010 and 2014, 55 novel biopharmaceuticals were approved in the United States or Europe, with almost one third of them being monoclonal antibodies (mAbs). Among others, further biopharmaceuticals approved included hormones, enzymes, vaccines, and fusion proteins [1]. In total, more than 200 biopharmaceuticals are currently on the market, typically for refrigerated storage (2–8 °C) and either in liquid or lyophilized dosage form [2].

This chapter is intended to discuss mechanisms of protein stabilization in liquid and dried formulations as well as the corresponding analytical methods. Furthermore, the impact of the drying process itself on protein stability is summarized.

4.1 Protein Stability

Protein stability is related to the primary sequence and the higher-order molecular structure (secondary, tertiary, and quaternary structure). Protein instabilities can be categorized as physical or chemical instabilities [3]. The latter includes the formation or the breakage of covalent bonds resulting in new chemical entities. Examples include deamidation, fragmentation, and oxidation. Physical instabilities, in contrast, are defined as altered physical state of the protein, including unfolded state, aggregation, and precipitation. In practice, both chemical and physical instability reactions occur simultaneously for proteins and can also lead to each other. For example, attractive protein–protein interactions may become stronger as a consequence of chemical changes such as oxidation or deamidation, and hence, oxidation or deamidation in combination with aggregation may be found.

External stresses are drivers for protein instability. In particular, these factors include interfaces (such as air–liquid and ice–liquid), temperature (heat), and light. Formulation parameters such as protein concentration, pH, ionic strength, and quality and quantity of excipients determine the stability and can – to some extent – stabilize (or destabilize) the protein against external stresses [4, 5].

Drying Technologies for Biotechnology and Pharmaceutical Applications, First Edition.
Edited by Satoshi Ohtake, Ken-ichi Izutsu, and David Lechuga-Ballesteros.

4.1.1 Physical Instability of Proteins

Physical instabilities can include changes in secondary or tertiary structure (conformational instability) or formation of multimers (aggregates, precipitation) (colloidal instability). Conformational and colloidal instability can be interconnected, as changes in higher-order structural change may expose structural elements such as hydrophobic parts of the protein previously buried within the fold, which may also change its aggregation propensity.

Important conformational instability pathways are thermal or chemical denaturation, and also cold denaturation has been discussed in this context [3]. Thermal denaturation is the unfolding of the protein upon increase of temperature. The melting temperature (T_m) at which half of the protein is denatured can be measured by differential scanning calorimetry (DSC). But also other methods that trace unfolding during a temperature ramp provide comparable information, such as Fourier transform infrared spectroscopy (FTIR) [6]. The T_m value of biopharmaceuticals should be well above the intended storage temperature, as well as accelerated conditions (higher temperature) that may occur temporarily during storage, processing, or shipment and during formulation development and/or stability testing. Cold denaturation, i.e. denaturation at low temperatures, is typically less relevant for the stability of biopharmaceuticals, but has been discussed being a concern during the freezing step in freeze drying (Section 4.3.1.1) [7]. Proteins can also be unfolded by chaotropic agents, called chemical denaturation. Guanidinium hydrochloride or urea concentration series has been used to gain information about the free energy of unfolding [8, 9].

Colloidal instability reflects the association of individual protein molecules to larger species. These protein molecules can be native or conformationally altered and thus more prone for association. Colloidal instability is mainly driven by repulsive and attractive forces that exist between protein molecules. The strength of these forces mainly depends on charge, charge distribution of the molecules, and surface hydrophobicity, which are impacted by pH, buffer composition, and ionic strength of the formulation. The net repulsion or attraction between protein molecules can be characterized by the osmotic second virial coefficient [10–12].

Aggregates can form as a result of the interplay between conformational and colloidal instability. These aggregates can be dimers, oligomers, soluble aggregates, and larger subvisible and visible particles and precipitates, recently also called protein particles or proteinaceous particles (Figure 4.1) [13].

4.1.2 Chemical Instability of Proteins

Various chemical changes in the protein primary sequence can occur. This includes breakage or formation of disulfide bonds, deamidation, oxidation, and glycation, which are described in more detail below, and also isomerization, hydrolysis, β-elimination, and racemization, for which the reader is referred to literature [3, 14, 15].

4.1.2.1 Disulfide Bond Formation

If cysteine residues are present in the primary protein sequence, oxidation of two cysteine residues may result in formation of a cystine linkage or disulfide

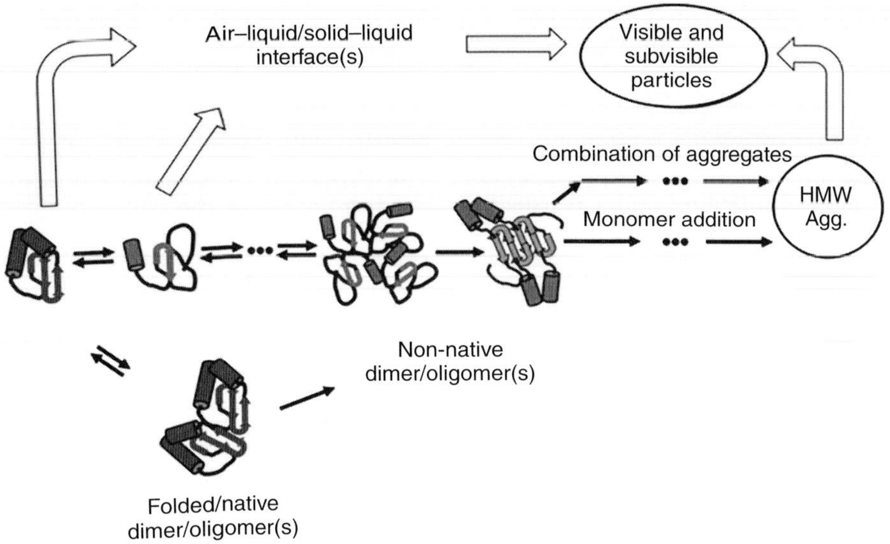

Figure 4.1 Scheme of possible aggregation mechanisms of proteins. Stress factors such as temperature, pH, or ionic strength may induce different aggregation pathways. Interfacial stress is mainly driven by air–liquid or solid–liquid interfaces such as the ice–liquid interface during freezing. Dark gray proteins represent native protein structure, whereas light gray proteins are partially or completely unfolded. Source: Amin et al. 2014 [13]. Reproduced with permission of Elsevier.

bond. This can occur (i) within one protein molecule leading to a different conformation or (ii) between two protein molecules inducing the formation of covalent aggregates [16, 17].

In case disulfide bonds are already present in a given molecule, there is also the risk that the bond may be reduced and disulfide bonds re-form in a different pattern. This can lead to (i) disulfide exchange in a given molecule (mispairing) leading to a different conformation, (ii) disulfide formation between two molecules leading to covalent aggregates, or (iii) a protein molecule retaining its reduced form. The latter has been a significant issue during fermentation of antibodies [18]. Copper sulfate can provide protection against this disulfide reduction by acting as an oxidizing agent [19]. It was shown for β-galactosidase that the freeze-dried formulation was more susceptible to the disulfide degradation pathway than the aqueous solution and in the freeze-dried samples covalent disulfide bonds were formed, whereas in solution noncovalent soluble aggregates resulted [20].

4.1.2.2 Deamidation

Deamidation is another common degradation pathway whereby an asparagine or glutamine amide side group is transformed into the corresponding carboxylic acid and the release of ammonium makes the reaction effectively irreversible [3]. The reaction is accelerated either at acidic ($pH < 4$) or at basic/neutral conditions ($pH > 6$) based on different mechanisms. The latter mechanism, via an intramolecular cyclization process forming a succinimide as intermediate, is more common in protein formulations. The pentacyclic intermediate of asparagine is more stable than the hexacyclic version of glutamine, and therefore asparagine reacts faster than glutamine. With more than just one asparagine or glutamine in the primary sequence, different deamidated protein species can result [3, 15, 21, 22]. Consequently, pH in the dried state is one of the key factors concerning this instability pathway. However, there is no clear definition of pH in solid formulations, and it is usually referred to the pH of the corresponding solution. Deamidation leads to changes in the charge heterogeneity of the molecule affecting charge based inter- and intramolecular interactions. In case deamidation occurs in the part of the molecule that relates to potency or binding, such as the complementarity-determining region (CDR) of a mAb, partial or full loss of efficacy may result [23].

4.1.2.3 Oxidation

Some amino acids are sensitive to oxidation including methionine, tryptophan as well as cysteine (see Section 4.1.2.1), histidine, and tyrosine. The oxidation process is usually mediated by reactive oxygen species and influenced by various intrinsic or extrinsic factors, such as protein structure and folding, pH, metals, and light. Reactive oxygen species can result from metal-induced Fenton reactions and side-chain oxidations of polymers such as excipients and contaminants, e.g. peroxides in excipients, light, and other sources [24].

4.1.2.4 Glycation

Glycation – also referred to as Browning or Maillard reaction – is the nonenzymatic reaction of a reducing sugar with a primary or secondary amine, e.g. lysine residues. The amine reacts with the carbonyl group to form a Schiff base, a reactive species that reacts further to the more stable *N*-glycosylated amines characterized by their brown color, which is the origin of the reaction's name. Sugars are frequently used as protein stabilizers in dried formulations, and the Maillard reaction is the reason why nonreducing sugars, such as sucrose or trehalose, are used instead of reducing sugars like glucose, lactose, fructose, or maltose. One also has to be aware of the fact that sucrose may invert into reducing sugars, glucose, and fructose, at elevated temperatures or acidic conditions [25, 26].

4.1.3 Analysis of Protein Stability

Protein drug stability is investigated in long-term stability studies at intended and accelerated storage conditions. Due to the various potential chemical and physical changes, a broad panel of analytical methods is recommended and typically applied. Stress parameters used in development to evaluate formulation parameters such as pH and type/amount of excipients are temperature, light, mechanical stress by shaking, and freeze/thaw stress [27, 28]. Typical standard analytical tools for routine stability testing include turbidity; color; pH; osmolality; subvisible particles; visible particles; purity methods, e.g. evaluating size-, charge-, or hydrophobicity-based separation; and measurement of content. Additional methods, such as spectroscopic techniques, can serve for biophysical characterization or extended characterization, and monitoring of other critical excipients may be employed to assess related changes.

4.1.3.1 Particle Analysis in Protein Formulations

Particle analysis has become very important given that aggregation and precipitation are typical instability pathways for most proteins. It has been speculated that protein aggregates/particles can lead to enhanced immune response to the protein drug molecules [29, 30]. Recently it has been suggested that protein aggregates/particles are only relevant for modulating the immune response if substantially chemically modified by oxidation [31, 32].

The amount or size of particles has to be evaluated by several different methods (e.g. light obscuration, nanoparticle tracking analysis [NTA], dynamic light scattering). Additionally, visual inspection should be performed during formulation development, since it is mandatory as in-process testing during manufacturing (100% inspection and culling drug product units with any visible particulate present) and quality control (release and stability). The size of particles visible to the human eye is a topic of debate. In fact, the size, type, number, color, refractive index of particulates, and the method of detection (unaided eye vs. magnification, color/type of background, light intensity, inspection duration, capability and ability of the operator) affect the outcome of the test. This is why it is not reasonable to define a "size" of visible particles. The number and size of smaller particles in the subvisible region (≥2 μm) are quantified by light obscuration or microscope methods (according to USP 788 and Ph Eur 2.9.19). Recently, micro-flow imaging has also been suggested for quantification, yet this method has significant shortcomings that currently render it to not be a viable option for quality control purposes.

The determination of particles in the nanometer region may provide an additional level of characterization. For example, NTA and resonance mass measurement (RMM) are emerging technologies used for detection of particles in the submicron (<1 μm) size range. High molecular weight species, i.e. soluble aggregates, are detected by size exclusion chromatography (SEC) (1–50 nm) (Section 4.1.3.2).

All the technologies mentioned above have their specific measurement (size) range and advantages and disadvantages and should be used complementarily. Some methods are generally used for quality control, such as light obscuration, visible particle inspection, and SEC, while others serve solely for extended characterization.

4.1.3.2 Other Purity Tests for Proteins

Chromatographic methods are widely used to identify physical and chemical changes of proteins. SEC is the analytical workhorse for the characterization and quantification of soluble higher molecular weight species (protein aggregates) and soluble fragments. Complementary methods to SEC are asymmetrical flow field-flow fractionation (AF4) or analytical ultracentrifugation (AUC). Purity testing also includes capillary electrophoresis sodium dodecyl sulfate (CE-SDS) or related gel-based methods, such as sodium dodecyl sulfate polyacrylamide gel electrophoresis (SDS-PAGE). Chemical changes can be monitored by reversed-phase, hydrophobic interaction, hydrophilic interaction, and ion exchange chromatography (IEC) or isoelectric focusing (IEF). IEC and IEF are well-established methods for the characterization of charge heterogeneity, but due to faster analysis and less complex method development, there is a preference toward the utilization of capillary electrophoresis (CE) techniques like capillary isoelectric focusing (cIEF) and capillary zone electrophoresis (CZE) [33, 34].

4.1.3.3 Analysis of Higher-Order Structure

Circular dichroism (CD) can be used to identify changes in secondary (far-UV CD, 190–250 nm, peptide bond conformation) and tertiary (near-UV CD, >250 nm, absorption of aromatic amino acids and cystine) protein structure based on the difference in absorption of left- and right-handed circularly polarized light. The location and intensity of characteristic bonds (α-helices, β-sheets, unordered structures) at certain wavelengths are used for analysis. Dry powders need to be rehydrated for CD analysis, ignoring the potential impact of reconstitution [35].

FTIR enables liquid and solid-state analysis of the secondary protein structure. It is based on the amide IC=O stretching band at 1700–1600 per cm. The drawback of this method is the low sensitivity that prohibits the detection of smallest changes to the protein structure, in particular if only single domains of the protein are affected [36]. Fluorescence-, UV-, and Raman-based methods may be used orthogonally. More innovative higher-order structure analytical methods include hydrogen–deuterium exchange (HDX).

4.2 Protein Stability in the Dried State

4.2.1 Theoretical Considerations

Compared with the aqueous solution, the dried state is characterized by a matrix that reduces protein mobility and less water (as residual moisture), which mediates many chemical reactions [37, 38]. The pharmaceutical industry developed various drying techniques suitable for protein stabilization, mainly adopted from the food industry [39, 40]. This includes vacuum drying [41, 42], fluid-bed drying [43], film drying [44], freeze drying [45], spray drying [46], or spray freeze drying [47], of which freeze drying is clearly dominant and preferred. All drying methods have in common that stabilizers are required to ensure protein stability.

Dry products that provide good protein stability are typically based on amorphous matrices. For the classic low molecular sugar, mostly sucrose matrices, two hypotheses regarding the stabilization mechanism are discussed [48, 49], which however cannot explain all cases of stabilization or destabilization. In some cases the water replacement theory helps explain the stabilization effect and in other cases the vitrification concept. The debate about the preferable hypothesis is still ongoing [49].

4.2.1.1 Water Replacement Hypothesis

As the name "water replacement theory" implies, the sugar molecules replace the hydrogen bonds of water at the surface of the protein. Thus, the sugar molecules stabilize the native conformation of the protein and thermodynamically stabilize against unfolding [50]. Theoretically, a sugar monolayer around the protein molecule should be adequate to retain complete protein activity replacing water at all hydrogen bonding sites. The fact that an increasing sugar to protein ratio leads to increased protein stability up to a saturation limit supports the water replacement theory. A similar molar ratio of sugar to protein of around 350–400 was shown to be sufficient for freeze- and spray-dried mAbs [51, 52]. Saturation was also shown for five different proteins at a similar or lower molar ratio [53]. Hydrogen bonding between sugar and protein can be assessed by FTIR [54].

4.2.1.2 Glass Dynamics Hypothesis and Vitrification

The second hypothesis on stabilization of proteins in the dried state is the so-called "glass dynamics" or "vitrification" hypothesis, which is based on kinetic considerations [55]. The mobility of the protein molecules is limited in the glassy matrix. As a consequence, reactions between protein molecules, as well as of protein molecules with water or oxygen, are slowed down, as the time scale of reactions is prolonged. This reduced mobility is reflected in α- and β-relaxations of the matrix [49]. It is not clear yet which of these relaxations is more relevant for protein stability or whether it is the combination of both. The α-relaxation, also called global or slow dynamics or primary motions, reflects slow translational and rotational motions on a second-to-month time scale. The motions correlate with the viscosity of the entire system and are therefore related to the glass transition [56, 57]. In contrast, β-relaxations, also named secondary motions or Johari–Goldstein relaxations [57], are local dynamics in spatial proximity that influence motions at a time scale of picoseconds. Since small distances between protein molecules drive protein aggregation, slowing down β-relaxations is suggested for improving protein stability [49, 56]. Low molecular weight excipients, e.g. glycerol and sorbitol, may be able to increase local β-relaxation times, but decrease global α-relaxation times, hence antiplasticizing β-motions and plasticizing α-motions at the same time [56, 58, 59].

4.2.2 Analysis of the Dried State

As described above, vitrification in an amorphous matrix with low mobility and hydrogen bonding is important to stabilize proteins in the dried state. To characterize these features, three basic routine tools can typically be utilized: DSC, X-ray powder diffraction (XRD), and residual moisture determination (Karl-Fischer or thermogravimetric analysis [TGA]). Also other more sophisticated tools have been applied, and the reader is referred to the primary literature on small-angle X-ray scattering (XRD), dielectric relaxation spectroscopy (DRS), dynamic mechanical analysis (DMA), fluorescence spectroscopy, nuclear magnetic resonance (NMR), positron annihilation lifetime spectroscopy (PALS), hydrogen–deuterium exchange mass spectroscopy (HDX MS) [60, 61] or solid-state NMR [62].

4.2.2.1 Investigation of Endo- and Exothermic Processes: Glass Transition and Crystallization

DSC is the standard tool for the determination of the glass transition temperatures (T_g) of amorphous solids. It can also be used to characterize crystallization events, polymorph variants, relaxation behaviors, T_g of the freeze concentrate (T_g'), and melting points [63]. DSC comparatively measures the heat capacities of a sample and a reference pan during cooling and heating cycles. Endothermic events (e.g. melting point) are characterized by a positive heat flow, hence energy input, whereas exothermic events (i.e. crystallizations, relaxations) set energy free and thus lead to a negative signal. The T_g characterizes the temperature at which amorphous solids transform from a glassy, rubbery state into a state with viscous flow accompanied by a distinct decrease in viscosity. This event is not related to a formal phase change, but a step in the DSC baseline occurs as the heat capacity changes. Storage temperatures of amorphous solids should not exceed T_g, as in this case macroscopic collapse of the formulation would result. Furthermore, protein stability can be drastically decreased upon storage above or close to T_g as the molecular mobility jumps up [64–66]. Furthermore, it is essential to assess the storage stability of amorphous solids since the metastable amorphous form tends to transform into a thermodynamically more stable crystalline polymorph, potentially indicated by an exothermic crystallization peak depending on kinetics. Crystallization comes along with the loss of the stabilizing amorphous matrix.

4.2.2.2 Sample Morphology: Crystalline or Amorphous Matrix?

XRD is the method of choice to gain information about sample morphology. The operation principle is the reflection of X-rays in an angle-dependent manner. Diffraction angles and patterns can be assigned to distinct structures based on Bragg's law. Thus the absence of peaks indicates an amorphous structure, and peak patterns allow for the differentiation of crystalline polymorphs. Mannitol, for example, forms at least four different polymorphs in addition to the amorphous form. Both the form itself and polymorphic transitions have to be considered regarding long-term storage stability. The hemihydrate form is prone to transform into one of the anhydrates (α-, β-, or δ-polymorph). The released crystal water is transferred into the amorphous phase acting as plasticizer. Ultimately T_g is decreased, the mobility of the system is increased, and instability reactions between protein molecules are enhanced. The released water may also be an important reaction partner itself, e.g. for hydrolytic reactions. The most stable crystalline mannitol form is the β-polymorph. It was shown that both spray drying and freeze drying rendered mainly the β-polymorph if no protein was present in the formulation. Increasing lysozyme concentrations stimulated the formation of α-mannitol during spray drying and of δ-mannitol upon freeze drying [67]. Formation of the δ-mannitol polymorph, which is unstable at room temperature, was related to the presence of the protein, but the mannitol–protein interactions requires further investigation for a better understanding. Thus, not only process differences but also formulation differences affect which polymorph forms.

4.2.2.3 Residual Moisture

The residual moisture content is an important quality attribute of the dried material. Higher water content may be directly related to reduced protein stability with water molecules acting as reaction partner or as plasticizer increasing molecular mobility. Thus, it is important to evaluate the impact of differently residual moisture levels on long-term stability. The duration and especially temperature of the secondary drying in freeze drying is the most decisive step for the amount of moisture remaining. Typically, a residual moisture content below 2% is being aimed for, considering many reactions would generally be slowed down below this level [68], although this clearly depends on the specific product (protein, formulation, etc.). Further drying to very low amounts of moisture may lead to so-called overdrying [69]. Karl-Fischer titration is the standard method for determination of the residual moisture. TGA could also be used, and recently spectroscopic analysis for nondestructive high throughput analysis has been introduced [70, 71].

4.2.3 Excipients Used to Stabilize Proteins in the Dried State

Most proteins require additional stabilizers to retain their activity during drying and subsequent storage. The amount of stabilizer that can be added may be limited by physiological considerations since parenterally applied solutions, obtained after reconstitution, should preferably be isotonic. The amount of stabilizer needed may follow different rules. On the one hand, the higher the ratio of stabilizing sugar to protein molecules, the better the stability and the increment of stability improvement levels off at higher ratios [51]. On the other hand, at higher protein concentration, less stabilizer may be needed due to a self-stabilization of the protein by steric repulsion of vicinal protein molecules and a reduced interface to protein molecule ratio at which denaturation could occur [72]. Although equal numbers of protein molecules are damaged, the relative fraction at higher protein concentration is lower [72, 73]. In freeze drying, one distinguishes between cryo- and lyoprotectants whereby some excipients combine both features. Cryoprotectants are known from nature as protectors against freezing-induced stress [74], and lyoprotectants protect against drying-induced stress. Stabilizers used for spray-dried products are comparable with the ones used in freeze drying [75–77]. More important in spray drying is the T_g of the excipients, which should be higher than the process temperature in order to prevent viscous flow. During spray drying it also needs to be considered that the water content of the formed particles and thus the product T_g depend on the moisture level of the drying environment and differ between the different stages of a spray dryer, as does the temperature. Thus, the situation may be rather complex. Since freeze drying is conducted at low temperatures, this factor is of minor importance, and secondary drying temperature, especially in the temperature ramp phase going into secondary drying, and storage temperature should not exceed the formulation T_g.

4.2.3.1 Sugars

Disaccharides are the most commonly used protein stabilizers. Due to their small size and flexibility, they are able to cover the protein surface acting directly on the protein. During drying, they typically form amorphous matrices as a key property for stabilization. They combine cryo- and lyoprotectant characteristics, and the mechanism of stabilization has been discussed above in more detail.

The most frequently utilized sugars in freeze and spray drying are sucrose and trehalose. Both of them are nonreducing sugars, hence not susceptible for Maillard reactions. Due to its less stable glycosidic bond, sucrose may invert into

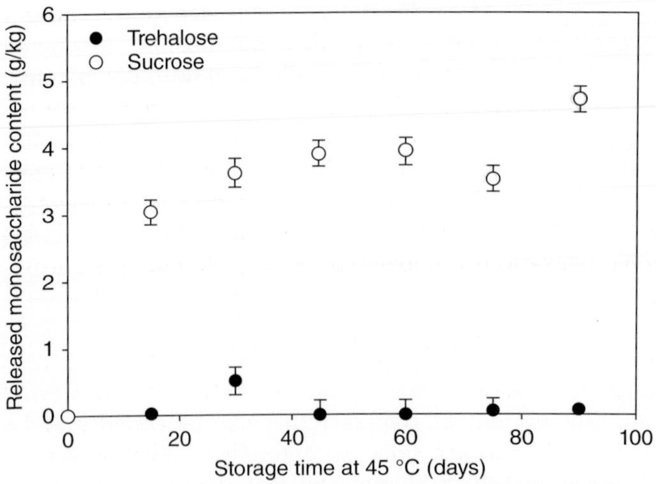

Figure 4.2 Progression of Maillard reaction in freeze-dried disaccharide matrices (2.5% m/V) determined by the release of the monosaccharide glucose via an enzymatic reaction. Trehalose (black) and sucrose (white) were lyophilized with bovine serum albumin (BSA) (1% m/m) and stored under controlled humidity conditions (22% RH) at 45 °C. Source: Schebor et al. 1999 [82]. Reproduced with permission of Elsevier.

the reducing monosaccharides glucose and fructose, even in freeze-drying studies, more markedly at low pH (Figure 4.2) and significantly high temperatures [78–82].

Both sucrose and trehalose show relatively high T_g values with 75 and 118 °C, respectively, which is advantageous for spray drying and for storage [83]. Particularly, trehalose shows one of the highest T_g values compared with other sugars, and also the relaxation time and the concluding fragility of the glass are important factors for its usage as stabilizing excipient [84, 85]. On the other hand, trehalose solutions showed a higher viscosity compared with sucrose solutions [86].

Trehalose is more prone to crystallization during freeze concentration [87], which could lead to a loss of cryoprotective function and protein stability problems. The crystalline modification may transform into the amorphous state in the course of the freeze-drying process and thus may not be obvious when only testing the final product [79, 88]. Upon spray drying of protein solutions, specifically with sugars as stabilizers, the plasticizing effect of moisture and thus stickiness of the resulting particles need to be carefully considered (see also Section 4.2.2.3) [89, 90]. Specifically for spray drying of proteins for inhalation use, other sugars can be considered as the drying behavior may be different; lactose and glucose, due to their ability to render aerodynamically more favorable particles, are preferred and approved for use in dry powder inhalers.

4.2.3.2 Polyols

The group of polyols that are frequently used for drying of proteins includes glycerol, sorbitol, and mannitol, showing different characteristics. The first two are plasticizing agents but may also improve protein stability in the dried state [58, 59, 91]. Due to their low T_g (glycerol −93 °C [92] and sorbitol 0 °C [93]), they are not suitable as the sole stabilizer for dried protein formulations as they do not render a solid material at room temperature. Thus, they need to be used in combination with other excipients having higher T_g [56]. Glycerol at low concentrations exhibits an antiplasticizing effect to the local motions of a protein formulation. The temperature needs to be below a critical antiplasticization temperature, which interestingly increases with lower glycerol concentrations [94]. Various studies explain an improved protein stability in the presence of glycerol by the increased relaxation time of local fast dynamics (β-relaxation), while the time scales for global relaxations are lowered [56, 58, 91, 95].The improved protein stability may also be explained differently by an increased density of the packing, reducing the free volume; small voids left by larger glass-forming molecules such as sucrose are filled by the plasticizer [56, 96]. In addition, the smaller glycerol molecules are sterically more suitable at gaining access to the surface of the protein molecules compared with larger excipients. Once the free volume is saturated by glycerol, the plasticizing characteristics dominate, and glycerol acts as a lubricant, accelerating the dynamics on all time scales [56].

Adding sorbitol to sucrose- or trehalose-based antibody formulations led to a decrease of the global relaxation time τ and, in some cases, improved stability. Sorbitol did not affect the native structure stability in combination with trehalose, but it did with sucrose. Thus, the global relaxation time τ could not predict stability adequately [59]. The combination of sucrose and sorbitol was beneficial for other proteins as well, and the effect may not be polyol specific as small amino acids were also found to be suitable [97]. Upon spray drying, the stabilizing effect of sorbitol on an IgG antibody was comparable with the effect of trehalose [89].

Polyols like mannitol do not have plasticizer properties, but are used as bulking agents in freeze drying. Bulking agents crystallize during the process and do not stabilize protein molecules but render robust scaffolds for good cake appearance (see also Section 4.2.2.2). It is important to achieve complete mannitol crystallization since amorphous mannitol leads to a low T_g of the formulation and only the crystalline form provides the scaffold. Spray-dried mannitol remains amorphous and is hence able to stabilize the protein in an amorphous matrix.

4.2.3.3 Polymers

Polymers can also stabilize proteins in the dried state. Usually, polymers show high T_g, which makes them suitable stabilizers by increasing the T_g of the whole formulation. The macromolecules differ in their stabilization mechanism from small molecules like sugars. Polymers hinder the protein interactions sterically; they increase the viscosity of the solution, hence slowing down the mobility; or they react via preferential exclusion [38]. Furthermore, they prevent pH decrease of phosphate buffers during freezing or crystallization of excipients. Commonly used polymers include serum albumins, polyvinylpyrrolidone, dextran, polyethylene glycol, or hydroxyethylcellulose at various molecular weights [38].

Polymers may not only be beneficial but can also negatively affect protein stability. Phase separation triggered by the polymer can be detrimental for proteins [98]. As a high T_g is not the only factor for a stable dried protein formulation, hydroxyethyl starch did not improve the protein stability compared with sucrose and trehalose [85]. One reason is the lower efficiency in forming hydrogen bonds with proteins as demonstrated for freeze-dried formulations of lactate dehydrogenase (LDH) containing dextran or trehalose [99]. Human serum albumin contains free sulfhydryl groups, which, thus, may lead to covalent aggregation (heteroaggregation) with cysteine-containing proteins. Also, the regulatory and safety status of the choice of excipients may in some cases be unfavorable for the choice of polymers for some parenteral products.

4.2.3.4 Amino Acids

A stabilizing effect of amino acids on proteins is still unclear. Forney-Stevens et al. screened 15 amino acids regarding the stabilization of two model proteins, rHA and alpha chymotrypsin (ACT), in the freeze-dried state [97]. It seems as if the positive amino acids, which are also larger in size than the other amino acids, have an advantageous stabilization effect. Added in small amount to sucrose, they formed amorphous lyophilizates. In contrast, glycine is a crystalline bulking agent, and phenylalanine also crystallizes during freeze drying, if the ratio of amino acid to sugar exceeds a certain limit [100]. Arginine also exhibited beneficial effects as amorphous stabilizer on freeze-dried protein formulations [101]. The arginine counterion plays an important role, of which chloride performed the best regarding stabilization [101]. Concerning spray drying, isoleucine was reported to improve flowability of the powder and protein stability of an IgG1 antibody [75].

4.2.3.5 Additional Excipients: Metal Ions/HP-β-CD/Surfactants/Buffers

Surfactants adsorb to interfaces with a higher tendency than proteins. Therefore, they keep protein molecules off the interface where proteins may unfold. The most critical interfaces are the ice–freeze concentrate interface formed during the freezing step in freeze drying and the air–liquid interface generated upon droplet formation during spray drying [102]. Stabilization of protein molecules by direct binding has been shown for albumin fusion proteins and albumin with a lipophilic binding pocket [103], whereas binding to other proteins is still up for debate. Typical surfactants used are the nonionic Polysorbate 20 and 80.

Cyclodextrins (CDs) are ring-shaped molecules consisting of at least six glucose molecules. They are amphiphilic with a hydrophilic outer surface and a rather hydrophobic interior. The CDs' limited solubility can be improved by substitution with hydroxypropyl or sulfobutyl groups. By incorporating hydrophobic moieties of a distinct size in their interior, CDs can improve solubility or reduce hydrophobic interactions. It was also shown that the CD derivatives have similar characteristics to surfactants, which make them suitable stabilizers against interface-induced stresses [104], however, probably acting via different mechanism than nonionic surfactants [105]. Concentrations higher than 1% lead to a lyoprotectant behavior, and also a good stability of spray-dried trypsin has been shown by CDs due to their glass-forming characteristics [106].

Buffers are added to protein formulations to keep the pH consistent. The pH is one of the most important parameters in protein formulations as it affects all degradation pathways, chemical reactions, and colloidal interactions, as well as conformational stability (see also Sections 4.1.1 and 4.1.2). Additionally the counterion effect has to be considered when comparing the typically negatively charged buffer salts, phosphate or citrate, to histidine or Tris. Concerning the dried state, histidine has been shown to be beneficial for protein stability [107] (see also Section 4.2.3.4). On the other hand, crystallization of buffer salts may have a detrimental effect on protein stability (see also Section 4.3.1.1).

Metal ions, specifically divalent cations like zinc, copper, or calcium, can bind to specific protein binding sites and may in some cases stabilize (but also destabilize) the native protein conformation. It was reported that phosphofructokinase stability was substantially improved if the divalent metal ions were added to a sucrose-based formulation [108]. Spray-dried formulations of recombinant human growth hormone were stabilized by zinc in combination with Polysorbate 20 without any sugar stabilizer by formation of a dimer complex [109].

4.3 How Does the Process Influence Protein Stability?

4.3.1 Process of Freeze Drying

The freeze-drying process can be separated into the steps of freezing (including annealing), primary drying at low product temperature under reduced pressure in order to remove ice from the frozen system by sublimation, and secondary drying at higher product temperature and reduced pressure to desorb water from the product. Each step requires special consideration in the context of drying protein products.

4.3.1.1 Freezing

Freezing is the first step after dispersing the liquid solution into the product containers and can already be detrimental for proteins. Several factors of influence are discussed. Cold denaturation describes the unfolding of proteins at low temperature due to a lower barrier in Gibbs free energy of unfolding [110]. It is difficult to determine the impact of cold denaturation on protein stability because ice formation and freeze concentration are two phenomena that influence protein stability and occur in parallel during freezing. Cold denaturation is assumed to be of minor relevance since the freezing step is rather short and often occurs at temperatures below the product temperature in freeze drying [7].

Another major critical effect during freezing is the formation of a freeze-concentrated liquid as a very densely structured hexagonal crystal lattice [111–113]. Both the protein concentration and the excipient concentrations increase. Especially for proteins sensitive to native-like aggregation, highly concentrated areas could promote particle formation during freezing [113].

Another phenomenon that may occur during freeze concentration is the crystallization of buffer components due to their limitation in solubility. In some cases, a pH shift of more than three pH units can occur. A famous example is sodium phosphate buffer in which the basic disodium salt is the less soluble component and precipitates during freezing. This shifts the acid–base balance toward the base since the base is removed from the equilibrium. Protons are set free and decrease the pH [110], which lead to denaturation of sensitive proteins, e.g. LDH [114]. Potassium phosphate in contrast leads to a pH increase since the monobasic salt precipitates during freezing [115, 116]. Additional pH shift-inducing buffers include succinate and tartrate. To prevent the occurrence of this phenomenon, low buffer concentrations or high protein concentrations can be used or buffers may be selected, which are not prone to pH shift, for example, histidine, glycine, citrate, or Tris. Addition of 0.25 M sucrose already prevented the pH shift to a large extent for both sodium and potassium phosphate buffer [116]. Thus the whole formulation composition influences the freezing behavior and hence the impact on protein stability. A recent article proposed the use of counterions that balance the pH shift of the buffer salt [117]. They investigated tetramethylammonium chloride (TMACl) whose anion is incorporated into the ice crystal structure during freezing, leading to a concentration-dependent basification. When used together with sodium phosphate buffer, the concluding acidification by the phosphate is diminished by the TMACl.

Freeze concentration concerns all excipients. For example a 0.9% sodium chloride solution concentrates 24-fold [92]. This enormous increase in ionic strength may influence the protein stability by reducing repulsive charge interactions. On the other hand, it was shown that sodium chloride could prevent aggregation of recombinant human albumin (rHA) upon lyophilization, which was correlated with a water uptake in short spatial proximity to rHA facilitating refolding into the native rHA [118]. The freeze concentration of sugars is one important factor for the cryopreservation of proteins. High sugar concentrations result in high viscosities, which slow down the molecular mobility of the system and hence prolong unfolding kinetics of the proteins [119].

In addition, the ice–liquid interface itself can be detrimental for the protein. Proteins adsorb to the ice surface, which promotes unfolding. The extent of unfolding at the ice–liquid interface is protein dependent. Infrared spectroscopy could show that the IgG and LDH structure changed at the ice–liquid interface leading to a higher β-sheet content, whereas the structure was unchanged in the freeze-concentrated liquid [120]. Regarding rhIFN-γ, aggregate formation could not be linked to the adsorption at the ice–liquid interface but most likely occurred at the air–liquid interface during reconstitution [102]. The ice–liquid interface may make the protein more susceptible for unfolding or structural perturbation. By addition of surfactants like polysorbates, interface-related damages can be prevented.

The amount of interfacial area and the ice crystal size depend on the chosen ice nucleation technique. The typically so-called uncontrolled nucleation technique is the shelf-ramped freezing, which leads to a high number of small ice crystals formed from the bottom to the top of the sample due to a high degree of supercooling. Overall the surface area may be rather heterogeneous as the degree of supercooling varies within a batch as crystallization occurs at random, but also affected by the position of the vial in the freeze dryer. Recently several different techniques to induce controlled ice nucleation were established [121]. Controlled nucleation techniques lead to nucleation at defined product temperature for the entire batch. Comparative studies of controlled nucleated and randomly nucleated protein formulations demonstrated changed physical characteristics, for example, faster reconstitution times for highly concentrated mAb formulations, although it did not correlate to enhanced protein stability [122, 123].

Annealing Annealing, also called thermal treatment, is the increase in temperature during the freezing step after the initial freezing prior to primary drying. Therefore, bulking agents like mannitol or glycine should crystallize completely. In addition, the ice crystal size should be increased, providing larger pores and thus lower cake resistance to vapor flow during primary drying. Potentially the lower specific surface area coming with annealing slows down secondary drying. The increase in temperature is recommended to be close to the T_g' of the solute in order to increase the mobility of the system [124]. Crystalline bulking agents should be fully crystalline after the freeze-drying process, since they are responsible for the formation of a mechanically stable cake structure. Furthermore, bulking agents usually exhibit a low T_g' (mannitol −35 °C [125]), causing difficulties in drying and storage stability. Additionally, during the annealing step, undesired crystallization of amorphous stabilizers like trehalose can occur. This crystallization resulted in an unfolding of BSA measured in freeze/thaw studies performed at typical mannitol annealing temperatures of −20 °C [126].

4.3.1.2 Drying

After freezing, the chamber pressure is reduced to initiate the drying process. Primary drying mainly removes the ice formed during freezing (80–90% of water), and during secondary drying operated at higher shelf temperature, the water kept in the freeze concentrate evaporates.

As the main part of the protein is phase-separated from the ice and located in the cryo-concentrated region, one could assume that primary drying is not the main stress on the protein. Nevertheless, if primary drying is carried out above T_g', the mobility of the amorphous phase is increased, which could enhance interactions between the protein molecules or protein molecules and reaction partners. Furthermore, product temperatures above T_g', e.g. induced by high chamber pressure or high shelf temperature, could induce macroscopic collapse. It was shown that collapse is not necessarily detrimental to protein stability [127], but other quality attributes like macroscopic appearance or reconstitution times may be affected.

The subsequent secondary drying to remove water that is bound stronger to the solids is commonly performed at 20 °C or higher. By desorption of water molecules, parts of the protein's hydration shell are removed. Many proteins require water in their active sites for their biologic function; hence removal of this water may induce loss of activity, which could be mitigated in the presence of suitable stabilizers that can replace hydrogen bonding initially provided by the surrounding water molecules [128].

Regarding the macroscopic appearance, the product temperature should stay below T_g during secondary drying in order to prevent macroscopic collapse. However, collapse does not need to be a drawback concerning protein stability [100, 127].

Currently many development projects focus on highly concentrated protein formulations mainly of mAbs. The solutions may exhibit high viscosity, and consequently a higher concentration of excipients like salts is required to reduce the viscosity. The formulations may also show a higher cake resistance to vapor flow and can exhibit very long reconstitution times. Additionally, the ratio of stabilizing excipient molecules to protein molecules may be lower compared with low protein concentration formulation as isotonicity limits the excipient concentrations. Colandene et al. demonstrated a marked increase in T_g' and T_c with increasing mAb concentration (0–100 mg/ml), which was much more pronounced for T_c (Δ12 °C) than for T_g' (Δ7 °C) [129]. Thus, drying above T_g', but below T_c, was easily possible, preserving cake structure as well as protein stability.

4.3.1.3 Typical Defects in Lyophilized Products Beyond Protein Stability

For marketed lyophilized drug products, appealing cake appearance is a critical factor. Defects like loose cake, large cracks, shrinkage, vial fogging, and meltdown or collapse may give rise to complaints or rejects, although not related to protein stability [130]. Meltdown and collapse are both related to high product temperatures commonly employed toward the end of primary drying [131]. Cracks on top of the cake or shrinkage usually occur when amorphous matrices are used as main excipient. This is due to tension within the cake when the desorbing water forces its way through the cake. As a result, the cake either cracks or shrinks by detaching from the vial wall, which both lead to relaxation [132–134]. Formulation creeping upward at the vial surface after filling and subsequent drying in this position is called vial fogging. Abdul-Fattah et al. showed that it can be reduced by several factors of formulation or process design. However, most effective was the use of hydrophobic vials [135].

4.3.2 Process of Spray Drying

In contrast to freeze drying, spray drying is a one-stage process. Two major stresses occur. Firstly, upon atomization, an enormous air–liquid interface is generated, which triggers protein adsorption and aggregation. Secondly, drying at higher temperature is performed, which can be critical for the conformational stability of the protein, possibly leading to aggregation and precipitation and/or oxidation [129].

4.3.2.1 Protein Stability During Droplet Formation

First, the solution is atomized into a spray. In this step, the main stress results from the newly generated enormous air–liquid interface, but also stresses provided by the nozzle play a role. Protein molecules adsorb to the air–liquid interface. This results in high local protein concentration fostering intermolecular interactions and potentially partial unfolding [136]. Ultimately soluble or insoluble aggregates can be formed. Addition of surfactants is the method of choice to protect the protein by preventing its adsorption. The addition of polysorbate was confirmed to reduce the extent of protein surface aggregation and increase protein stability, e.g. for BSA, recombinant human growth hormone (rHGH), LDH, and recombinant IL-11 by electron spectroscopy for chemical analysis (ESCA) and stability assays [76, 109, 137, 138]. Different nozzle types are available, and the stress induced by the shear or temperature effect of the nozzle itself needs to be considered [77, 139].

4.3.2.2 Protein Stability During the Drying Phase

During the drying phase, as the water evaporates, temperature is a highly critical factor [76]. It requires a careful balance. The droplet temperature must not exceed the protein melting temperature as long as the protein is still in solution. At the same time, the temperature has to be high enough to ensure drying results in a non-sticking powder with adequate residual moisture [140]. The temperature setting needs to be decided against the background of the ongoing endothermal drying process that keeps the droplet temperature low as long as substantial evaporation proceeds close to inlet air temperature conditions for a short time. The dried particles ultimately face the outlet temperature conditions for longer time. The residual moisture typically is higher as compared with freeze-dried products and may be reduced in an additional drying step at higher temperature and vacuum similar to secondary drying in freeze drying [75, 141]. This may also help to reduce the risk of recrystallization of amorphous excipients. Amorphous excipients like sucrose, trehalose, or CDs been demonstrated to be essential for protein stabilization during the drying phase [89, 142–144]. During spray drying, oxidation can occur as air is used as the typical drying gas. Addition of methionine has been shown to prevent rhIL-11 from oxidation and formation of related species [138].

4.4 Summary

Drying can significantly improve the stability of protein drugs compared with liquid formulation. Almost exclusively, freeze drying is employed for protein drug products for this purpose. However, chemical instability like formation of disulfide bonds, oxidation, deamidation, or glycation and physical instability such as conformational instability or aggregation also occur in the dried state. Due to the complexity of the protein molecules, comprehensive analyses with a multitude of methods such as particle analysis, chromatography, CD, or infrared spectroscopy are necessary. Typical excipients in drying include sugars, surfactants, polyols, or polymers. The two leading hypotheses for their ability to stabilize proteins in the dried state are water replacement and immobilization in an amorphous glass. Each step during the freeze- or spray-drying process affects protein stability in different ways. Interfacial-related stress occurs in almost all process steps, whereas concentration effects are important during freeze concentration or droplet formation.

References

1 Walsh, G. (2014). Biopharmaceuticals benchmarks. *Nature Biotechnology* 32: 992–1000. https://doi.org/10.1038/nbt.3040.

2 Pharma Circle. (2016). https://www.pharmacircle.com (accessed March 2016).

3 Manning, M.C., Chou, D.K., Murphy, B.M. et al. (2010). Stability of protein pharmaceuticals: an update. *Pharmaceutical Research* 27: 544–575. https://doi.org/10.1007/s11095-009-0045-6.
4 Mahler, H.-C., Friess, W., Grauschopf, U., and Kiese, S. (2009). Protein aggregation: pathways, induction factors and analysis. *Journal of Pharmaceutical Sciences* 98: 2909–2934. https://doi.org/10.1002/jps.21566.
5 Wang, W. (2005). Protein aggregation and its inhibition in biopharmaceutics. *International Journal of Pharmaceutics* 289: 1–30. https://doi.org/10.1016/j.ijpharm.2004.11.014.
6 Matheus, S., Friess, W., and Mahler, H.-C. (2006). FTIR and nDSC as analytical tools for high-concentration protein formulations. *Pharmaceutical Research* 23: 1350–1363. https://doi.org/10.1007/s11095-006-0142-8.
7 Kasper, J.C. and Friess, W. (2011). The freezing step in lyophilization: physico-chemical fundamentals, freezing methods and consequences on process performance and quality attributes of biopharmaceuticals. *European Journal of Pharmaceutics and Biopharmaceutics* 78: 248–263. https://doi.org/10.1016/j.ejpb.2011.03.010.
8 Schön, A. and Freire, E. (2016). Three easy pieces. *Biochimica et Biophysica Acta - General Subjects* 1860: 975–980. https://doi.org/10.1016/j.bbagen.2015.12.003.
9 Clarkson, B.R., Schön, A., and Freire, E. (2016). Conformational stability and self-association equilibrium in biologics. *Drug Discovery Today* 21: 342–347. https://doi.org/10.1016/j.drudis.2015.11.007.
10 Rubin, J., Linden, L., Coco, W.M. et al. (2013). Salt-induced aggregation of a monoclonal human immunoglobulin G1. *Journal of Pharmaceutical Sciences* 102: 377–386. https://doi.org/10.1002/jps.23363.
11 Chi, E.Y., Krishnan, S., Randolph, T.W., and Carpenter, J.F. (2003). Physical stability of proteins in aqueous solution: mechanism and driving forces in nonnative protein aggregation. *Pharmaceutical Research* 20: 1325–1336. https://doi.org/10.1023/A:1025771421906.
12 Frka-Petesic, B., Zanchi, D., Martin, N. et al. (2016). Aggregation of antibody drug conjugates at room temperature: SAXS and light scattering evidence for colloidal instability of a specific subpopulation. *Langmuir* 32: 4848–4861. https://doi.org/10.1021/acs.langmuir.6b00653.
13 Amin, S., Barnett, G.V., Pathak, J.A. et al. (2014). Protein aggregation, particle formation, characterization & rheology. *Current Opinion in Colloid & Interface Science* 19: 438–449. https://doi.org/10.1016/j.cocis.2014.10.002.
14 Wang, W., Singh, S., Zeng, D.L. et al. (2009). Antibody structure, instability, and formulation. *Journal of Pharmaceutical Sciences* 96: 1–26. https://doi.org/10.1002/jps.
15 Lai, M.C. and Topp, E.M. (1999). Solid-state chemical stability of proteins and peptides. *Journal of Pharmaceutical Sciences* 88: 489–500. https://doi.org/10.1021/js980374e.
16 Dillon, T.M., Ricci, M.S., Vezina, C. et al. (2008). Structural and functional characterization of disulfide isoforms of the human IgG2 subclass. *The Journal of Biological Chemistry* 283: 16206–16215. https://doi.org/10.1074/jbc.M709988200.

17 Wypych, J., Li, M., Guo, A. et al. (2008). Human IgG2 antibodies display disulfide-mediated structural isoforms. *The Journal of Biological Chemistry* 283: 16194–16205. https://doi.org/10.1074/jbc.M709987200.

18 Hutterer, K.M., Hong, R.W., Lull, J. et al. (2013). Monoclonal antibody disulfide reduction during manufacturing untangling process effects from product effects. *MAbs* 5: 608–613. https://doi.org/10.4161/mabs.2475.

19 Chaderjian, W.B., Chin, E.T., Harris, R.J., and Etcheverry, T.M. (2008). Effect of copper sulfate on performance of a serum-free cho cell culture process and the level of free thiol in the recombinant antibody expressed. *Biotechnology Progress* 21: 550–553. https://doi.org/10.1021/bp0497029.

20 Yoshioka, S., Aso, Y., Izutsu, K.-I., and Terao, T. (1993). Aggregates formed during storage of β-galactosidase in solution and in the freeze-dried state. *Pharmaceutical Research* 10: 687–691. https://doi.org/10.1023/A:1018951530927.

21 Li, B., Schowen, R.L., Topp, E.M., and Borchardt, R.T. (2006). Effect of N-1 and N-2 residues on peptide deamidation rate in solution and solid state. *The AAPS Journal* 8: E166–E173. https://doi.org/10.1208/aapsj080120.

22 Manning, M.C., Patel, K., and Borchardt, R.T. (1989). Stability of protein pharmaceuticals. *Pharmaceutical Development and Technology* 6: 903–918.

23 Harris, R.J., Kabakoff, B., Macchi, F.D. et al. (2001). Identification of multiple sources of charge heterogeneity in a recombinant antibody. *Journal of Chromatography. B, Biomedical Sciences and Applications* 752: 233–245. https://doi.org/10.1016/S0378-4347(00)00548-X.

24 Hovorka, S.W. and Schoenneich, C. (2001). Oxidative degradation of pharmaceuticals: theory, mechanisms and inhibition. *Journal of Pharmaceutical Sciences* 90: 253–269. https://doi.org/10.1002/1520-6017(200103)90:3<253::AID-JPS1>3.0.CO;2-W.

25 Fischer, S., Hoernschemeyer, J., and Mahler, H.C. (2008). Glycation during storage and administration of monoclonal antibody formulations. *European Journal of Pharmaceutics and Biopharmaceutics* 70: 42–50. https://doi.org/10.1016/j.ejpb.2008.04.021.

26 Hawe, A. and Friess, W. (2008). Development of HSA-free formulations for a hydrophobic cytokine with improved stability. *European Journal of Pharmaceutics and Biopharmaceutics* 68: 169–182. https://doi.org/10.1016/j.ejpb.2007.04.018.

27 Hawe, A., Wiggenhorn, M., van de Weert, M. et al. (2012). Forced degradation of therapeutic proteins. *Journal of Pharmaceutical Sciences* 101: 895–913. https://doi.org/10.1002/jps.22812.

28 Tamizi, E. and Jouyban, A. (2015). Forced degradation studies of biopharmaceuticals: selection of stress conditions. *European Journal of Pharmaceutics and Biopharmaceutics* 98: 26–46. https://doi.org/10.1016/j.ejpb.2015.10.016.

29 Carpenter, J.F., Randolph, T.W., Jiskoot, W. et al. (2009). Overlooking subvisible particles in therapeutic protein products: gaps that may compromise product quality. *Journal of Pharmaceutical Sciences* 98: 1201–1205. https://doi.org/10.1002/jps.

30 Moussa, E.M., Panchal, J.P., Moorthy, B.S. et al. (2016). Immunogenicity of therapeutic protein aggregates. *Journal of Pharmaceutical Sciences* 105: 417–430. https://doi.org/10.1016/j.xphs.2015.11.002.

31 Bessa, J., Boeckle, S., Beck, H. et al. (2015). The immunogenicity of antibody aggregates in a novel transgenic mouse model. *Pharmaceutical Research* 32: 2344–2359. https://doi.org/10.1007/s11095-015-1627-0.

32 Boll, B., Bessa, J., Folzer, E. et al. (2017). Extensive chemical modifications in the primary protein structure of IgG1 subvisible particles are necessary for breaking immune tolerance. *Molecular Pharmaceutics* 14: 1292–1299. https://doi.org/10.1021/acs.molpharmaceut.6b00816.

33 Tamizi, E. and Jouyban, A. (2015). The potential of the capillary electrophoresis techniques for quality control of biopharmaceuticals: a review. *Electrophoresis* 36: 831–858. https://doi.org/10.1002/elps.201400343.

34 Sosic, Z., Houde, D., Blum, A. et al. (2008). Application of imaging capillary IEF for characterization and quantitative analysis of recombinant protein charge heterogeneity. *Electrophoresis* 29: 4368–4376. https://doi.org/10.1002/elps.200800157.

35 Bloemendal, M. and Jiskoot, W. (2005). Circular dichroism spectroscopy. In: *Methods for Structural Analysis of Protein Pharmaceuticals* (eds. W. Jiskoot and D.J.A. Crommelin), 83–130. Arlington, TX: AAPS Press.

36 Van der Weert, M., Hering, J.A., and Haris, P.I. (2005). Fourier transform infrared spectroscopy. In: *Methods for Structural Analysis of Protein Pharmaceuticals* (eds. W. Jiskoot and D.J.A. Crommelin), 131–166.

37 Wang, W. (1999). Instability, stabilization, and formulation of liquid protein pharmaceuticals. *International Journal of Pharmaceutics* 185: 129–188. https://doi.org/10.1016/S0378-5173(99)00152-0.

38 Wang, W. (2000). Lyophilization and development of solid protein pharmaceuticals. *International Journal of Pharmaceutics* 203: 1–60. https://doi.org/10.1016/S0378-5173(00)00423-3.

39 Roser, B. (1991). Trehalose, a new approach to premium dried foods. *Trends in Food Science and Technology* 2: 166–169. https://doi.org/10.1016/0924-2244(91)90671-5.

40 Chen, X.D. and Mujumdar, A.S. (2008). *Drying Technologies in Food Processing*. New York: Wiley.

41 Mattern, M., Winter, G., Kohnert, U., and Lee, G. (1999). Formulation of proteins in vacuum-dried glasses. II. Process and storage stability in sugar-free amino acid systems. *Pharmaceutical Development and Technology* 4: 199–208. https://doi.org/10.1081/PDT-100101354.

42 Kumar, V., Sharma, V.K., and Kalonia, D.S. (2009). In situ precipitation and vacuum drying of interferon alpha-2a: development of a single-step process for obtaining dry, stable protein formulation. *International Journal of Pharmaceutics* 366: 88–98. https://doi.org/10.1016/j.ijpharm.2008.09.001.

43 Wildfong, P.L.D., Samy, A.S., Corfa, J. et al. (2002). Accelerated fluid bed drying using NIR monitoring and phenomenological modeling: method assessment and formulation suitability. *Journal of Pharmaceutical Sciences* 91: 631–639. https://doi.org/10.1002/jps.10070.

44 Abdul-Fattah, A.M., Lechuga-Ballesteros, D., Kalonia, D.S., and Pikal, M.J. (2008). The impact of drying method and formulation on the physical properties and stability of methionyl human growth hormone in the amorphous solid state. *Journal of Pharmaceutical Sciences* 97: 163–184. https://doi.org/10.1002/jps.21085.

45 Rey, L. and May, J.C. (2010). *Freeze Drying/Lyophilization of Pharmaceutical and Biological Products*. New York: Informa Healthcare.

46 Bowen, M., Turok, R., and Maa, Y.-F. (2013). Spray drying of monoclonal antibodies: investigating powder-based biologic drug substance bulk storage. *Drying Technology* 31: 1441–1450. https://doi.org/10.1080/07373937.2013.796968.

47 Wanning, S., Süverkrüp, R., and Lamprecht, A. (2015). Pharmaceutical spray freeze drying. *International Journal of Pharmaceutics* 488: 136–153. https://doi.org/10.1016/j.ijpharm.2015.04.053.

48 Chang, L.L., Shepherd, D., Sun, J. et al. (2005). Mechanism of protein stabilization by sugars during freeze-drying and storage: native structure preservation, specific interaction, and/or immobilization in a glassy matrix? *Journal of Pharmaceutical Sciences* 94: 1427–1444. https://doi.org/10.1002/jps.20364.

49 Cicerone, M.T., Pikal, M.J., and Qian, K.K. (2015). Stabilization of proteins in solid form. *Advanced Drug Delivery Reviews* 93: 14–24. https://doi.org/10.1016/j.addr.2015.05.006.

50 Prestrelski, S.J., Tedeschi, N., Arakawa, T., and Carpenter, J.F. (1993). Dehydration-induced conformational transitions in proteins and their inhibition by stabilizers. *Biophysical Journal* 65: 661–671. https://doi.org/10.1016/S0006-3495(93)81120-2.

51 Cleland, J.L., Lam, X., Kendrick, B. et al. (2001). A specific molar ratio of stabilizer to protein is required for storage stability of a lyophilized monoclonal antibody. *Journal of Pharmaceutical Sciences* 90: 310–321. https://doi.org/10.1002/1520-6017(200103)90:3<310::AID-JPS6>3.0.CO;2-R.

52 Andya, J.D., Maa, Y.F., Costantino, H.R. et al. (1999). The effect of formulation excipients on protein stability and aerosol performance of spray-dried powders of a recombinant humanized anti-IgE monoclonal antibody. *Pharmaceutical Research* 16: 350–358. https://doi.org/10.1023/A:1018805232453.

53 Wang, B., Tchessalov, S., Warne, N.W., and Pikal, M.J. (2009). Impact of sucrose level on storage stability of proteins in freeze-dried solids: I. Correlation of protein-sugar interaction with native structure preservation. *Journal of Pharmaceutical Sciences* 98: 3131–3144.

54 Allison, S.D., Chang, B.S., Randolph, T.W., and Carpenter, J.F. (1999). Hydrogen bonding between sugar and protein is responsible for inhibition of dehydration-induced protein unfolding. *Archives of Biochemistry and Biophysics* 365: 289–298. https://doi.org/10.1006/abbi.1999.1175.

55 Yoshioka, S. and Aso, Y. (2007). Correlations between molecular mobility and chemical stability during storage of amorphous pharmaceuticals. *Journal of Pharmaceutical Sciences* 96: 960–981. https://doi.org/10.1002/jps.20926.

56 Cicerone, M.T., Tellington, A., Trost, L., and Sokolov, A.P. (2003). Substantially improved stability of biological agents in dried form - the role of glassy

dynamics in preservation of biopharmaceuticals. *Bioprocess Technical* 1: 36–47. http://www.bioprocessintl.com/manufacturing/fill-finish/substantially-improved-stability-of-biological-agents-in-dried-form-1120036 (accessed 19 November 2019).

57 Zografi, G. and Newman, A. (2017). Interrelationships between structure and the properties of amorphous solids of pharmaceutical interest. *Journal of Pharmaceutical Sciences* 106: 5–27. https://doi.org/10.1016/j.xphs.2016.05.001.

58 Cicerone, M.T. and Soles, C.L. (2004). Fast dynamics and stabilization of proteins: binary glasses of trehalose and glycerol. *Biophysical Journal* 86: 3836–3845. https://doi.org/10.1529/biophysj.103.035519.

59 Chang, L.L., Shepherd, D., Sun, J. et al. (2005). Effect of sorbitol and residual moisture on the stability of lyophilized antibodies: implications for the mechanism of protein stabilization in the solid state. *Journal of Pharmaceutical Sciences* 94: 1445–1455. https://doi.org/10.1002/jps.20363.

60 Wahl, V., Khinast, J., and Paudel, A. (2016). Lyophilized protein powders: a review of analytical tools for root cause analysis of lot-to-lot variability. *TrAC Trends in Analytical Chemistry* 82: 468–491. https://doi.org/10.1016/j.trac.2016.05.012.

61 Wahl, V., Scheibelhofer, O., Roessl, U. et al. (2015). The influence of residual water on the secondary structure and crystallinity of freeze-dried fibrinogen. *International Journal of Pharmaceutics* 484: 95–102. https://doi.org/10.1016/j.ijpharm.2015.02.010.

62 Suihko, E.J., Forbes, R.T., and Apperley, D.C. (2005). A solid-state NMR study of molecular mobility and phase separation in co-spray-dried protein–sugar particles. *European Journal of Pharmaceutical Sciences* 25: 105–112. https://doi.org/10.1016/j.ejps.2005.02.002.

63 Clas, S., Dalton, C., and Hancock, B. (1999). Differential scanning calorimetry: applications in drug development. *Pharmaceutical Science & Technology Today* 2: 311–320. https://doi.org/10.1016/S1461-5347(99)00181-9.

64 Duddu, S.P. and Dal Monte, P.R. (1997). Effect of glass transition temperature on the stability of lyophilized formulations containing a chimeric therapeutic monoclonal antibody. *Pharmaceutical Research* 14: 591–595. http://www.ncbi.nlm.nih.gov/pubmed/9165528.

65 Carpenter, J.F., Chang, B.S., Garzon-Rodriguez, W., and Randolph, T.W. (2002). *Rational Design of Stable Lyophilized Protein Formulations: Theory and Practice*, 109–133. Boston, MA: Springer.

66 Fang, R., Grobelny, P.J., Bogner, R.H., and Pikal, M.J. (2016). Protein internal dynamics associated with pre-system glass transition temperature endothermic events: investigation of insulin and human growth hormone by solid state hydrogen/deuterium exchange. *Journal of Pharmaceutical Sciences* 105: 3290–3295. https://doi.org/10.1016/j.xphs.2016.07.028.

67 Grohganz, H., Lee, Y.Y., Rantanen, J., and Yang, M. (2013). The influence of lysozyme on mannitol polymorphism in freeze-dried and spray-dried formulations depends on the selection of the drying process. *International Journal of Pharmaceutics* 447: 224–230. https://doi.org/10.1016/j.ijpharm.2013.03.003.

68 Pikal, M.J. (1990). Freeze-drying of proteins. Part I: process design. *Biopharm.* 3: 18–23.

69 Pikal, M.J. and Shah, S. (1997). Intravial distribution of moisture during the secondary drying stage of freeze drying. *PDA Journal of Pharmaceutical Science and Technology* 51: 17–24. http://www.ncbi.nlm.nih.gov/pubmed/9099060.

70 Lin, T.P. and Hsu, C.C. (2002). Determination of residual moisture in lyophilized protein pharmaceuticals using a rapid and non-invasive method: near infrared spectroscopy. *PDA Journal of Pharmaceutical Science and Technology* 56: 196–205. http://www.ncbi.nlm.nih.gov/pubmed/12181804 (accessed 7 February 2017).

71 Duncan, D.I., Veale, J.R., Cook, I., and Ward, K. (2015). Using laser-based headspace moisture analysis for rapid nondestructive moisture determination of sterile freeze-dried product. 1–12. http://www.lighthouseinstruments.com/uploads/New_documents_9Jan2015/Brochure_Whitepaper_2009_2015_PRINT.pdf (accessed 19 November 2019).

72 Mozhaev, V.V. and Martinek, K. (1984). Structure-stability relationships in proteins: new approaches to stabilizing enzymes. *Enzyme and Microbial Technology* 6: 50–59. https://doi.org/10.1016/0141-0229(84)90034-6.

73 Allison, S.D., Dong, A., and Carpenter, J.F. (1996). Counteracting effects of thiocyanate and sucrose on chymotrypsinogen secondary structure and aggregation during freezing, drying, and rehydration. *Biophysical Journal* 71: 2022–2032. https://doi.org/10.1016/S0006-3495(96)79400-6.

74 Crowe, J.H., Carpenter, J.F., and Crowe, L.M. (1998). The role of vitrification in anhydrobiosis. *Annual Review of Physiology* 60: 73–103. https://doi.org/10.1146/annurev.physiol.60.1.73.

75 Schüle, S., Schulz-Fademrecht, T., Garidel, P. et al. (2008). Stabilization of IgG1 in spray-dried powders for inhalation. *European Journal of Pharmaceutics and Biopharmaceutics* 69: 793–807. https://doi.org/10.1016/j.ejpb.2008.02.010.

76 Adler, M. and Lee, G. (1999). Stability and surface activity of lactate dehydrogenase in spray-dried trehalose. *Journal of Pharmaceutical Sciences* 88: 199–208. https://doi.org/10.1021/js980321x.

77 Schmid, K., Arpagaus, C., and Friess, W. (2011). Evaluation of the nano spray dryer B-90 for pharmaceutical applications. *Pharmaceutical Development and Technology* 16: 287–294. https://doi.org/10.3109/10837450.2010.485320.

78 O'brien, J. (1996). Stability of trehalose, sucrose and glucose to nonenzymatic browning in model systems. *Journal of Food Science* 61: 679–682. https://doi.org/10.1111/j.1365-2621.1996.tb12180.x.

79 Sundaramurthi, P. and Suryanarayanan, R. (2010). Trehalose crystallization during freeze-drying: implications on lyoprotection. *Journal of Physical Chemistry Letters* 1: 510–514. https://doi.org/10.1021/jz900338m.

80 Ohtake, S. and Wang, Y.J. (2011). Trehalose: current use and future applications. *Journal of Pharmaceutical Sciences* 100: 2020–2053. https://doi.org/10.1002/jps.22458.

81 Colaço, C. and Roser, B. (1994). Trehalose-a multifunctional additive for food preservation. In: *Food Packaging and Preservation* (ed. M. Mathlouthi), 123–140. Boston, MA: Springer https://doi.org/10.1007/978-1-4615-2173-0_7.

82 Schebor, C., Burin, L., del P. Buera, M., and Chirife, J. (1999). Stability to hydrolysis and browning of trehalose, sucrose and raffinose in low-moisture systems in relation to their use as protectants of dry biomaterials. *LWT - Food Science and Technology* 32: 481–485. https://doi.org/10.1006/fstl.1999.0576.

83 Taylor, L.S. and Zografi, G. (1998). Sugar-polymer hydrogen bond interactions in lyophilized amorphous mixtures. *Journal of Pharmaceutical Sciences* 87: 1615–1621. https://doi.org/10.1021/js9800174.

84 Chieng, N., Cicerone, M.T., Zhong, Q. et al. (2013). Characterization of dynamics in complex lyophilized formulations: II. Analysis of density variations in terms of glass dynamics and comparisons with global mobility, fast dynamics, and Positron Annihilation Lifetime Spectroscopy (PALS). *European Journal of Pharmaceutics and Biopharmaceutics* 85: 197–206. https://doi.org/10.1016/j.ejpb.2013.03.036.

85 Xu, Y., Carpenter, J.F., Cicerone, M.T., and Randolph, T.W. (2013). Contributions of local mobility and degree of retention of native secondary structure to the stability of recombinant human growth hormone (rhGH) in glassy lyophilized formulations. *Soft Matter* 9: 7855. https://doi.org/10.1039/c3sm51251g.

86 Sola-Penna, M. and Meyer-Fernandes, J.R. (1998). Stabilization against thermal inactivation promoted by sugars on enzyme structure and function: why is trehalose more effective than other sugars? *Archives of Biochemistry and Biophysics* 360: 10–14. https://doi.org/10.1006/abbi.1998.0906.

87 Jena, S., Suryanarayanan, R., and Aksan, A. (2016). Mutual influence of mannitol and trehalose on crystallization behavior in frozen solutions. *Pharmaceutical Research* 33: 1413–1425. https://doi.org/10.1007/s11095-016-1883-7.

88 Sundaramurthi, P., Patapoff, T.W., and Suryanarayanan, R. (2010). Crystallization of trehalose in frozen solutions and its phase behavior during drying. *Pharmaceutical Research* 27: 2374–2383. https://doi.org/10.1007/s11095-010-0243-2.

89 Maury, M., Murphy, K., Kumar, S. et al. (2005). Spray-drying of proteins: effects of sorbitol and trehalose on aggregation and FT-IR amide I spectrum of an immunoglobulin G. *European Journal of Pharmaceutics and Biopharmaceutics* 59: 251–261. https://doi.org/10.1016/j.ejpb.2004.07.010.

90 Gikanga, B., Turok, R., Hui, A. et al. (2015). Manufacturing of high-concentration monoclonal antibody formulations via spray drying-the road to manufacturing scale. *PDA Journal of Pharmaceutical Science and Technology* 69: 59–73. https://doi.org/10.5731/pdajpst.2015.01003.

91 Cicerone, M.T. and Douglas, J.F. (2012). β-Relaxation governs protein stability in sugar-glass matrices. *Soft Matter* 8: 2983. https://doi.org/10.1039/c2sm06979b.

92 Franks, F. (1990). Freeze-drying: from empiricism to predictability. *Cryo Letters* 11: 93–110.

93 Yu, L., Mishra, D.S., and Rigsbee, D.R. (1998). Determination of the glass properties of D-Mannitol using sorbitol as an impurity. *Journal of Pharmaceutical Sciences* 87: 774–777. https://doi.org/10.1021/js970224o.

94 Obrzut, J., Anopchenko, A., Douglas, J.F., and Rust, B.W. (2010). Relaxation and antiplasticization measurements in trehalose–glycerol mixtures: a model formulation for protein preservation. *Journal of Non-Crystalline Solids* 356: 777–781. https://doi.org/10.1016/j.jnoncrysol.2009.07.045.

95 Bhattacharya, S. and Suryanarayanan, R. (2009). Local mobility in amorphous pharmaceuticals: characterization and implications on stability. *Journal of Pharmaceutical Sciences* 98: 2935–2953. https://doi.org/10.1002/jps.21728.

96 Roussenova, M., Andrieux, J.-C., Alam, M.A., and Ubbink, J. (2014). Hydrogen bonding in maltooligomer-glycerol-water matrices: relation to physical state and molecular free volume. *Carbohydrate Polymers* 102: 566–575. https://doi.org/10.1016/j.carbpol.2013.12.003.

97 Forney-Stevens, K.M., Bogner, R.H., and Pikal, M.J. (2016). Addition of amino acids to further stabilize lyophilized sucrose-based protein formulations: I. Screening of 15 Amino acids in two model proteins. *Journal of Pharmaceutical Sciences* 105: 697–704. https://doi.org/10.1002/jps.24655.

98 Heller, M.C., Carpenter, J.F., and Randolph, T.W. (1996). Effects of phase separating systems on lyophilized hemoglobin. *Journal of Pharmaceutical Sciences* 85: 1358–1362. https://doi.org/10.1021/js960019t.

99 Mensink, M.A., Van Bockstal, P.-J., Pieters, S. et al. (2015). In-line near infrared spectroscopy during freeze-drying as a tool to measure efficiency of hydrogen bond formation between protein and sugar, predictive of protein storage stability. *International Journal of Pharmaceutics* 496: 792–800. https://doi.org/10.1016/j.ijpharm.2015.11.030.

100 Bosch, T. (2014). *Aggressive freeze-drying: a fast and suitable method to stabilize biopharmaceuticals*. München: Ludwig-Maximilians Universität München.

101 Stärtzel, P., Gieseler, H., Gieseler, M. et al. (2015). Freeze drying of l-Arginine/sucrose-based protein formulations, part I: influence of formulation and arginine counter ion on the critical formulation temperature, product performance and protein stability. *Journal of Pharmaceutical Sciences* 104: 2345–2358. https://doi.org/10.1002/jps.24501.

102 Webb, S.D., Golledge, S.L., Cleland, J.L. et al. (2002). Surface adsorption of recombinant human interferon-γ in lyophilized and spray-lyophilized formulations. *Journal of Pharmaceutical Sciences* 91: 1474–1487. https://doi.org/10.1002/jps.10135.

103 Bam, N.B., Randolph, T.W., and Cleland, J.L. (1995). Stability of protein formulations: investigation of surfactant effects by a novel EPR spectroscopic technique. *Pharmaceutical Research* 12: 2–11. https://doi.org/10.1023/A:1016286600229.

104 Serno, T., Geidobler, R., and Winter, G. (2011). Protein stabilization by cyclodextrins in the liquid and dried state. *Advanced Drug Delivery Reviews* 63: 1086–1106. https://doi.org/10.1016/j.addr.2011.08.003.

105 Serno, T., Härtl, E., Besheer, A. et al. (2013). The role of polysorbate 80 and HPβCD at the air-water interface of IgG solutions. *Pharmaceutical Research* 30: 117–130. https://doi.org/10.1007/s11095-012-0854-x.

106 Millqvist-Fureby, A., Malmsten, M., and Bergenståhl, B. (1999). Spray-drying of trypsin: surface characterisation and activity preservation. *International Journal of Pharmaceutics* 188: 243–253. https://doi.org/10.1016/S0378-5173(99)00226-4.

107 Chen, B., Bautista, R., Yu, K. et al. (2003). Influence of histidine on the stability and physical properties of a fully human antibody in aqueous and solid forms. *Pharmaceutical Research* 20: 1952–1960. https://doi.org/10.1023/B:PHAM.0000008042.15988.c0.

108 Carpenter, J.F., Crowe, L.M., and Crowe, J.H. (1987). Stabilization of phosphofructokinase with sugars during freeze-drying: characterization of enhanced protection in the presence of divalent cations. *Biochimica et Biophysica Acta (BBA) - General Subjects* 923: 109–115. https://doi.org/10.1016/0304-4165(87)90133-4.

109 Maa, Y.-F., Nguyen, P.-A.T., and Hsu, S.W. (1998). Spray-drying of air–liquid interface sensitive recombinant human growth hormone. *Journal of Pharmaceutical Sciences* 87: 152–159. https://doi.org/10.1021/js970308x.

110 Bhatnagar, B.S., Bogner, R.H., and Pikal, M.J. (2007). Protein stability during freezing: separation of stresses and mechanisms of protein stabilization. *Pharmaceutical Development and Technology* 12: 505–523. https://doi.org/10.1080/10837450701481157.

111 Jennings, T.A. (1999). The importance of process water. In: *Lyophilization: Introduction and Basic Principles*. Englewood: Interpharm Press.

112 Twomey, A., Kurata, K., Nagare, Y. et al. (2015). Microheterogeneity in frozen protein solutions. *International Journal of Pharmaceutics* 487: 91–100. https://doi.org/10.1016/j.ijpharm.2015.04.032.

113 Roessl, U., Leitgeb, S., and Nidetzky, B. (2015). Protein freeze concentration and micro-segregation analysed in a temperature-controlled freeze container. *Biotechnology Reports* 6: 108–111. https://doi.org/10.1016/j.btre.2015.03.004.

114 Anchordoquy, T.J. and Carpenter, J.F. (1996). Polymers protect lactate dehydrogenase during freeze-drying by inhibiting dissociation in the frozen state. *Archives of Biochemistry and Biophysics* 332: 231–238. https://doi.org/10.1006/abbi.1996.0337.

115 Bhatnagar, B.S., Pikal, M.J., and Bogner, R.H. (2008). Study of the individual contributions of ice formation and freeze-concentration on isothermal stability of lactate dehydrogenase during freezing. *Journal of Pharmaceutical Sciences* 97: 798–814. https://doi.org/10.1002/jps.21017.

116 Szkudlarek, B.A. (1997). *Selective crystallization of phosphate buffer components and pH changes during freezing: implications to protein stability*. Ann Arbor, MI: University of Michigan.

117 Krausková, Ľ., Procházková, J., Klašková, M. et al. (2016). Suppression of protein inactivation during freezing by minimizing pH changes using ionic

cryoprotectants. *International Journal of Pharmaceutics* 509: 41–49. https://doi.org/10.1016/j.ijpharm.2016.05.031.

118 Costantino, H.R., Griebenow, K., Mishra, P. et al. (1995). Fourier-transform infrared spectroscopic investigation of protein stability in the lyophilized form. *Biochimica et Biophysica Acta, Protein Structure and Molecular Enzymology* 1253: 69–74. https://doi.org/10.1016/0167-4838(95)00156-O.

119 (Charlie) Tang, X. and Pikal, M.J. (2005). Measurement of the kinetics of protein unfolding in viscous systems and implications for protein stability in freeze-drying. *Pharmaceutical Research* 22: 1176–1185. https://doi.org/10.1007/s11095-005-6036-3.

120 Schwegman, J.J., Carpenter, J.F., and Nail, S.L. (2009). Evidence of partial unfolding of proteins at the ice/freeze-concentrate interface by infrared microscopy. *Journal of Pharmaceutical Sciences* 98: 3239–3246. https://doi.org/10.1002/jps.21843.

121 Geidobler, R. and Winter, G. (2013). Controlled ice nucleation in the field of freeze-drying: fundamentals and technology review. *European Journal of Pharmaceutics and Biopharmaceutics* 85: 214–222. https://doi.org/10.1016/j.ejpb.2013.04.014.

122 Geidobler, R., Konrad, I., and Winter, G. (2013). Can controlled ice nucleation improve freeze-drying of highly-concentrated protein formulations? *Journal of Pharmaceutical Sciences* 102: 3915–3919. https://doi.org/10.1002/jps.23704.

123 Winter, G., Vollrath, I., Hawe, A. et al. (2016). Controlled ice nucleation in freeze-drying. Freeze-Drying of Pharmaceutics and Biologics, July 12–15, Breckenridge, CO, USA.

124 Esfandiary, R., Gattu, S.K., Stewart, J.M., and Patel, S.M. (2016). Effect of freezing on lyophilization process performance and drug product cake appearance. *Journal of Pharmaceutical Sciences* 105: 1427–1433. https://doi.org/10.1016/j.xphs.2016.02.003.

125 Chang, B.S. and Randall, C.S. (1992). Use of subambient thermal analysis to optimize protein lyophilization. *Cryobiology* 29: 632–656. https://doi.org/10.1016/0011-2240(92)90067-C.

126 Jena, S., Horn, J., Suryanarayanan, R. et al. (2017). Effects of excipient interactions on the state of the freeze-concentrate and protein stability. *Pharmaceutical Research* 34: 462–478. https://doi.org/10.1007/s11095-016-2078-y.

127 Schersch, K., Betz, O., Garidel, P. et al. (2013). Systematic investigation of the effect of lyophilizate collapse on pharmaceutically relevant proteins, part 2: stability during storage at elevated temperatures. *European Journal of Pharmaceutics and Biopharmaceutics* 85: 240–252. https://doi.org/10.1002/jps.23121.

128 Barman, A., Smitherman, C., Souffrant, M. et al. (2016). Conserved hydration sites in PIN1 reveal a distinctive water recognition motif in proteins. *Journal of Chemical Information and Modeling* 56: 139–147. https://doi.org/10.1021/acs.jcim.5b00560.

129 Colandene, J.D., Maldonado, L.M., Creagh, A.T. et al. (2007). Lyophilization cycle development for a high-concentration monoclonal antibody formulation lacking a crystalline bulking agent. *Journal of Pharmaceutical Sciences* 96: 1598–1608. https://doi.org/10.1002/jps.20812.

130 Depaz, R.A., Pansare, S., and Patel, S.M. (2016). Freeze-drying above the glass transition temperature in amorphous protein formulations while maintaining product quality and improving process efficiency. *Journal of Pharmaceutical Sciences* 105: 40–49. https://doi.org/10.1002/jps.24705.

131 Tang, X. and Pikal, M.J. (2004). Design of freeze-drying processes for pharmaceuticals: practical advice. *Pharmaceutical Research* 21: 191–200. https://doi.org/10.1023/B:PHAM.0000016234.73023.75.

132 Ullrich, S., Seyferth, S., and Lee, G. (2015). Measurement of shrinkage and cracking in lyophilized amorphous cakes part 3: hydrophobic vials and the question of adhesion. *Journal of Pharmaceutical Sciences* 104: 2040–2046. https://doi.org/10.1002/jps.24441.

133 Ullrich, S., Seyferth, S., and Lee, G. (2015). Measurement of shrinkage and cracking in lyophilized amorphous cakes part 4: effects of freezing protocol. *International Journal of Pharmaceutics* 495: 52–57. https://doi.org/10.1016/j.ijpharm.2015.08.091.

134 Rambhatla, S., Obert, J.P., Luthra, S. et al. (2005). Cake shrinkage during freeze drying: a combined experimental and theoretical study. *Pharmaceutical Development and Technology* 10: 33–40. https://doi.org/10.1081/PDT-35871.

135 Abdul-Fattah, A.M., Oeschger, R., Roehl, H. et al. (2013). Investigating factors leading to fogging of glass vials in lyophilized drug products. *European Journal of Pharmaceutics and Biopharmaceutics* 85: 314–326. https://doi.org/10.1016/j.ejpb.2013.06.007.

136 Koepf, E., Schroeder, R., Brezesinski, G., and Friess, W. (2017). The film tells the story: physical-chemical characteristics of IgG at the liquid-air interface. *European Journal of Pharmaceutics and Biopharmaceutics* 119: 396–407. https://doi.org/10.1016/j.ejpb.2017.07.006.

137 Adler, M., Unger, M., and Lee, G. (2000). Surface composition of spray-dried particles of bovine serum albumin/trehalose/surfactant. *Pharmaceutical Research* 17: 863–870. https://doi.org/10.1023/A:1007568511399.

138 Fitzner, M. (2003). *Chemical and physiochemical stability of spray dried rhIL-11 formulations*. Bravia, Germany: Friedrich-Alexander Universität Erlangen-Nürnberg.

139 Schaefer, J. and Lee, G. (2015). Arrhenius activation energy of damage to catalase during spray-drying. *International Journal of Pharmaceutics* 489: 124–130. https://doi.org/10.1016/j.ijpharm.2015.04.078.

140 Maury, M., Murphy, K., Kumar, S. et al. (2005). Effects of process variables on the powder yield of spray-dried trehalose on a laboratory spray-dryer. *European Journal of Pharmaceutics and Biopharmaceutics* 59: 565–573. https://doi.org/10.1016/j.ejpb.2004.10.002.

141 Maa, Y.F., Nguyen, P.A., Andya, J.D. et al. (1998). Effect of spray drying and subsequent processing conditions on residual moisture content and physical/biochemical stability of protein inhalation powders. *Pharmaceutical Research* 15: 768–775. https://doi.org/10.1023/A:1011983322594.

142 Lassner, P., Adler, M., and Lee, G. (2014). Formation of insoluble particulates in a spray-dried f(ab′)2 fragment. *Journal of Pharmaceutical Sciences* 103: 1021–1031. https://doi.org/10.1002/jps.23891.

143 Broadhead, J., Rouan, S.K., Hau, I., and Rhodes, C.T. (1994). The effect of process and formulation variables on the properties of spray-dried beta-galactosidase. *The Journal of Pharmacy and Pharmacology* 46: 458–467. https://doi.org/10.1111/j.2042-7158.1994.tb03828.x.

144 Branchu, S., Forbes, R.T., York, P. et al. (1999). Hydroxypropyl-β-cyclodextrin inhibits spray-drying-induced inactivation of β-galactosidase. *Journal of Pharmaceutical Sciences* 88: 905–911. https://doi.org/10.1021/js9804819.

5

Vaccines and Microorganisms

Akhilesh Bhambhani and Valentyn Antochshuk

Merck & Co. Inc, New Technology-Drug Product Development, 770 Sumneytown Pike, West Point, PA 19446, USA

5.1 Introduction

Vaccines lessen the overall healthcare burden by preventing diseases either by controlling or in some cases totally eliminating the disease. Smallpox, for example, has been globally eradicated, while the burden of diphtheria, tetanus, measles, mumps, and rubella has been substantially reduced [1]. For continuous improvement of public health, research and development of new vaccines for new or emerging infectious diseases (e.g. Ebola, Zika, etc.) remains a high priority [2, 3]. Despite the benefit and desire to advance vaccine development, vaccine development remains a challenging task. This is attributed to a combination of factors, including but not limited to lack of a true biomarker as an immune correlate for protection, lack of structure/function correlation for analytical characterization and in some cases lack of a suitable *in vitro*/*in vivo* model. The aforementioned issues along with the fact that vaccines are administered to a healthy population (i.e. lacking the disease state) often result in large clinical studies required to establish safety and efficacy of novel vaccines.

Additionally, expansion of existing vaccines to emerging markets is further complicated by the intrinsic instability of vaccines and the lack of an established cold-chain footprint in certain markets. It is therefore critical for a product development scientist to develop not only a safe, efficacious, and stable formulation for the intended shelf life of the product but also one that is capable of withstanding the typical stresses (e.g. thermal, shear, etc.) associated with manufacturing, packaging, storage, shipping, and distribution. It is also essential that the vaccine can be successfully produced under the specific regulatory guidance that meets the local manufacturing requirement for the vaccine. This section is not meant to be exhaustive but a brief overview of drug product development with key considerations involved in both early- and late-stage vaccine development, and it is shared as per authors' perspective along with some case studies.

Drying Technologies for Biotechnology and Pharmaceutical Applications, First Edition.
Edited by Satoshi Ohtake, Ken-ichi Izutsu, and David Lechuga-Ballesteros.

5.2 Vaccine Drug Product Development

The objective of this section is to share general approaches, authors' experiences and developmental guidelines for various drug product development stages. The specific approach used is determined based on the particular antigen in question. Often the approach used for a vaccine drug product development is derived from the initially proposed target product profile, which in turn depends on the vaccine candidate in question (e.g. bacterial-derived antigen vs. live virus vaccines [LVVs]), previous experiences, and program needs (e.g. intended storage/shipping/market needs) among other business drivers. For example, development of LVVs often requires lyophilization to achieve desired stability profiles. Thus, the proposed approaches and guidelines shared below may not be applicable to all vaccine candidates and must be evaluated on a case-by-case basis as per the desired product profile for a given market and the developmental stage of the program.

5.2.1 Early Development to Phase I

During the very early developmental stage of a program, the process optimization activities are often focused on the speed to clinic and limited by the drug substance/antigen availability (amount as well as purity). This is further complicated by lack of well-defined stability indicating assays, thereby prompting an up-front investment in the developability assessment. The goal of the developability assessment is to assist in the evolution of the candidate's target product profile through strain selection and providing information regarding the stability profile of the candidate and in some cases identification of predominant degradation pathways through biophysical characterization (wherever applicable). In cases where biophysical characterization is not possible, animal studies often serve as a means for lead candidate identification and/or optimization. Developability studies allow optimization of discovery as well as process activities and form the basis for conducting pre-formulation studies, analytical characterization studies, and formulation development activities, leading to a "fit-for-purpose" phase I formulation. This is further described in details below.

5.2.1.1 Developability

It is generally agreed that developability is an exercise intended to provide rapid assessment of the risks associated with specific product candidate and probability of progressing through clinical development. Such an assessment is typically conducted utilizing a limited set of key metrics and limited resources. The goal of developability is a rigorous evaluation with a minimal amount of material to gain an understanding of product properties to make informed decisions about candidates and guide development activities. The outcome of the developability exercise is a risk profile that can be used to define the scope of activities once a preclinical candidate is selected. Hence, developability data and the resulting early risk profile can serve as basis for critical quality attributes (CQA) assessment and enable a rapid progression through development.

Developability or manufacturability assessment has been reported in the literature and at scientific conferences as a tool to rank-order candidates [4]. Such assessment is typically conducted prior to significant resource commitment associated with the candidate nomination and commitment to process development and material production.

The strategy and implementation of developability can vary, but the productive outcome increases probability of success by identifying underlying risks associated with each candidate. The timing for developability studies is typically within discovery–development interface. When a recombinant protein is used as a vaccine antigen, some examples of primary liabilities can include deamidation sites Asn-Gly (NG), glycosylation sites, free cysteine, methionine oxidation, and isomerization Asp-Gly (DG). Examples of secondary liabilities include deamidation sites (NS and NA), tryptophan oxidation, glycation on lysine, clipping between Asp and Pro, isomerization (DS), and deamidation (QG and QS). While not strictly a liability, compatibility with the standard or platform purification processes and formulations is one of the factors that can propel or slow down development timelines.

Typical developability approaches for protein antigens include multistep targeted screening utilizing functional assays to narrow down the pool of candidates, followed by sequence liabilities evaluation and subsequent testing of the transiently produced materials with a subset of biophysical tools to identify lead candidates. Such approaches require not only high throughput tools, but more importantly it relies on the understanding of critical attributes and their acceptance ranges. The key challenge is the availability of material to support analytics and process assessment early in the program. Options for material production in the Chinese hamster ovary (CHO) expression system include transient expression and transfection pool or stable pool production. Transiently expressed material could afford rapid production. However, if this approach is undertaken, it is recommended to directly compare the results from high throughput screening efforts between transient and stably expressed antigen across several projects to confirm that the results are consistent. As mentioned above, in contrast to protein antigens, lead identification/optimization for LVV candidates involves greater dependence on animal models with complementary support from cell-based assays for strain selection.

As result of the exercise (and within the constraints of intended product profile, DS availability, program timeline, and process and analytical capabilities), the candidate should meet minimum requirements to trigger the desired immune response and generate potency/efficacy, species cross-reactivity, tissue cross-reactivity, and/or minimum biochemical/biophysical characterization prior to candidate nomination and start of development. During biologics candidate selection, for example, epitope immunogenicity prediction is often used for rank ordering and selection of potential candidates using relative immunogenicity. Furthermore, the complexity of vaccine development requires considerations of other attributes besides antigen such as adjuvants and immune modulators, delivery routes, and formulations. In summary, developability is a disciplined decision-making process and informed prioritization of the candidates is required. Once the lead candidate is identified, the program advances into the pre-formulation stage.

5.2.1.2 Pre-formulation

The goal of pre-formulation development is to provide an initial assessment of product stability as a function of excipient screening and adjuvant selection (if required). Pre-formulation screening builds on the developability data and often involves extensive biophysical, biochemical, and/or potency/immunogenicity characterization to elicit mechanistic understanding of potential degradation pathways (i.e. establishing structure/ function correlations by coupling potency/stability with analytical changes) for the given vaccine candidate (wherever possible). It should be noted that during the pre-formulation stages, an animal models may serve as a screening tool for evaluating gross changes in the final drug product (or process) and its corresponding impact to immunogenicity. Given the breadth of approaches for characterizing the antigen structure, a dedicated section on biophysical characterization is provided below.

Biophysical Characterization Similar to protein pre-formulation/formulation work, biophysical characterization of vaccines and adjuvants provides the foundation for rational product design and optimization. These biophysical attributes can be divided into the following common types: thermal stability, structural stability, antigen/adjuvant interaction, and protein/protein or protein/adjuvant interaction evaluation.

Differential scanning calorimetry (DSC), differential scanning fluorimetry (DSF), and various versions of thermal melts (circular dichroism [CD], dynamic light scattering [DLS], etc.) serve as common approaches to characterize thermal stability of the antigens and complexes through the melting temperature (T_m) that is dependent upon secondary and tertiary structures. Thermal stress is one of the most common tools utilized by a formulator or process developer to "quickly" evaluate the impact of attributes/processes on the material. The measured thermal events are associated with significant structural perturbations of antigen and its subsequent degradation and are utilized to judge/predict the relative stability of the protein or selected formulation condition.

A variety of spectroscopic tools (CD, Fourier transform infrared [FTIR], UV, fluorescence, etc.) is typically used for structural stability evaluation. CD and FTIR spectroscopy are the most common tools for secondary structure evaluation. Intrinsic fluorescence spectroscopy of tryptophan residues is typically utilized for assessment of tertiary structure through evaluation of conformational and oxidation state of tryptophan residues. Extrinsic fluorescence measurements using hydrophobic probes (e.g. bis-ANS) provide additional information about local structural environments and their perturbations under a variety of formulation conditions.

Similarly, the size of the antigen particles (free as well as bound) is often a critical attribute optimized during development and can be measured using size exclusion chromatography (SEC), high accuracy particle counter (HIAC), micro-flow imaging (MFI), FlowCam, NanoSight, transmission electron microscopy (TEM), or scanning electron microscopy (SEM). Sizing tools (SEC,

MFI, HIAC, TEM, SEM) are often important to control morphology and size distribution of the product, and evolution of these parameters (or change in particle size distribution) is frequently associated with product changes or degradation.

For adjuvanted vaccines, evaluation of antigen/adjuvant interaction is important to understand the stability of adsorbed antigen and impact of the local microenvironment (pH, surface interactions). Electrostatic charge modulation using formulation conditions (pH and ionic strength) are frequently utilized to optimize the stability of the adjuvant/antigen complexes. Zeta potential, isothermal titration calorimetry (ITC), static light scattering (SLS), and DLS techniques are commonly used to study such interactions. For screening adjuvants, optimum pH is determined as per the point of zero charge (pzc) of adjuvant and the pI (isoelectric point) of the antigen followed by an evaluation of adsorption efficiency. Further in-depth characterization of antigen/adjuvant interactions (e.g. binding capacity and affinity) may be warranted to determine the impact of adjuvant on antigen stability as well as antigenicity.

Biophysical tools, as mentioned above, are helpful beyond formulation screening/optimization and process development; they can be utilized for product monitoring during manufacturing, stability studies, forced degradation data analysis, and lot-to-lot comparability. Such extensive characterization often results in a significant amount of data that requires visualization in a simple format for rank ordering formulations. Given the importance of data presentation and visualization, a brief overview of commonly used visualization approaches is provided below. The reader is advised to refer to the associated literature for additional details.

Data Visualization Developability and pre-formulation screening frequently utilize high throughput tools and generate a significant body of data. Multiple sequence/construct screening, using a number of assays and array of pre-formulation conditions, can lead to thousands of data points that need to be evaluated, sorted, and rank-ordered to select the best candidate. Data visualization and data reduction and processing are increasingly becoming a bottleneck especially for multiparameter systems. There are a few commonly used approaches that generally involve charts creation with a high "data–ink ratio" [5] using a variety of statistical/data analysis software.

A few examples of successful multivariate data visualization to mention are empirical phase diagrams for interpretation and presentation of biophysical data [6–8], surface plots for purification process evaluation [9], and radar charts [10] to demonstrate formulation impact on particle formation.

The aforementioned data interpretation and presentation tools enable high throughput workflows that allow screening and multivariate data interpretation at a fast pace. Furthermore, the approach provides tolerance for data/sample loss while providing information on the formulation/process design space. The abovementioned methods are best used for screening purposes (developability, pre-formulation, manufacturability) when the speed and ability to process a significant number of samples is fully supported by appropriately selected analytical methods. Such extensive characterization (whenever possible) also

Table 5.1 Potential benefits and limitations of liquid drug product vs. lyophilized drug product presentation development.

	Benefits	Limitations
Liquid	Ease of marketing/manufacturing, convenience to end user, lower cost of goods compared with dried formulation	Liquid formulation is more prone to degradation during storage, agitation, and shear and may suffer from material compatibility issues
Freeze-dried	Improved stability; shipping; reduced clinical timelines early in developmental stages render freeze drying preferable over liquid formulations	Freeze drying, compared with liquid form/fill process, is both capital and energy intensive with process stress and involves a reconstitution step by the end user

allows a greater understanding of the stability profile of the candidate and may prompt the need to consider a dried formulation for inherently unstable molecules.

Consideration for Development of Liquid vs. Freeze-Dried Dosage Forms The stability, storage, and/or shipping requirements often make freeze drying the method of choice over a liquid formulation. Lyophilization is a time-, energy-, and capital-intensive process and induces freezing and drying stress that could be detrimental for the product. Table 5.1 documents the key drivers for choosing freeze drying over the conventional liquid form/fill process.

As mentioned above, the predominant factor for choosing lyophilization is the poor stability profile of the candidate vaccine in the liquid state. This is especially true for LVVs due to their highly labile nature, rendering them unstable in the liquid state. For example, degradation rates for some vaccines could be ≥10% per hour in the liquid state, thereby necessitating the use of freeze drying to deliver a safe and efficacious vaccine over its intended shelf life [11]. In addition, the process of freeze drying (also known as lyophilization) meets the product sterility assurance requirement by virtue of the fact that vials can be stoppered in the freeze-drying chamber prior to unloading, thereby making it a trusted aseptic unit operation during the form/fill process. Other cost-saving advantages such as early entry into the clinic by utilizing platform approaches, improved thermal stability with reduced cold chain needs for improving vaccine access, and decreased bulk storage requirement through stockpiling of vaccine antigen through bulk drying could also influence the choice between a liquid and lyophilized development.

Some of the disadvantages of freeze drying include higher cost of manufacturing due to significant up-front capital investment along with the additional energy-intensive drying unit operation. Furthermore, in contrast to a liquid dosage, the technology transfer for a freeze-dried process from laboratory scale to pilot to commercialization is a complex process. Equipment differences, for example, between lab-scale, pilot-scale, and commercial lyophilizers, require systematic characterization of heat and mass transfer differences between the different scales to maintain critical product attributes (e.g. moisture, potency, etc.). Thus it is critical to develop a robust lyophilization process during the various stages of development with scale-up considerations. Furthermore, incompatibility of lyophilization with aluminum adjuvant containing vaccines, freezing and drying stress from the lyophilization process itself, and the additional need for a reconstitution step prompt careful considerations in establishing the drug product development roadmap. As per the outcome of risk assessment and candidate's stability profile in the initial pre-formulation development stages, the program is then advanced to formulation development for clinical readiness, evaluation, and eventually commercial launch.

5.2.1.3 Formulation Development

Key learning from the pre-formulation studies forms the basis of formulation development for safety assessment to phase I readiness and eventually establishing a line of sight for a robust, scalable, and manufacturable formulation/process that results in a safe and efficacious product during the intended shelf life of the vaccine. Due to resource/time constraints and/or other technical challenges, multiple key activities (e.g. characterization assay development, pre-formulation development, process optimization, etc.) are often performed in parallel and could result in suboptimal formulation/processes. Phase I marks a key milestone in defining the formulation and processes, while safety assessment batch preparation may also enable the initiation of real-time probe stability. The significance of these activities along with key considerations for early- and late-stage development is described briefly below.

Safety assessment toxicology (SA Tox) formulation allows evaluation of potential phase I formulations against target product profile and often includes antigen $\pm$ adjuvant (both identity and dose) and drug product image (liquid, frozen, and/or freeze-dried) along with the desired excipients (buffer, pH, stabilizers such as cryo- and lyoprotectant in a freeze-dried formulation, etc.). Real-time probe stability studies can be initiated once the safety assessment formulation has been identified to enable clinical supply dating for the phase I clinical program. For a phase I freeze-dried product, a formal probe stability initiation may only be accomplished post phase I good manufacturing practice (GMP) manufacturing due to lack of GMP lyophilizers for generating probe stability samples. The laboratory-scale lyophilizers, however, may be used to complement formal stability studies. Additionally, frozen formulations may be used for SA Tox study. This is often the case for labile LVVs. In contrast, liquid stability is likely achievable for subunit vaccines. For frozen SA Tox samples, feasibility assessment is performed by characterizing vaccine pre- and post-multiple freeze/thaw cycles. For freeze-dried phase I formulations, often due to time and resource constraints, a suboptimum lyophilization cycle is used. Similarly, based on the intended clinical study design, additional factors may be studied. For adjuvanted vaccines, for example, it is critical to determine the impact of adjuvant on antigen stability as well as antigenicity during real-time and in-use condition to determine single-vial vs. field-mix approach. Similarly, time-out-of-refrigeration (TOR), post-reconstitution stability, and material compatibility along with recommendations for types of syringes and needles to be used for supporting SA Tox studies must be provided.

Generally, a phase I formulation is similar to SA Tox formulation (but not always) and in some cases may include a reduced concentration of an excipient, an altered fill volume, and/or a modified image (e.g. frozen SA Tox with lyophilized phase I) or a different sequence of excipient (or adjuvant) addition than SA Tox formulation. Changes, if any, are often derived from the ongoing stability assessment, characterization activities, a technology transfer change due to equipment and/or process difference in the GMP setting, or a new competitive knowledge that prohibits use of a given excipient and/or process. Additionally, criteria that are essential for ensuring a successful phase I campaign may include inputs from various studies such as TOR, time in solution (TIS), freeze/thaw stability, field-mix stability or settling study and its impact on the fill process (for adjuvanted formulations), and material compatibility studies for product contact surfaces and impact of process conditions (e.g. stirring, pumping and filtration) on the vaccine modality [12]. Given the vast diversity of vaccines (e.g. inactivated vs. live attenuated viruses, polysaccharide vs. conjugated vaccines, adjuvanted vs. unadjuvanted vaccines), a platform approach may not be available, and the studies required to support the phase I campaign must be vaccine specific.

This is further complicated for a lyophilized vaccine, as the additional unit operation further adds to the inherent complexity of vaccine drug product development. Lyophilization requires development of a robust scalable process while maintaining the target product profile characteristics of these highly labile vaccine formulations along with necessary quality attributes desired from the lyophilized products (i.e. cake appearance, moisture content, reconstitution time, etc.). Zostavax®, a live enveloped virus vaccine, for example, is a Merck product that is stored frozen or refrigerated post-lyophilization [13]. Similarly, respiratory syncytial virus (RSV) data suggests that the best stability condition, even at high sucrose concentrations, requires storage at sub-zero condition (reportedly at −70 °C) [14]. Furthermore, any additional unit operation causes potential for more failure modes during the form/fill and inspection process. A few high-level issues/considerations relevant to lyophilization of vaccines and microorganisms as experienced by the authors are showcased below.

Pre-formulation and formulation development of vaccines, in some cases, revealed the need for salt (e.g. sodium chloride, calcium chloride, etc.) and/or polyols (e.g. glycerol, sorbitol, etc.) as a stabilizer (in certain cases tonicity modifiers) besides commonly used excipients (e.g. buffers, sugar, amino acids, surfactants, polymers, and other bulking agents). Presence of high salt or a plasticizer such as sorbitol, even though necessary for stability, resulted in a formulation with low T_g', thereby impacting the lyophilization cycle. Based on our experience and given the interdependent nature of formulation and lyophilization [15–18], it is our recommendation that the significance of formulation and its corresponding impact on lyophilization process parameters must be assessed early in the development to avoid delays during the late stages of program development [19]. Furthermore, if the vaccine is intended for the global market, care must be taken to satisfy regulatory requirements for all market needs. For example, use of animal-derived excipients and/or raw materials must be avoided to meet China and Japan regulatory requirements. Besides formulation selection, additional process parameters that may impact scale-up and/or tech transfer delays must also be considered to establish a successful technology transfer package and eventually develop a line of sight to commercialization. For example, to mitigate the high degradation rates in solution, LVVs are often blast frozen to minimize their TIS. Faster freezing often results in an increased mass resistance due to smaller ice crystals, eventually resulting in long primary drying. Similarly, since rate of desorption is dependent on specific surface area (besides K_v – apparent heat transfer coefficient and T_{shelf} – Shelf temperature), secondary drying needs to be optimized to achieve a shorter duration of time over higher temperature to achieve the desired moisture content. Based on authors' experience, some LVVs benefit from optimal moisture level over intended storage/stability, and lower moisture may not "always" be the best choice.

5.2.2 Late-Stage Development (Phase II and Beyond)

Similar to early-stage development, the primary goal of the late-stage development (defined here as phase II and beyond) is to preserve and improve (wherever possible) the quality attributes that enables the desired product efficacy and safety. Additionally, late-stage efforts focus on streamlining the process for attaining operational excellence by integrating technical process (e.g. lyophilization cycle parameters) and production workflows (e.g. operator shifts) with the existing operational attributes of the facility (e.g. automation) as per the relevant quality and GMP guidance. Compared with other modalities (i.e. small molecule and biologics), vaccines may require clinical bridging studies when substantial formulation and/or process changes are made post phase II especially when there is a lack of a well-defined *in vitro* immune marker as an immune correlate of protection (as is often the case with LVVs). Thus, it is critical to optimize the formulation as well as process conditions prior to phase II initiation.

Vaccines, especially LVVs, often rely on process consistency and release assays (cell-based assays) to define vaccine CQAs, and it is, therefore, often justifiably stated that in vaccine production, "process is the product." Within the small molecule space, process analytical testing (PAT) [20] and quality by design (QbD) [21] tools are often employed to build quality into the process. PAT enables product quality by "designing, analyzing and controlling the manufacturing process through timely measurements of CQAs and critical performance attributes (CPAs) (critical performance attributes) of material (raw and in-process) and process" [20]. Integration of PAT and QbD with the manufacturing process is in line with the regulatory expectation that suggests that quality should not be tested into product and must be built into the process itself [22]. In vaccine drug product development, however, the application of PAT and/or QbD is often restricted to specific unit operations (e.g. lyophilization) and applied appropriately to ensure final product quality. Integration of PAT and/or QbD is based on structure/function, or a cause-and-effect correlation, however, for many vaccines establishing this relationship is a challenging task due to their intrinsic complexity and inherent stability. Lack of an end-to-end QbD approach during vaccine development is often attributed to inherent complexity of vaccines either due to large size, heterogeneity and/or multicomponent nature of the vaccine itself, complexity of raw materials or the form/fill process used for vaccine manufacturing, or lack of clear understanding of the link between product attributes with clinical safety/efficacy [23–25].

Optimizing critical process parameters, as the vaccine program advances to late-stage development, thus rely on modeling/experimentation for evaluating the impact of scale on form/fill process differences (e.g. small-scale benchtop freeze/thaw or TIS vs. large volume freeze/thaw or TIS during scale-up) either due to equipment (e.g. use of thermocouple to monitor end of lyophilization cycle in lab vs. use of pressure sensors during scale-up) or facility constraints (e.g. manual stoppering in laboratory vs. automated stoppering in scale-up) on product quality. Since technology transfer/scale-up is one of the most challenging areas as vaccine programs advance from early stage to late phase, a dedicated subsection documenting scale-up considerations is described below using lyophilization as an illustrative unit operation.

5.2.2.1 Scale-Up Considerations and Case Studies

Freeze drying, a controlled mass and heat transfer process, relies on driving sublimation (rate and amount) and controlling product temperature by leveraging chamber pressure, shelf temperature, and time. Numerous studies and articles documenting the freeze-drying process transfer already exist in the literature [26–28], and only a brief summary is provided here. Successful scale-up requires evaluation of mass and heat transfer at intended scales (e.g. range of batch sizes) for a given freeze dryer, and adjustments may be required to address any equipment and/or environmental differences between the uncontrolled laboratory and aseptic production suite. Lack of cycle adjustments, as per scale-up requirements, may not only result in suboptimal processes but may also impact the final product quality. Differences in scale, equipment, and/or environment, for example, may result in suboptimal product quality with variances in cake appearance (at macroscopic and microscopic levels), moisture inconsistencies leading to stability impact, or batch failure due to equipment limitations such as choke flow, inconsistency within and between runs, and/or amplified edge effects. Impact of process conditions and differences in radiation effect, chamber pressure, shelf temperature, and process monitoring differences must be, therefore, evaluated to account for differences in scale-up between lab- and scaled-up (pilot- and commercial-scale) freeze dryer, and corresponding mitigation strategies must be designed [29]. Freezing inhomogeneity between lab and pilot scale due to the presence of particulate differences between lab-scale (uncontrolled) and GMP-scale (class 100) manufacturing, for example, may be minimized by incorporating an annealing step [30]. It should be noted that an annealing step may add value to a subunit vaccine lyophilization process and may not always be applicable to LVV lyophilization as most LVVs are often flash frozen and may not be suitable for an annealing process. Similarly, certain LVV drying processes rely on the use of different trays in pilot and commercial dryers to facilitate transfer post flash freezing. Thus, it is critical not only to develop the drying cycle at laboratory scale with the use of such alternate systems such as tray type (e.g. perforated aluminum trays vs. stainless steel trays) but also to evaluate the impact of repeated cleaning and sterilization on the tray itself. Slight warping of the tray, for example, may result in collapsed product due to suboptimal contact with the freeze-dryer shelf. It is recommended to evaluate these factors early in the drug product development stages to establish clear line of sight to commercial and to minimize/avoid scale-up and technology transfer delays.

Open communication between the formulation scientist, analytical lead, and process engineer is considered key component for successful development of a "well-characterized" process with appropriate design space (often done by executing range-finding studies with identification of failure modes) and corresponding control strategy for establishing a robust scalable manufacturing process for commercialization. Additionally, during this optimization process, timely input from the quality and regulatory team is desired to establish a clear line of sight to commercialization for the intended vaccine market. The Center for Biologics Evaluation and Research (CBER) is responsible, for example, for releasing all commercial vaccine lots. Thus, it is critical to incorporate quality and regulatory feedback to remain compliant with the agency guidance and to ensure vaccine quality is met for use within the United States.

Manufacturing process development for vaccines and scale-up and transfer of such process require special considerations for lyophilized products. Such attention is warranted due to inherent complexity of aforementioned manufacturing processes and subsequent risk of product heterogeneity, which may result in performance inconsistency or reduced stability of the product. Complexity and risks associated with vaccine lyophilization process implementation are often compounded by inherent instability and thermal lability of antigens. While the commonly known challenges associated with freeze-drying cycle scale-up and transfer are typically well understood and no different from other product modalities manufactured in glass vials, several nuances pertinent to vaccines are worthy of mentioning [31, 32].

Whereas annealing is frequently used during the lyophilization processes to improve porosity and homogeneity of the product, the associated increase in product temperature may create unexpected detrimental effects during manufacturing of heat-labile antigens. A practical example of freeze-dryer loading process impact on the defect levels is discussed for flash-frozen complex biological product [31]. While the flash-freeze process is not commonly utilized in industry, the particular antigen required a rapid freezing process to maintain product yields. The standard method to load the product into the lyo cabinet impacted the rate of product collapse during the lyophilization process. The authors were able to correlate increased collapse levels with onset of unwanted annealing happening [31] during loading of a liquid nitrogen flash-frozen formulation into the lyo unit. Following the detailed investigation, the loading process was successfully modified to prevent unwanted annealing. The proposed nonstandard loading method had the majority of the shelves collapsed during loading, and shelves were indexed up during loading. Such loading led to a successful process with low level of defects. Proper temperature mapping studies and engineering runs prior to active runs for process qualification and validation are the best investment that one can make to reduce the risks during transfer between sites and cabinets.

Another practical example that illustrates the importance of thorough process characterization is a study of heat and mass transfer within pilot and production units [32]. Theoretical models can be constructed to evaluate lyophilization cycle robustness at full scale and further optimize parameters and set points using a limited number of runs with the production units. Success of the studies could be improved when combined with several measuring techniques such as wireless thermocouples, temperature loggers, pressure rise testing, and in-line moisture control. When properly constructed, such models allow the simulation of ice temperature profiles and duration of primary drying as well as minimize the number of production runs.

The data modeling [33] established that the critical parameters for heat transfer are the shelf temperature (most critical) and cabinet pressure. Further analysis confirmed differences in heat transfer characteristics of pilot and production freeze dryers. Success of the engineering batches (similarity of moisture levels, slightly longer primary drying but within safety margin, and acceptable vial reject rates) served as the basis to continue process validation. It is our recommendation that the risks associated with scale-up and unit operations (worst-case scenarios) critical to the product quality must be assessed and determined on a case-by-case basis [31, 32].

The aforementioned challenges and limitation with the lyophilization process itself have driven interest to alternative faster drying technologies such as spray drying (SD) and microwave vacuum drying. These technologies are considered as viable alternatives to established lyophilization processes, and they have potential to provide flexible and continuous manufacturing. Specifically, these drying technologies have potential to improve drying time without compromising product quality but suffer from lack of a well-established aseptic manufacturing platform and require additional proof-of-concept studies for successful commercialization.

5.3 Spray Drying: An Alternate to Lyophilization

SD is often considered as an alternative to lyophilization for manufacturing of biologics and vaccines [33]. This drying approach, similar to lyophilization, provides the potential for retaining protein conformational, biophysical, and biochemical properties stabilized via employment of the solid state. Lyophilization and SD both rely on the solid matrix and low moisture content as stabilizing factors, thereby limiting ion mobility via controlled drying. In contrast to lyophilization, SD is an evaporative process with drying stresses that are different from lyophilization. The addition of sugars, however, has been shown to stabilize some pharmaceutical proteins upon being spray-dried. Furthermore, the typical spray-dried formulations of biologics and vaccines utilize standard bulking agents such as sucrose, trehalose, and mannitol [34].

The spray-drying process is a relatively simple process that has significant advantages over lyophilization. The most frequently discussed benefits of spray-dried vaccines are improved stability profile, drying speed (hours vs. days), improved throughput, high solids content processing, increased dissolution rate, customizable doses (powder dispensing), and dosage manufacturing for alternative delivery routes (without reconstitution via the gastrointestinal tract, respiratory mucosa, skin, or implant).

The spray-drying process consists of rapid drying of liquid microdroplets (liquid, suspension, emulsion) and bulk powder collection. There are several variants of spray-drying processes that have been developed to improve vaccine product stability profiles. The spray-freeze-drying (SFD) process avoids high temperatures via utilization of low pressure for drying processes [35]. The bubble dryer is used during carbon dioxide-assisted nebulization (CAN-BD) of liquids in another variant of the SD process [36].

The desirable product characteristics are controlled during SD via feed rate, drying air temperature, and aspiration capacity [35]. The drying air temperature is a critical product parameter that governs stability in several ways. Too low temperature can result in higher moisture and poor long-term stability, while too high temperature can result in significant product degradation during manufacturing and eventually lead to poor stability profile. Process analytical technology (PAT) is often used to monitor the temperature of the dry cylinder, high performance cyclone, and collecting tube over time during process development.

High moisture content in spray-dried formulations is known to cause protein instability. Increased feed rate and decreased inlet temperature, for example, result in a significant increase in moisture content [37]. As the feed rate increases, moisture content increases because more water needs to be evaporated and may lead to inefficient drying. As the inlet temperature increases, moisture content in the dried product may decrease because of low relative humidity in drying air. The interactions between inlet temperature with aspiration and feed rate with aspiration also significantly affect the moisture content. Moisture content is directly proportional to outlet temperature; increase in outlet temperature causes decrease in sample moisture. Thus, similar to lyophilization process, the critical process parameters may be altered to impact the desired CQAs. However, in contrast to lyophilization, SD relies on drying product outside the primary container/closure, thereby increasing the burden for dry product handling, dispending, equipment cleanability, and turnaround. Thus, the choice of SD vs. lyophilization depends not only on the intrinsic property (or stability) of the molecule or additional unit operations requirements for powder handling but relies on all aspects of QbD principles.

5.4 Summary and Path Forward

Vaccines have substantially improved human health in the past century and efforts are underway to develop new products for unmet medical needs including new and emerging infectious diseases. The recent measles, Ebola, and Zika outbreaks further emphasize the importance of vaccine products and vaccination in disease management. A brief overview of the vaccine product development stages including candidate selection, development, and scale-up is presented here. Special considerations are given to critical steps of lead identification and optimization (i.e. developability), pre-formulation development (i.e. thorough biophysical characterization), and data visualization (i.e. decision making). Such approaches combined with stage-appropriate formulation development allow accelerated program advancement from SA Tox to development and commercialization. The fundamental instability of vaccines often renders lyophilization as the method of choice for product stabilization to achieve the shelf life and provide distribution chain flexibility. Specific case studies further illustrate challenges and opportunities associated with lyophilization development and some failure modes during the technology transfer from lab to pilot to commercial scale. Alternate drying technologies such as SD and microwave vacuum drying are currently in various stages of evaluation and development. These technologies are considered as viable alternatives to established lyophilization processes and may provide continuous and flexible manufacturing options with higher throughput than currently attainable with conventional lyophilization. The interested reader is referred to Chapters 7 and 9, respectively, for further detail.

References

1 Center for Disease Control and Prevention (1999). Ten great public health achievements—United States 1900-1999. *Morbidity and Mortality Weekly Report*: 241–243.

2 Cohen, J. (2016). Unfilled vials. *Science* 351: 16–19.

3 Meulen, J., Casimiro, D., Coller, B.A. et al. (2015). Winning a race against evolving pathogens with novel platforms and universal vaccines. In: *Novel Approaches and Strategies for Biologics, Vaccines and Cancer Therapies* (eds. M. Salnikova and M. Singh), 251–287. Amsterdam, Netherlands: Elsevier Inc.

4 Ambrogelly, A., Antochshuk, V., Shi, S. et al. (2015). A path to building quality during monoclonal antibody candidate selection. In: *Monoclonal Antibodies: Development, Delivery and Applications* (ed. L. Zheng), 6–22. London: Future Science Ltd.

5 Tufte, E.R. (2001). *The Visual Display of Quantitative Information*. Cheshire, CT: Graphics Press.

6 Joshi, B.S., Bhambhani, A., Zheng, Y., and Middaugh, C.R. (2010). An empirical phase diagram/high throughput screening approach to the characterization and formulation of biopharmaceuticals. In: *Formulation and Process Development Strategies for Manufacturing Biopharmaceuticals* (eds. F. Jameel and S. Hershenson), 173–204. New York, Wiley.

7 Maddux, N.R., Joshi, S.B., Volkin, D.B. et al. (2011). Multidimensional methods for the formulation of biopharmaceuticals and vaccines. *Journal of Pharmaceutical Sciences* 100 (10): 4171–4197.

8 Bhambhani, A., Thakkar, S., Joshi, S.B., and Middaugh, C.R. (2012). A formulation method to improve the physical stability of macromolecular-based drug products. In: *Therapeutic Protein Formulation: Practical Approaches*

in the Laboratory, Manufacturing and the Clinic (ed. B.K. Meyer), 13–45. Philadelphia, PA: Woodhead Publishing.

9 Welsh, J.P., Petroff, M.G., Rowicki, P. et al. (2014). A practical strategy for using miniature chromatography columns in a standardized high-throughput workflow for purification development of monoclonal antibodies. *Biotechnology Progress* 30: 626–635.

10 Kalonia, C., Kumru, O.S., Kim, J.H. et al. (2013). Radar chart array analysis to visualize effects of formulation variables on IgG1 particle formation as measured by multiple analytical techniques. *Journal of Pharmaceutical Sciences* 102: 4256–4267.

11 Burke, C.B., Hsu, T., and Volkin, D.B. (1999). Formulation, stability, and delivery of live attenuated vaccines for human use. *Critical Reviews in Therapeutic Drug Carrier Systems* 16 (1): 1–83.

12 Morefield, G.L. (2011). A rational, systematic approach for the development of vaccine formulations. *The AAPS Journal* 13 (2): 191–200.

13 Merck. (2019). Zostavax® product [package insert]. www.merck.com

14 Gupta, C.K., Leszczynski, J., Gupta, R.K., and Siber, G.R. (1996). Stabilization of respiratory syncytial virus (RSV) against thermal inactivation and freeze-thaw cycles for development and control of RSV vaccines and immune globulin. *Vaccine* 14: 1417–1420.

15 Harris, J.H., Shire, S.J., and Winter, C. (2004). Commercial manufacturing scale formulation and analytical characterization of therapeutic recombinant antibodies. *Drug Development Research* 61: 137–154.

16 Sarciaux, J.M., Mansour, S., Hageman, M.J., and Nail, S.L. (1999). Effects of buffer conditions on aggregation of bovine IgG during freeze-drying. *Journal of Pharmaceutical Sciences* 12: 1354–1361.

17 Chang, B.S., Kendrick, B.S., and Carpenter, J.F. (1996). Surface-induced denaturation of proteins during freezing and its inhibition by surfactants. *Journal of Pharmaceutical Sciences* 12: 1325–1330.

18 Blue, J. and Yoder, H. (2009). Successful lyophilization development of protein therapeutics. *American Pharmaceutical Review*: 40–44.

19 Bhambhani, A. and Blue, J.T. (2010). Lyophilization strategies for development of a high-concentration monoclonal antibody formulation: benefits and pitfalls. *American Pharmaceutical Review*: 31–38.

20 U.S. Department of Health and Human Services, Food and Drug Administration. (2004). Guidance for industry: PAT—a framework for innovative pharmaceutical development, manufacturing and quality assurance. https://www.fda.gov/regulatory-information/search-fda-guidance-documents/pat-framework-innovative-pharmaceutical-development-manufacturing-and-quality-assurance.

21 Rathore, A.S. and Winkle, H. (2009). Quality by design for biopharmaceuticals. *Nature Biotechnology* 27: 26–34.

22 U.S. Department of Health and Human Services, Food and Drug Administration. (2009). Guidance for industry: Q8(R2) pharmaceutical development. https://www.fda.gov/regulatory-information/search-fda-guidance-documents/q8r2-pharmaceutical-development.

23 Schellekens, H. (2009). Biosimilar therapeutics-what do we need to consider? *Nephrology, Dialysis, Transplantation* 2 (Suppl 1): i27–i36.

24 Rathore, A.S. (2009). Follow-on protein products: scientific issues, developments and challenges. *Trends in Biotechnology* 27 (12): 698–705.

25 Kirdar, A.O., Chen, G., and Rathore, A.S. (2010). Application of near-infrared (NIR) spectroscopy for screening of raw materials used in the cell culture medium for the production of a recombinant therapeutic protein. *Biotechnology Progress* 26: 527–531.

26 Blue, J.T., Sinacola, J., and Bhambhani, A. (2015). Process scale-up and optimization of lyophilized vaccine products in lyophilized biologics. In: *Vaccines and Cancer Drugs Modality Based Approaches* (eds. D. Varshney and M. Singh), 179–210. New York: Springer.

27 Rambhatla, S. and Pikal, M.J. (2003). Heat and mass transfer scale up issues during freeze-drying. Part I. Atypical radiation and the edge-vial effect. *AAPS PharmSciTech* 4: e14.

28 Rambhatla, S., Ramo, R.T., Bhugra, C., and Pikal, M.J. (2004). Heat and mass transfer scale up issues during freeze drying, II: control and characterization of the degree of supercooling. *AAPS PharmSciTech* 5: e58.

29 Rambhatla, S., Tchessalov, S., and Pikal, M.J. (2006). Heat and mass transfer scale up issues during freeze drying, III: control and characterization of dryer differences via operational qualification tests. *AAPS PharmSciTech* 7 (2): e1.

30 Patel, S.M., Jameel, F., and Pikal, M.J. (2010). The effect of dryer load on freeze drying process design. *Journal of Pharmaceutical Sciences* 99 (10): 4363–4379.

31 Searles, J.A., Carpenter, J.F., and Randolph, T.W. (2001). Annealing to optimize the primary drying rate, reduce freezing-induced drying rate heterogeneity, and determine T_g' in pharmaceutical lyophilization. *Journal of Pharmaceutical Sciences* 90: 872–887.

32 Wallen, A.J., Susan, H.V.O., Sinacola, J.R., and Phillips, B.R. (2009). The effect of loading process on product collapse during large-scale lyophilization. *Journal of Pharmaceutical Sciences* 98 (3): 997–1004.

33 Tsinontides, S.C., Rajniak, P., Pham, D. et al. (2014). Freeze drying principles and practice for successful scale-up to manufacturing. *International Journal of Pharmaceutics* 280: 1–16.

34 McAdams, D., Chen, D., and Kristensen, D. (2012). Spray drying and vaccine stabilization. *Expert Review of Vaccines* 11: 1211–1219.

35 Ingvarsson, P.T., Schmidt, S.T., Christensen, D. et al. (2013). Designing CAF-adjuvanted dry powder vaccines: spray drying preserves the adjuvant activity of CAF01. *Journal of Controlled Release* 167: 256–264.

36 Maa, Y.F., Ameri, M., Shu, C. et al. (2004). Influenza vaccine powder formulation development: spray-freeze-drying and stability evaluation. *Journal of Pharmaceutical Sciences* 93: 1912–1923.

37 Cape, S.P., Villa, J.A., Huang, E.T.S. et al. (2008). Preparation of active proteins, vaccines and pharmaceuticals as fine powders using supercritical or near-critical fluids. *Pharmaceutical Research* 25: 1967–1990.

Part II

Common Drying Technologies

6

Advances in Freeze Drying of Biologics and Future Challenges and Opportunities

Bakul Bhatnagar and Serguei Tchessalov

Pfizer Inc., BioTherapeutics, Pharmaceutical Sciences, 1 Burtt Road, Andover, MA 01810, USA

6.1 Introduction

Freeze drying, also termed lyophilization, has been utilized for desiccation and stabilization of compounds (pharmaceuticals and biopharmaceuticals) for several decades [1, 2]. One of the earliest references to freeze drying of labile compounds can be found in the context of serum and biologics in 1935 by Flosdorf and coworkers [3], which were subsequently followed by numerous publications of drying of plasma, viruses, bacterial cultures, etc. [4–10]. Several examples of the application of freeze drying of foods (fish, meat, potatoes, tofu, etc.) have been actually dated to several centuries earlier than drying of pharmaceuticals. Freeze drying is the most widely employed technique for drying of pharmaceuticals and represents the gold standard to which other drying technologies are compared. A number of reviews on freeze drying can be found in the literature for practitioners engaged in formulation, process development, and scale-up of pharmaceutical compounds [11–15]. The focus of this commentary is to provide a summary of the evolution and advances in pharmaceutical freeze drying, with an emphasis on the drying of biologics. We will review the approaches ("best practices") for the stabilization, tools for process monitoring and control, and methods for characterization of the physical matrix and the active compounds in the dried state and current challenges and future opportunities in freeze drying.

6.2 Where Are We Now?

At least 475 prescription medicines (new molecular entities and biologics) have been approved by the US FDA since 2000 [16]. Based on our analysis of drug products in development vs. commercially available (using PharmaCircle), over 650 marketed drug products are lyophilized. There are hundreds of biologics in development for several therapeutic indications that include monoclonal antibodies (mAbs), antibody drug conjugates (ADCs), enzymes, clotting factors, fusion proteins, and emerging modalities in the areas of cell and gene therapy. A significant fraction of biologics in development exhibit instability in aqueous

Drying Technologies for Biotechnology and Pharmaceutical Applications, First Edition.
Edited by Satoshi Ohtake, Ken-ichi Izutsu, and David Lechuga-Ballesteros.

environments, thereby presenting the need for the removal of water to improve their shelf life. Biologic drug substances and drug products are lyophilized in a variety of containers, including glass bottles, vials, dual-chamber systems (syringes, cartridges), and trays [2].

During freeze drying, water is converted to ice during the freezing step, ice is removed via sublimation during the primary drying step, and the unfrozen water is removed by desorption during the secondary drying step. Typically, freezing, primary drying, and secondary drying are conducted at different shelf temperatures. In addition, during the drying steps, the chamber pressure within the freeze dryer is controlled to a predetermined set point. There are also examples of lyophilization processes where both primary and secondary drying could be combined into a single step. While lyophilization is intended to preserve and stabilize a biologic, freezing and drying lead to dramatic alternations in the environment of a protein, thereby causing the development of a variety of stresses, which can compromise the pharmaceutical stability of the protein [17–20]. The stresses during freezing include low temperature, ice, and freeze concentration. The low temperature has been implicated in protein unfolding during cooling/freezing and is described as cold denaturation [21–25]. Ice formation leads to the greatest change in the physical environment and leads to concentration of the solutes, a process known as freeze concentration (or cryo-concentration). Freeze concentration, in turn, could lead to separation of the amorphous phases [26, 27] and/or crystallization of solutes from the cryo-concentrate [28–31]. Solute crystallization of components, specifically bulking agents such as mannitol or glycine, is intended and advantageous and utilized to reduce the duration of the drying [11, 15]. The unintended crystallization of formulation components such as buffer salts [32–34] or cryoprotectants [35, 36] can be damaging and are often encountered in the case of poorly formulated biologics. Ice crystallization presents a new interface (ice–freeze concentrate interface) and has been shown to cause protein unfolding [37, 38]. The overall effect of ice is governed by the degree of supercooling and the freezing rate, which in turn affect the size and number of ice crystals. The structure of the frozen matrix leaves its imprint on the dried matrix and determines the rate of drying [39]. Larger ice crystals are formed during slow cooling, which lead to larger pores on ice sublimation and facilitate faster drying. Fast cooling leads to the formation of smaller ice crystals and consequently smaller pores during primary drying and poses a greater resistance to water vapor transport during drying. In addition, the appearance of ice has been thought to also impose a mechanical stress on proteins [40, 41]. Removal of the unfrozen water during drying further stresses proteins and leads to additional degradation during drying [19].

6.3 Current State

6.3.1 Rational Formulation Design: Keeping It Simple

Over the years, several guidelines have been described for rational/systematic formulation development as opposed to trial-and-error (or empirical) approaches [2, 11, 42]. A general approach is to include a buffer (*to maintain the pH*), a cryo-/lyoprotectant (*to ensure stabilization during freezing and drying*), and a surfactant (to protect from ice–aqueous interface) in a protein formulation and can be easily extended to a number of modalities ranging from mAbs to ADCs to vaccines. In such a scenario, the choice of components and composition should be such that the buffer salt and stabilizer do not crystallize during freezing and drying. Examples of formulation platforms based on a thorough understanding of factors causing protein destabilization (physical and chemical) as well as thermal and phase behavior of the formulation exist across the pharmaceutical industry, with the approach being to keep formulations "simple" and "lyophilization friendly." Poorly designed formulations can significantly extend the duration of drying from a couple of days to a week or longer. In addition, the use of trial-and-error or empirical approaches in formulation and/process development can lead to conservative and less efficient processes.

A buffer is included to control the pH during freeze drying and in the reconstituted solution. Commonly utilized buffer systems in biopharmaceuticals include glutamate, histidine, sodium citrate, sodium (or potassium) phosphate, succinate, and Tris buffers [43, 44]. Acetate-, carbonate-, or imidazole-based buffers are avoided due to their volatile nature. Since buffer crystallization during freezing is well documented in the literature for the more commonly utilized buffers such as phosphate and succinate buffers [32, 45, 46], an understanding of the phase behavior can be utilized in the design of the formulation such that the required buffer capacity and pH are maintained during processing. A recommended strategy is to utilize a high weight ratio of the non-crystallizable (that is, the cryo-/lyoprotectants such as sucrose and trehalose) formulation components to that of the buffer [11, 15].

Freeze-dried formulations of biologics containing a low solids content (1%) also include a bulking agent to increase the cake mass and to prevent blowout during drying. Bulking agents could be crystallizable such as glycine and mannitol, which crystallize during either freezing or subsequent annealing and provide a scaffold on which the amorphous formulation components can be dried above the critical temperature (collapse temperature) [1, 2]. Widely utilized bulking agents, one example being the disaccharide sucrose, remain amorphous during freeze drying. Bulking agents can confer stabilizing effects and prevent protein instability if they remain in the amorphous state. Amino acids (glycine), disaccharides (sucrose, trehalose), polyols (mannitol, sorbitol), and polymers (dextran, Ficoll, polyethylene glycol, polyvinylpyrrolidone) exhibit protection during freezing (cryoprotectant) and drying (lyoprotectant). Crystallization during processing can cause destabilization (by the removal of the stabilizer from the same phase as the protein) and has been observed in the case of trehalose [35, 36] and sorbitol [47, 48], which have been shown to crystallize during prolonged annealing or storage at temperatures above the glass transition temperature of the freeze concentrate (T_g'). Mannitol is not recommended as a stabilizer due to the risk of crystallization either during processing or on storage. The crystallization behavior of mannitol is influenced by a formulation composition (inclusion of salts, ratio of mannitol to non-crystallizable component) and processing conditions (rate of cooling, freezing temperature, annealing temperature and time).

In the context of cryoprotection by sugars such as sucrose, it appears that the extent of stabilization is dependent on the pre-freeze solution concentration of the sugar, with 0.2–0.5 M providing effective stabilization [1, 11, 49]. A weight ratio of the stabilizer to protein of at least 1 : 1 is recommended for ensuring good stability during drying and/or storage and ~5 : 1 for optimal stability. In a study on aggregation during storage of several protein (recombinant cytokines and fusion proteins, molecular weights between 19 and 185 kDa), the physical stability increased monotonically with an increase in the disaccharide concentration over a sugar to protein mass ratio (R) of 0.5 : 4 (or a molar ratio of 56 : 541). The authors also observed that when the sugar to protein weight ratio was ~1, the native structure retention and structural relaxation time (indicator of global mobility in the dried matrix) reached a maximum. Local mobility measurements based on the mean-square amplitude of motion using neutron backscattering correlated with aggregation rate constants at all the compositions [50, 51]. Sucrose and trehalose are widely utilized as stabilizers in protein formulations. While there are reports of no differences in protein stability in sucrose vs. trehalose formulations, there are also reports where sucrose-based formulations exhibited greater stability (by a factor of two) than in trehalose-containing formulations. Even though a greater global mobility was associated with the sucrose-based formulations than in trehalose formulations, a greater decrease in the fast dynamics (a measure of local mobility) was observed in the sucrose formulations when compared with the trehalose systems [52]. Local mobility may exhibit better coupling with stability during storage at temperatures far below the T_g. Similar effects on local mobility were observed in observed in protein–sugar systems containing small amounts of antiplasticizer (glycerol or sorbitol). It is hypothesized that the inclusion of glycerol decreased the free volume in the protein–sucrose glasses, limiting motion and thereby slowing down local mobility [53]. Similar observations have been documented in disaccharide glasses containing sorbitol [54]. The inclusion of plasticizers presents an additional option in the design of freeze-dried formulations.

Very often, other salts in addition to the buffer salts are included as formulation excipients to prevent precipitation of the protein or to reduce the viscosity of highly concentrated proteins. The overall effect of solubility and viscosity is dependent on the nature of the ionic species and the protein/protein interactions. Examples of salts included in the formulations include sodium chloride and arginine hydrochloride, among others [55, 56]. In addition, salts have been shown to decrease the collapse temperature [57, 58] and can also exacerbate the pH shifts in the event of buffer crystallization [32, 34]. While the inclusion of salts results in a formulation that could need conservative processing, there are approaches one could utilize to counter the reduction in the collapse temperature of salt-containing system. In such scenarios, it is advised to utilize a sucrose–mannitol combination such that sucrose provides the necessary stabilization during processing and storage, while mannitol can crystallize and enable drying at higher temperatures, thereby reducing processing times. Such a strategy based on the use of mannitol–sucrose combination at mannitol to sucrose ratios ranging from 2 to 4 ensures mannitol crystallization and can be of practical benefit in the lyophilization of low protein concentration formulations (≤50 mg/ml) in the absence or presence of salts.

Since proteins are prone to adsorption and aggregation at interfaces (air–liquid, air–solid, ice–freeze concentrate), surfactants are included to ensure protein stability during formulation, fill, and finish operations as well as during freeze/thawing and reconstitution. Nonionic surfactants (fatty acid esters of sorbitan polyethoxylates such as Polysorbate 20 and 80) are commonly included at low concentrations (0.01–0.1% w/v, which is above the chemistry, manufacturing, and controls (CMCs) value) to prevent surface denaturation [59]. Polysorbates are prone to oxidative or hydrolytic degradation. Oxidative degradation in polysorbates can be mitigated by the inclusion of an antioxidant, chelator, or radical scavenger (ethylenediaminetetraacetic acid (EDTA) or methionine) [60, 61]. An alternate surfactant to polysorbate is poloxamer 188 (Pluronic F68), which is also approved for parenteral administration by the FDA [62]. We note that platform-based formulations may not always provide optimal stabilization for biologics such as cell-based and viral vector-based therapies and would require more extensive pre-formulation and formulation prescreening.

6.3.2 Process Design and Monitoring

6.3.2.1 Freezing

There is a common agreement that freezing step defines the properties of lyophilized material [2]. The temperature at which ice crystallization occurs (ice nucleation temperature), the rate of conversion of water into ice, formulation composition, and the ratio of stabilizer to the active ingredient dictate post-lyophilization stability of drug product. Due to the stochastic nature of ice nucleation, the thermal history of each individual vial may be different, leading to potential variability in product quality.

Annealing, as was demonstrated by Searles et al. [63], could minimize the differences in thermal history, increase the pore size (determined by the ice crystal size), and increase the sublimation rate [64]. During annealing, the product temperature is increased above the T_g', thereby facilitating ice crystal growth (that is, increasing in the size of the larger ice crystals at the expense of smaller ice crystals, and the number of ice crystals, described as Ostwald ripening). The farther the product temperature from the glass transition temperature, the faster the annealing process. In the case of systems where the bulking agent is crystallizable, the eutectic melting (or secondary melting) temperature defines the upper limit for the annealing process. Thus, annealing may not be applicable to formulations exhibiting a high T_g'. Besides ice recrystallization (devitrification), annealing also promotes crystallization of the bulking agent(s) and significantly improves sublimation rates by enabling more aggressive drying [65]. An increase in the mobility during annealing could, however, induce phase separation, which may not be favorable for some products, limiting application of the annealing process [63, 66].

An alternative method of "erasing" the difference in structure due to ice nucleation variability is through the application of controlled ice nucleation. During controlled ice nucleation, product temperature is reduced below the melting temperature of the formulation, and after a predetermined equilibration, ice nucleation is induced by an "ice fog" injection [39, 67–69], quick depressurization of the drying chamber post-pressurization [70], reduction of the chamber pressure [71, 72], or ultrasound [73–76]. Similar to annealing, controlled ice nucleation has been shown to reduce heterogeneity in drying rates across a shelf of vials, typically resulting in the reduction of primary drying duration.

There are differences in the ice structure that forms on freezing induced via controlled ice nucleation vs. annealing post uncontrolled/spontaneous freezing. During stochastic freezing, ice typically nucleates at the bottom of a vial, and the ice front propagates from the bottom toward the top of the solution. It is, therefore, not unusual to observe a "concentrated film/layer" at the surface of the lyophilized cake because of the freezing process suggesting phase separation. Annealing, performed after initial ice crystallization, could promote additional phase separation. It is not surprising, therefore, that the initial resistance of a cake generated from a process utilizing annealing is higher than that of the cake formed during stochastic freezing. During controlled nucleation, ice typically forms at the surface of the liquid material (top of the vial) and propagates toward the bottom of the vial, pushing freeze concentrate to the bottom of vial. Therefore, it is not unusual to observe a ring of more dense material at the bottom of the cake produced using controlled nucleation. One can expect some differences in the distribution of formulation components within the cakes produced using annealing vs. controlled ice nucleation methods. In theory, some differences in the stability behavior could be result of differences due to the freezing method. Therefore, both methods should be utilized during freezing process design to identify the most suitable method for the product.

To the best of the knowledge of the authors, annealing is more often employed during freezing than controlled ice nucleation. The reason for this is quite simple. The commercial dryer design does not need to be modified for implementation of annealing as long as the software allows inclusion of multiple steps for freezing. The implementation of controlled ice nucleation requires either modification of the dryer to enlarge the port for quick depressurization (in the case of pressurization/depressurization-induced freezing) or the purchase of a separate unit to generate a sterile ice fog. Controlled ice nucleation is available in laboratory and large-scale dryers available from most lyophilizer manufacturers. The potential benefits, challenges, and costs of the technology must be considered in determining the implementation of the technology. The biggest obstacle is the finding the "right product," which could not be manufactured without the use of controlled nucleation. Examples of such products exist: virus as an active ingredient in animal vaccines [77], whose survival could be only guaranteed by utilization of controlled nucleation (as opposed to annealing). The implementation of controlled nucleation for freeze drying of biologics appears to be limited in at least two scenarios. The first example is of products containing high potency drugs (low-concentration active pharmaceutical ingredient (API)) in a formulation consisting of a crystallizable bulking agent with a stabilizer and where annealing can be successfully utilized. Crystallization of the bulking agent creates a matrix that can withstand significantly higher temperatures (up to 40 °C during primary drying) without any negative impact on product quality.

Thus, faster drying is available without the need for modification to the dryer (as would be needed for controlled ice nucleation). The other scenario exists in the case of formulations containing high protein concentrations where aggressive drying can be utilized (typically above the T_g') [78]. In this case, freeze drying above the T_g' or even above the microscopic collapse temperature could reduce drying heterogeneity without affecting the product quality. There appears to be a limited need for application of controlled ice nucleation for lyophilization of such products. Thus, due to the limited number of products that could significantly benefit from controlled nucleation, implementation costs, additional validation activities, and regulatory implications, implementation of controlled nucleation method has not progressed as fast as one would assume despite the obvious benefits of the technology. In the opinion of the authors, it may be another decade before controlled ice nucleation is routinely employed for commercial manufacturing.

6.3.2.2 Product Temperature Measurement

Product temperature measurement is likely the oldest and is most directly linked to product quality. Thermocouples and resistance temperature detectors (RTDs) were the preferred tools for the measurement of product temperature [79]. In the experience of the authors, RTDs were mostly employed for monitoring of bulk freeze drying (product filled in trays) since the measuring element is typically >3 mm and is not suitable for temperature measurement in small volumes. Thermocouples were more suited for vial-based freeze drying. Both types of sensors are easy to calibrate and provide important information on process status (product temperature) at the point of contact. Since measurements are limited to the location of temperature sensors, the use of multiple sensors at critical locations (identified from the experience, for example, corners and center of the shelf) is a typical strategy for successful process control. If the sensors are positioned accurately, they provide information on product temperature relative to the critical temperature and also enable detection of the end point of freezing and primary drying. Product temperature sensors in combination with batch monitoring systems (discussed below) are powerful tools for the process control. While they are useful tools in process monitoring and control, the misuse of temperature sensors, due to wrong placement, could lead to variability in temperature measurement, which could complicate operator's decision on the state of process. Temperature sensors are invasive and influence the drying behavior in vial being monitored [64] since they could serve as nucleation sites. This results in the nucleation of ice at higher temperature in sensor-containing vials during the freezing ramp, lowest cake resistance, and shorter drying duration when compared with most vials (non-sensor-containing vials). Controlled nucleation or annealing could minimize the differences in product resistance, but sensor-containing vials may still not be representative due to the additional heat received by product from the sensors (encountered to a greater degree in the edge vials). During commercial manufacturing, product temperature placement is typically utilized in only edge vials due to sterility concerns. Since edge vials are not representative of the entire batch (due to the additional radiant heat received by the product from the chamber walls and door), the determination of the primary drying end point could be challenging. For these reasons, temperature measurement devices were abandoned for the most commercial processes, especially when automatic loading systems were introduced into manufacturing. Wireless sensors, especially those that do not introduce heat into the product (for example, Tempris® probes) [79], could reintroduce direct temperature measurement as a valuable tool for the process monitoring. Since product temperature history is directly linked to product quality, temperature sensors could serve as "true" process analytical technology (PAT) tools. Miniaturization of wireless sensors, addition of robotic systems for sensor placement in commercial lines, and modification of existing control systems allowing process decision making based on sensor feedback in combination could increase the probability of implementation of temperature measurement into routine commercial processes.

6.3.2.3 Pressure Rise Test/Manometric Temperature Measurement

The pressure rise test (PRT) is a batch monitoring processes that has been well known for decades, but is also a test whose potential was never completely utilized. PRT is performed, both during primary and secondary drying, by the closing valve between the chamber and condenser and monitoring the resulting chamber pressure increase. The shape of the pressure increase curve could provide very valuable information about the product as well as the process: the average batch product temperature at the sublimation surface, vial heat transfer coefficient, cake resistance, sublimation rate, and end point of primary drying [80]. Manometric temperature measurement (MTM) was one of the first PAT tools for process control at the time of its introduction in 1997. The lack of reliability of fast response valves (that is, fast or quickly closing valves) limited the application of MTM for process control. MTM, however, is still considered a valuable method for the detection of end points of primary and secondary drying. In the opinion of the authors, multiple factors such as availability of software, experience of drug product manufacturers with PRT, and availability of hardware (which is typically built into the design of modern freeze dryers) will help maintain PRT as a valuable option for the process control.

6.3.2.4 SMART Freeze-Dryer™ Technology

The introduction of the SMART™ freeze dryer was a revolutionary step in freeze-drying process control [81]. It provided an inexperienced operator the tool(s) to conduct close to optimal freeze drying. The starting point of process design using SMART technology is providing information about the product (solids content, critical product temperature, nature of product [amorphous or crystalline]), container closure (internal and external vial diameters), and number of vials and initiating the process without providing the exact set points for process parameters. Based on the product properties, the software selects or identifies an appropriate freezing process by introducing an annealing step, if needed, and maintaining the product below the T_g' during the vacuum initiation step. During primary drying, by periodically closing the valve between the chamber and condenser for a short duration coupled with application of the MTM method, the product temperature at the sublimation surface is estimated, and cycle parameters are adjusted to maintain product below the critical temperature. By integrating the sublimation rate, estimated at each point of MTM test, the software predicts the end point of primary drying and moves process from primary to secondary drying. During secondary drying, the program continues testing the status of drying by comparing the increase in the pressure during PRT to a predetermined value, which is linked to target residual water content of product. Once the estimated water content is less than the target water content, the software moves process to the final holding step. Thus, there is no interaction between the operator and freeze dryer during entire process. In theory, each step of the process could be the optimal as long as the input parameter (such as pressure increase during testing) is accurate. In reality, it has been reported that [82] the predictions of sublimation rate and product temperature are not accurate after completion of approx. 50% of primary drying, especially for high solids content formulations. In the experience of the authors, product temperature predictions become less reliable after the completion of approx. about 65% of primary drying and is accompanied with underestimated of primary drying durations for high protein concentration formulations. In addition, pressure increase during PRT results in a small (up to 1 °C) increase in the product temperature, which could be critical if the cycle is operating at the edge of failure. Again, fast-closing valves (necessary for the successful execution of PRT) are still not available for the commercial dryers. A combination of the multiple factors listed above (*less accurate sublimation rate and product temperature predictions, pressure increased coupled with product temperature increase, and unavailability of fast-closing valves at commercial scale*) may be responsible for the lack of implementation of the SMART technology for commercial manufacturing. In addition, the current "rule of thumb" (or do we say, requirements?) for lyophilization process description in the regulatory submissions and batch records does not provide the flexibility that is built into the SMART approach.

6.3.2.5 Application of Pirani Gauge for the Control of Primary Drying

In the past, Pirani and similar thermal conductivity-type gauges were popular for pressure monitoring and process control in laboratory and commercial freeze dryers. While some of these gauges were stable to steam sterilization, the other failed after being subjected to only a few sterilization cycles [79]. Due to their sensitivity to gas composition in the dryer chamber, Pirani sensors were replaced by capacitance manometers (CM), which are currently the preferred pressure sensors for process control. The sensitivity of the Pirani gauge to water vapor is the basis for the "comparative" pressure measurement method. In this method, the difference between Pirani and CM readings is constantly compared and serves as a major input in determination of the drying end point. In theory, at the end of primary drying, when there is no water vapor in the drying chamber, the pressure difference should be zero at all pressure set points. This, in turn, could be utilized to advance to the secondary drying step. In reality, there is always an offset between Pirani gauge and CM sensor reading, which can be determined during an initial calibration in a dry and empty chamber. The midpoint of the Pirani decay curve has been identified as the point at which almost all primary drying could be considered complete [83]. The algorithm for the "comparative" pressure method is well developed and tested, at least, on laboratory-scale dryers. The Pirani sensors are inexpensive and relatively robust, thereby providing a reliable tool for process control. In the opinion of the authors, the lack of flexibility in the description of lyophilization processes based on the regulatory submission requirements limits the use of comparative pressure measurement for routine commercial manufacturing. Since the primary drying duration in regulatory dossiers and batch records is typically fixed, any change in the primary drying duration is considered as a deviation.

6.3.2.6 Application of Mass Spectroscopy for Process Control

The benefits of application of mass spectroscopy (MS) to lyophilization process control have been known for at least a few decades [84]. It is an accurate method for the detection of gas composition in the drying chamber, which could be employed for the detection of end points of primary and secondary drying steps. However, the technology was not routinely used due to high cost of equipment and the footprint. Recent advances in miniaturization of mass spectrometers as well as the associated cost reduction have enabled the installation of mass spectrometers, or of the lesser expensive residual gas analyzers (RGAs), on commercial freeze dryers. To the author's knowledge, several RGAs are currently installed on large-scale dryers. The purpose of an RGA is to enable the detection of silicone oil leaks [85]. The authors believe that in the near future, RGAs will be routine utilized in freeze-drying process control. One application of RGAs is in the measurement of sublimation rate. In principle, if the molar ratios of gases in the chamber during primary drying are measured by an RGA, one could estimate the rate of generation of water molecules due to sublimation at a known flow rate of nitrogen (used for the pressure control). By estimating the sublimation rate, one could then calculate the average product temperature at the sublimation surface, which could then serve as an input parameter for process control. Unlike PRT/MTM, this method does not require periodic interruption of the process, and therefore, in theory, it could be more suitable for implementation in combination with the SMART technology.

6.3.2.7 Heat Flux Sensors as PAT Tools

Heat flux sensors (HFSs) have been recently proposed as PAT tools for lyophilization process control [79]. The sensors are attached to the shelf surface at certain locations and allow measurement of the vial heat transfer coefficient, product temperature, and sublimation rate without direct contact with the product. When placed at representative locations across the freeze dryer, the inclusion of HFSs presents the opportunity to control each step of lyophilization. For example, they could be employed for the detection of crystallization end point of excipients during freezing [86] or of the end points of primary and secondary drying (will require extremely sensitive of sensors). HFSs can also be utilized for the control of heat flux from the shelf to the product during freezing to manipulate the ice structure (and consequently specific surface area) to form larger pores. Linked to the programmable logic controller (PLC), information from all HFSs could serve as inputs into process control and potentially used for the development of the next generation of SMART technology. In spite of their potential, it appears, to the best of our knowledge, that HFSs are currently not yet installed on any commercial dryers due to incompatibility with automatic loading systems. If HFSs can be embedded into the shelves at certain locations during shelf fabrication process (to minimize interference during operations), they could serve as powerful tools for process monitoring and control.

6.3.2.8 Pressure Decrease Method

Recently Pisano and coworkers [87] described a method for control of primary drying by periodically closing the controlled leakage valve and applying the algorithm for data extraction, termed as a pressure decrease test (PDT). During this test, the valve that controls chamber pressure by nitrogen injection is shut off for a short duration, resulting in a decrease in the chamber pressure. The PDT algorithm enables calculation of the vapor flow rate produced by sublimation, cake resistance, and vial heat transfer coefficient. A steady-state primary drying model is utilized to calculation of the product temperature. The decision to move the process to the next step is facilitated by these inputs. Thus, unlike the PRT/MTM method, a slight drop in the product temperature during PDT allows more effective execution of the process at the edge of failure. While the input parameters for the primary drying model generated from the PDT method are similar to those from the MTM method, it appears to be more easily implemented in commercial dryers. The leakage valve is fast closing and relatively cheap, and implementation of the method does not require dryer modification since it is currently an included feature in most modern dryers. Incorporation of the PDT method into SMART approach, in the author's opinion, appears to be more reliable when compared with the MTM method. The authors, however, are not aware of any successful commercial implementation of PDT to date.

6.3.2.9 Tunable Diode Laser Absorption Spectroscopy (TDLAS)

Tunable diode laser absorption spectroscopy (TDLAS) [88] is a near-IR (NIR)-based optical method for the measurement of mass flow rate during drying. The optical hardware is placed in the duct between the chamber and condenser with the laser beam positioned at a 45° angle to the direction of the flow. In the opinion of the authors, TDLAS is currently the only reliable noninvasive methodology that has been tested on large-scale dryers. However, it requires modification of existing freeze dryers in order to mount the hardware. TDLAS has been demonstrated to be very useful tool for calculation of the product temperature at the sublimation surface [89], vial heat transfer coefficients [90], and cake resistance [91]. Generation of these input parameters during an active process without any intervention and the subsequent application of the algorithm based on the steady-state primary drying model enable process control process in a similar manner to the SMART technology. The implementation of TDLAS into SMART will bring lyophilization process control to the next level.

6.3.2.10 Emerging Analytical Tools for Process Monitoring and Control

Raman and infrared (IR) spectroscopy have been utilized for monitoring of the entire freeze-drying process. While this approach provides important information on the state of excipients (phase behavior) [92, 93] or in estimation of the product temperature without contact [94], these technologies are limited to observation of the edge vials, which are not representative of an entire batch. In the past decade, IR cameras have been integrated into freeze dryers to enable online process monitoring [95]. One must track the advances in these technologies, which in the future may provide options that could be applied in development of a new generation of process control.

6.3.2.11 Modeling of Freeze-Drying Process

When efficient process monitoring and control based on critical attribute such as product temperature are not available, modeling of the freeze-drying process could assist in design of optimal drying process. To the best of our knowledge, no reliable models exist for freezing in vials at laboratory and commercial scales. Robust primary drying models have existed at least three decades and are routinely utilized for process design, scale-up, and analyses of deviations [96]. The most accessible (user-friendly) secondary drying model was published recently [97] and can be easily implemented into the existing control systems (if input parameters are known). In the author's opinion, the use of modeling is essential for the process design. However, modeling efforts must be coupled with advanced PAT tools and advanced algorithms to design and transfer the most efficient lyophilization process.

6.3.3 Tools to Monitor Dried Products

Characterization of the formulation prior to and post freeze drying is critical for formulation and process development. The discussion on characterization here is limited to the dried state. Several tools are available to monitor the physical and chemical stability of the biologic along with the matrix into which the drug is lyophilized.

6.3.3.1 Structure of the Biologic

Chemical degradation of proteins during processing and on storage is determined using liquid chromatography-mass spectrometry (LC-MS) [98]. Physical degradation (non-covalent aggregation) is investigated using UV spectrometry, light scattering, size exclusion chromatography, analytical centrifugation, and IR spectroscopy. Fourier transform infra-red (FTIR) has been widely utilized to assess the secondary structure during storage for at least two decades [52, 99]. Raman spectroscopy is utilized to characterize the phase behavior of the matrix (containing crystallizable components) [100] as well was the secondary structure of proteins during storage [101, 102]. More recently, solid-state hydrogen–deuterium exchange mass spectrometry (ssHDX-MS) and solid-state photolytic labeling mass spectrometry (ssPL-MS) were employed for the characterization of formulation and process-induced conformational changes in lyophilized proteins [103, 104]. Deuterium uptake using ssHDX-MS of several mAb formulations determined post-lyophilization correlated with the physical (aggregation) and chemical instability storage. The authors of the study presented ssHDX-MS as promising approach to obtain an early readout of differences in long-term stability between several formulations and therefore accelerate formulation screening and selection [105]. In the past several years, the range of modalities with the biologics portfolios has expanded with the introduction of cell and gene therapy-based formulations. The arrival of new modalities presents new challenges for formulation and analytical scientists to develop tools to monitor structural changes in cells and viral vectors in the dried state and the consequent impact on product properties.

6.3.3.2 Characterizing Matrix Contributions to Stability

The toolbox for the analytical characterization of the excipient matrix continues to expand. Calorimetric (*differential scanning calorimetry, isothermal microcalorimetry*), spectroscopic (*IR, Raman, frequency modulation spectroscopy for headspace water analysis*), diffractometric (*ambient and variable temperature X-ray diffractometric*), gravimetric (*dynamic vapor sorption*), chemical, and combinations thereof (X-ray diffractometry- differential scanning calorimetry (*XRD-DSC), thermogravimetry, DVS-Raman*) are routinely utilized for the characterization of product quality attributes (thermal, water content and uptake, phase behavior, etc.) [106]. Scanning electron microscopy, Brunauer-Emmett-Teller (BET)-based N2 or Kr sorption–desorption measurements, and mercury porosimetry enable assessment of drying behavior and product morphology. A number of recent publications on the use of X-ray CT illustrates the growing interest in understanding cake structure and morphology and their relationship with product properties (drying behavior, appearance, reconstitution) [107, 108]. Combination of data generated using specific tools (BET analysis of nitrogen or krypton adsorption isotherms + electron spectroscopy for chemical analysis, ESCA/X-ray photoelectron spectroscopy (XPS)) can also help resolve the contribution of the specific surface to the overall degradation in the dried state [109, 110].

While lyophilization provides a great improvement in the stability of proteins by reducing molecular motion in the dried state relative to that in solution, there is still sufficient molecular mobility (global and local, as a function of temperature, water content, formulation composition) for degradation to occur [111]. Consequently, characterization of molecular mobility has been a topic of great interest for at least three decades. Specifically, there have been efforts to understand if there exists coupling between dynamics (primary or α-relaxations vs. secondary or β-relaxations) in the amorphous glasses and pharmaceutical stability [112, 113]. Motions directly coupled with viscosity are described as global, primary, or α-relaxations where a structural relaxation time, τ, is utilized to describe the time constant for such motions. The reciprocal of the structural relaxation time provides an estimate of global mobility. Such relaxations slow greatly below the glass transition temperature. The stability of several proteins was determined above and below the glass transition temperature where optimal stability was observed far below the T_g. Co-lyophilization of proteins with a high-T_g glass-forming solute appeared to provide good stability, though in other cases it did not yield optimal stabilization [50]. Therefore, there is a consensus that a high T_g is not a sufficient predictor of molecular mobility [114]. Dynamics in glasses are governed by fragility, thermal history, and T_g. The difference between the T_g and the storage temperature is not directly related to molecular mobility since a high-T_g formulation could exhibit higher mobility due to a difference in fragility. While α-relaxations greatly slow down at temperatures well below the T_g, molecular mobility is determined by secondary or β-relaxations, which represent fast dynamics. Local mobility characterized using neutron scattering [52, 112, 115] or solid-state nuclear magnetic resonance (NMR) [116, 117] has been implicated in degradation of human growth hormone (hGH), insulin, mAbs, and other proteins. Several techniques are employed to characterize the molecular mobility and include differential scanning calorimetry (DSC), dielectric analysis (DEA), thermally stimulated current (TSC), isothermal microcalorimetry (IMC), NMR, and neutron backscattering. In some of the cases, the limitation to the use of the techniques may either be due to lack of easy access or long measurement times (days). There have also been efforts to develop surrogate measurements to neutron backscattering such as low frequency Raman scattering [118], which appears to rank-order formulations and therefore distinguish between even slightly different formulations.

There are also other contributors to stability beyond molecular mobility and include phase separation [119, 120], effective solid-state pH (characterized via Hammett acidity function) [121, 122], and specific surface area [109, 110]. Traditionally DSC is utilized for detection of phase separation in polymer-based systems but is of limited use in protein-rich systems. Instead, Raman line mapping and solid-state NMR have been utilized to detect phase separation, where ssNMR has been successful at detecting phase separation in domain sizes smaller than the Raman line mapping capability [111]. A combination of ESCA and BET was utilized to evaluate dried proteins (mAbs and vaccines) covering a 30-fold range of specific surface areas, generated through foam drying, freeze drying, and spray drying [109, 123]. A strong correlation is observed between degradation rate and fraction of protein available at the surface when compared with surfactant-containing systems. In a subsequent study using hGH, aggregation on storage correlated with percentage protein at the surface in formulations containing sucrose, trehalose, or hydroxyethyl starch (HES) as stabilizers, suggesting that surface degradation accounted for significant fraction of total degradation [110]. One must exercise caution in interpreting stability data for freeze-dried products or those containing lower or higher specific surface areas (SSAs) (foam dried, spray dried, spray freeze dried, etc.) and consider the contribution of surface degradation and others to overall destabilization.

6.3.3.3 Looking Beyond the Biologic and the Formulation Matrix

In addition to monitoring and characterizing the drug product, the volume of the container above the drug product (headspace) is also monitored [124, 125]. Headspace analysis, based on laser absorption spectroscopy, is utilized for nondestructive measurement of gases (oxygen, carbon dioxide, water vapor) during container-closure/packaging development, during stability study, and for in-line testing during manufacturing. In addition, foreign particles (examples: metal, glass) are detected via X-ray-based analysis and aid in the identification of non-formulation components/contamination during visual inspection.

6.4 Current Challenges

6.4.1 Understanding Protein Degradation in the Frozen State and Dried States

The physical environment of a protein undergoes dramatic changes leading to the development of several stresses that affect protein stability. The three key stresses include low/cold temperature, ice formation, and freeze concentration [18]. Freeze concentration, in turn, could facilitate second-order reactions, crystallization of solute (buffer or cryo-/lyoprotectants), phase separation (amorphous–amorphous separation), and redistribution of solutes. The formation of ice leads to the development of a large ice–aqueous interfacial area. Proteins have also been shown to adsorb and unfold at the ice–freeze concentrate interface.

The formation and growth of ice crystals could also lead to entrapment of the solution (freeze concentrate) phase, which is dependent on the conditions of freezing (geometry of the crystallization front, progression rate of the ice–freeze concentrate interface, and macroscopic viscosity) [126]. A concentration gradient at the ice–freeze concentrate interface as opposed to the bulk environment could create heterogeneity in composition and could have implications on protein stability. One could invoke ice-induced solution entrapment as an alternate mechanism for protein degradation. Entrapment of the freeze concentrate could cause partitioning of proteins into a quasi-liquid layer (QLL) on the ice crystal surface (also described as a liquid-like layer below the ice melting temperature) as opposed to the bulk freeze concentrate. The microenvironment experienced by the proteins in the QLL (could be different w.r.t. local acidity) when compared to the bulk freeze concentrate. While entrapment of solutes by ice has been investigated in binary and ternary systems using optical refractometry, FTIR, and confocal Raman microscopy, its effect on protein degradation is unknown. Typical protein formulations are multicomponent systems containing protein, buffer salt, cryoprotectant, and surfactant. The evolution of the freeze concentrate and consequently the spatial heterogeneity would be much more complex than in the "simpler" binary and ternary systems. Lastly, the phase transformation of water to ice also leads to a volume expansion and presents the potential role of mechanical stresses and elevated local pressure in protein destabilization. Additional ice crystallization (also described as devitrification) occurs during warming above the T_g' of the frozen solution. Thus, proteins could experience a dual stress imposed by ice formation during freezing and warming. We note that only limited information exists on the contribution of mechanical stresses to protein degradation during freeze/thawing [40, 41]. Considering the diversity of biologics modalities that formulation scientists are currently encountering (mAbs, fusion proteins, cell and gene therapy-based therapeutics), there are numerous future opportunities to improve our understanding of the freezing stresses on protein stability.

Addition of excipients such as disaccharides provides stabilization in the frozen state (cryoprotection) as well during and post-drying (lyoprotection). Components such as surfactants minimize degradation during freezing and reconstitution. Chemical stabilization is achieved through appropriate selection of pH, buffer, and antioxidant. Some formulation components can also provide protection from physical and chemical degradation. In the context of degradation and stabilization in the dried state, thermodynamic and/or kinetic stabilization mechanisms are invoked. The "water substitute hypothesis" is a thermodynamic stabilization mechanism, and the "glass dynamics hypothesis" offers kinetic stabilization [114]. Several commentaries are available invoking either mechanism or making the case for thermodynamic vs. kinetic stabilization [54, 112, 115, 127–130]. It has been argued that stability data can be interpreted via either mechanism and remains a hot topic for investigators. It has been pointed out that the lack of agreement on stabilization mechanism(s) could be attributed to either incomplete analyses of the stability data or to inadequate characterization tools. The use of H/D exchange, solid-state tryptophan fluorescence spectroscopy, low frequency Raman scattering, and solid-state NMR may help resolve contributions to degradation and stabilization. Furthermore, in several cases, experiments may not be appropriately designed to investigate the contributions of thermodynamic vs. kinetic stabilization where both mechanisms could be in play [114]. The identification of other contributors to instability such as degradation at the solid–air interface points to the complex nature of solid-state protein degradation/stabilization.

6.4.2 Process Inefficiency

In organizations engaged in the manufacture of a large number of lyophilized products, there may be very often limited capacity for bringing new products onboard. In such cases, optimization of legacy processes, which are often empirical, inefficient, and suboptimal, becomes a critical activity. The key reason for this inefficiency is likely due to utilization of conservative approaches (an accepted tradition in the past and sometimes even in the current times) to develop robust process. In such conservative approaches, the product temperature during drying was typically maintained below the T_g', and soak time during primary drying was of extended duration to account for any unexpected process variations, thereby resulting in long process durations. Freeze drying above collapse temperature (microscopic or visual) was mostly uncommon. Recent advances in freeze drying above the collapse temperature [65, 131–134] suggest that formulations (of both biologics and small molecules) can be freeze-dried well above the T_g', microscopic collapse temperature, and even above visual collapse temperature with retention of quality during the shelf life. The key benefit of freeze drying above the collapse temperature is the short drying duration, which in turn helps bring down operational and utility costs and creates additional manufacturing capacity.

We provide a few critical activities to ensure design of efficient processes:

(i) Determine maximum allowable product temperature (not always collapse temperature) drying above which could affect long-term stability and other critical quality attribute (CQAs) (such as reconstitution time).
(ii) Determine freeze-dryer capabilities (minimum controllable pressure and maximum sublimation rate) as a part of equipment qualification.

(iii) Implement reliable PAT tools to make timely decision on the process (freezing, primary drying, and secondary drying end-point determination).
The outputs of these activities when combined with modeling enables the design of the most efficient cycle, possibly executed at the edge failure. The risk of failure, however, could be reduced by implementing the best PAT tools available to date (TDLAS, Tempris, PRT, comparative pressure measurement, mass spectrometry, etc.). As discussed earlier, poorly designed formulations, at least in our view, is a key contributor for the design inefficient drying processes. Formulations with $T_g' < -40\,°C$ were not that uncommon in the past. Even the best efforts and tools for process optimization would yield relatively long freeze-drying processes. In such cases, reformulation based on best freeze-drying practices may be the best option for operational efficiency.

6.5 Vision for the Future

While lyophilization remains the gold standard for the preservation of biopharmaceuticals, it must continue to evolve and innovate to provide process monitoring and control options and support the needs presented by new modalities.

6.5.1 Advances in Container-Closure Systems

The majority of current container systems, used for lyophilization, are glass vials, typically type 1. They exhibit a low extractable and leachable profile and are relatively inexpensive. It appears that fogging (or hazing) behavior could be associated with less expensive glass vials and was eliminated with the use of (more expensive) vials with a hydrophobic coating [135, 136]. Vial breakage poses serious challenges when considering possible product contamination due to broken glass and consequently with the cleaning of drying chamber. Crystallization of excipients such as mannitol [137–139], sodium chloride [140], and dibasic sodium phosphate [141] during freezing or drying was implicated. A modified freezing protocol (slower cooling) or reduction of fill volume could minimize this negative phenomenon. The introduction of mechanically strong and chemically durable Valor® vial enables the use of larger fill volumes. In addition, it could possibly facilitate faster filling rates and therefore reduce the ambient temperature hold of temperature-sensitive drugs, unless shear stress induced by accelerated presents stability challenges. Despite higher cost, superior mechanical strength, and chemical inertness, glass containers with hydrophobic surfaces may become more popular in freeze drying of biopharmaceuticals for more expensive drug products.

Convenience in administration of drugs presents a critical driver for the use of dual-chamber systems (vials, syringes, cartridges) in spite of the additional processing challenges (presented by the need for siliconization, stopper assembly, loading and unloading, stoppering in more controlled environments, filling of the diluent, etc.). The market share of dual-chamber-based systems has increased steadily and is expected to continue to grow unless processing costs and costs of goods exceed projected costs. Plastic containers present an alternative to glass-based systems and could be of practical benefit if the challenges associated with the diffusion of water vapor and oxygen during storage could be resolved.

Stoppers with vent(s), to facilitate water vapor removal during drying, will continue to remain the most popular closure systems for use in lyophilization. Most likely, igloo-type stoppers will prevail over two-leg stoppers due to reported better machinability and handling behavior during filling at commercial scale [142, 143]. Advances in rubber formulations will continue to evolve to ensure elasticity for handling, limit permeability to water and oxygen, and also target the lowest extractable and leachable profiles. In the opinion of the authors, stoppers with hydrophobic coatings will become more common due to two advantages: (i) reduction in the sticking of stoppers to the shelf during stoppering process and (ii) decrease in leachables.

6.5.2 Dryer Design

6.5.2.1 Laboratory-Scale Dryers

Currently, modern laboratory-scale freeze dryers can be equipped with a variety of tools, including wireless temperature sensors (for example, Tempris), HFSs, TDLAS, mass spectrometer, and comparative pressure measurement to control the process based on the critical temperature(s) and detection of the end points of primary and secondary drying. In addition, as described earlier, a few technologies are available to control ice nucleation during freezing and to minimize the differences in product resistance between laboratory and commercial products. Some manufacturers also offer freeze dryers fabricated with large ducts between the chamber and condenser, thereby minimizing the resistance to mass flow and facilitating a relatively robust pressure control at high sublimation rates. The edge effect, typical for current design of freeze dryers [144], can be also minimized by controlling the chamber wall and door temperatures, an option that is also offered by manufacturers. Refrigeration systems are designed to maintain low shelf temperatures during freezing (for example, to crystallize sodium chloride, if needed) or maintain low condenser temperatures (<−60 °C) even at the peak of sublimation. SMART Freeze-Dryer technology [81] is also available and aids in optimal process control based on critical temperature(s) and desired product properties. The next generation of SMART Freeze-Dryer-like process control software could become available in the recent future, thereby providing the option(s) for most efficient process design at laboratory scale, available for users with a range of lyophilization experiences. A typical laboratory-scale freeze dryer can process up to 2000 × 2 ml vials (or 500 × 20 ml vials). In addition, some of laboratory-scale dryers can be converted into steam sterilized units with clean in place (CIP) capabilities. For very low batch size products (for examples, cell and gene therapy, personalized medicines), advanced laboratory-size dryers can be used to conduct the manufacture of clinical materials.

In summary, one can conclude that development scientists have access to most advanced and well-equipped dryers to deliver the most optimal lyophilization cycles. The energy efficiency of process, however, is very low (<2%), which should be a target for the future improvements of laboratory dryers at reasonable acquisition costs for the end user [145].

Due to the high costs associated with production of biologics, very often only limited quantities of drug substance/drug product may be available in the early stages of product development. Therefore, process development could be challenging and could be alleviated by the use of appropriate replacement materials (surrogates) with similar thermal properties, drying behavior, and cake resistance such that 10% of the vials could contain the active material, with the remainder being the mimic material-containing vials. An alternate option has been provided by freeze-dryer manufacturers through the development of miniaturized versions of laboratory-scale freeze dryers. LyoCapsule and Micro Freeze dryer are examples of commercially available units and are equipped with a variety of options (HFSs, TDLAS, controlled ice nucleation, etc.) depending on the manufacturer. With this option, cycle development and scale-up activities can be conducted using a few vials [146]. The drying chamber is small, which allows accurate measurement of thermal events, such as crystallization of excipients, which is easily monitored in dryers equipped with the HFS [86]. One could expect an increase in sensitivity of analytical tools (HFSs) used in micro freeze dryers in near future. With continued innovation in the design of the next-generation miniaturized dryers, one could foresee dryers combining the capabilities of HFSs (as in differential scanning calorimeters), computational fluid dynamics (CFD) modeling, and conventional dryers. The best-case scenario would be such that a small batch of vials could be lyophilized with the ability to accurately detect and characterize thermal events during freeze and drying. If controlled nucleation becomes widely used at commercial scales, micro freeze dryers may become essential tools for the process development and scale-up.

6.5.2.2 Commercial-Scale Freeze Dryers

The conceptual design of currently available commercial freeze dryers has not significantly evolved in the past four decades. The large chambers are reinforced to withstand pressures up to 2 bar (1500 Torr, 0.2 MPa) and operate in vacuum as low as 1 Pa (1E-5 bar, 7.5E-3 Torr) and temperatures from −60 °C to 127 °C. The chamber is heated to >120 °C during steam sterilization, vacuum dried, and tested for leaks. Cooling post steam sterilization could be a rate-limiting step toward initiation of loading of the dryer. Some commercial freeze dryers are equipped with a jacket through which a heat transfer fluid (typically water) is circulated to expedite the cooling from the sterilization temperature. In most cases, the lowest temperature that wall could support is the temperature above the freezing point of water. To the best of our knowledge, jacket cooling does not appear to be utilized during freeze drying. Thus, during the drying of low collapse products (shelf temperature is typically <−25 °C), the wall and door temperatures are in equilibrium with the ambient temperature outside the dryer and the shelf temperatures causing a significant edge effect. In the experience of the authors, the edge effect (defined as the ratio of heat received by edge vials to the heat received by center vials) could reach 1.5, at least at the beginning of drying process [147]. Calculations performed using the primary drying model [96] with the cake resistance values taken for 10% sucrose [148] revealed that edge effect of 1.5 could result in differences in primary drying time between edge and center vials in a range from 20% (collapse temperature of $T_c = -38\,°C$) to 35% ($T_c = -15\,°C$). The shelf temperature and pressure were varied between −34.5 to 23.0 °C and 30 to 50 mTorr, respectively. In theory, edge effect could be eliminated if wall and door temperature would be held close to the product temperature during the drying process. While currently it is very expensive to maintain jacket temperature below 0 °C, technology innovations may enable, in near future, the design of freeze dryers with the minimal edge effect.

The consistency of product quality attributes strongly depends on uniformity of heat transfer through the shelves of freeze dryer. In current commercial freeze dryers, the difference in the shelf surface temperature is typically within 3 °C. Some of current freeze-dryer manufacturers already produce relatively thin shelves with heat transfer coefficient similar to those in laboratory dryers [149]. Improvements in shelf design targeting enhancement of heat transfer could minimize challenges in process scale-up from laboratory to the commercial dryers.

Condenser design is critical to the performance of lyophilizer. Suboptimal condenser design could limit achievable sublimation rates [150]. For many years, manufacturers have utilized a "rule of thumb" in designing condensers such that the ratio of the condenser surface to the shelf surface should be at least 1. Using low condenser temperatures ($\leq -70\,°C$) [150] may not necessarily be beneficial since it creates a heterogeneity in ice distribution across the condenser (with greater ice deposition at the entrance to the condenser). Ideally, ice distribution should be uniform within the condenser. Specially designed baffles can be utilized to direct the water vapor flow within the condenser. An alternate option is to section off the condenser to create surfaces with different temperatures and could be assessed in future designs. The direct simulation Monte Carlo (DSMC) technique could be applied to model vapor flow in the condenser chamber and predict ice deposition on the condenser surface [151].

The geometry of duct between chamber and condenser is critical, and it could impact the flow rate from the chamber to condenser. For example, modifications of location of the baffles increased the flow rate by at least 50% [152]. On the other hand, introduction of a CIP pipe into the duct resulted in notable (about 20%) decrease in the mass flow rate [153]. Basic engineering principles suggest that longer and smaller duct requires a larger pressure gradient to maintain a certain sublimation rate. Recent advances in CFD enable tuning of duct geometry (diameter, length, valve configuration) and condenser performance (temperature) based on the target sublimation rate [154]. While TDLAS is a valuable PAT tool, it requires an increase in the duct length to position the sensors. Dryer manufacturers also offer a very short duct equipped with a mushroom valve that enables very high sublimation rates. As an alternative to TDLAS, one can also employ differential pressure measurement across the duct for the estimation of sublimation rate [155].

Three process parameters are typically controlled during commercial manufacturing: shelf temperature (inlet temperature of heat transfer fluid, in most cases), chamber pressure, and time. Conventional commercial freeze dryers are equipped with CM, Pirani gauge, flow meter to control pressure by injecting nitrogen, and valve between the condenser and chamber providing the capability to conduct the PRT. Some "modern" freeze dryers are also equipped with mass spectrometer, TDLAS, or internal antennas for wireless temperature measurement. All tools described here are readily available and provided as customizable feature/options on the acquisition of new dryers.

While shelf temperature control is typically ±3 °C, chamber pressure control may not be so accurate. The pressure can vary from the set point by 1 mTorr or could be as high as 30 mTorr depending on the load and stage of drying. The parameters for proportional–integral–derivative (PID) controller are typically set by manufacturer for the empty and clean dryer during or prior factory acceptance test. Due to significant differences in the gas composition during drying, constant values of PID input parameters may not be suitable for all stages of process, causing large pressure fluctuations either at the initial stage (when sublimation rate is the highest) or toward the end of primary drying depending on the tuning of the controller. To cover these fluctuations and assure achievable process tolerances for the commercial process, one would need to perform robustness study targeting a wide product temperature design space, which could lead to unnecessarily conservative process [156].

Another variable during lyophilization process is the condenser temperature, which could peak during initial sublimation step, resulting in pressure control failure. Manufacturers account for the potential of such an occurrence and typically overengineer a refrigeration system adding cost to the dryer.

Given current experience in manufacture of freeze dryers as well as advances in computational modeling and PAT tools, one could expect, in near future, that equipment manufacturers could offer following improvements to the design of commercial lyophilizers:

- Temperature-controlled walls and doors of freeze dryers.
- CFD-led design to optimize configuration of duct/condenser for higher throughput.
- Flexible PID inputs, adjustable to sublimation rate, to drastically reduce pressure fluctuations (ideally, to keep pressure within 1 mTorr from the set point).
- Adjustable refrigeration system to match peak (or maximum) sublimation and reduce power consumption.

In addition, an ideal freeze dryer could be equipped with all available PAT tools to date: *comparative pressure measurement (Pirani vs. capacitance manometer), PRT, mass spectrometer, tool for direct or indirect sublimation rate measurement (TDLAS, PDT, pressure gradient through the duct etc.), wireless temperature sensors, and IR camera.* The combined cost of all listed tools could be less than the cost of a single drug product lot, given the cost of biologics and other parenteral products. With the target to design the most efficient process and based on current experience and equipment capabilities, the ideal freeze dryer should be able to deliver normalized sublimation rate >1.5 kg/m^2. A combination of all tools listed above would be of practical benefit only if the freeze-drying cycle duration can be flexible and most optimal for every single product lot. The combination of inputs from variety of sensors will ensure that the cycle yields a product with the required quality. Implementation of product temperature sensors would also assist in the analysis of process deviations when other methods fail to assess the actual product temperature during cycle in relevance to the proven product temperature design space and will, potentially, enable real-time product release.

6.5.3 Redefining Product Appearance/Elegance

The appearance of the lyophilized drug product (cake, powder, etc.) is the one of most important quality attributes. Since freeze drying is performed at low temperatures, an educated customer expects uniform elegant cylinder, which in most cases is a white cake. This is probably fair expectation if manufacturers include mannitol or glycine as bulking agents and the concentration of active ingredient in formulations is smaller relative to the other excipients. Nonuniform cakes in such formulations are usually evidence of inefficient manufacturing process that could be accompanied with elevated moisture and exhibit faster degradation. In most cases, however, the presence of bulking agent enables the use of very aggressive cycles without affecting product quality [65, 134]. Moreover, systematic investigation of effect of collapse on protein stability [132, 157, 158] revealed greater protein stability in collapsed cakes where collapse had occurred during drying when compared with that in the cakes that collapsed during storage. A recent commentary describes scenarios where a nonideal (an inelegant) cake appearance has no impact on product quality and is an inherent characteristic of the product (either due to formulation, drug product presentation, or freeze-drying process) [159]. It has also been previously documented that product appearance may not play a significant role in product stability if the residual water content is within specification and other attributes such as reconstitution time are not affected [133].

Recent advances in analytical techniques provide the capability to conduct of 100% inspection by NIR or headspace analysis at the commercial scale. This, in turn, could provide the opportunity/flexibility for real-time product release if the PAT tools demonstrate that process was within the validated design space and that the residual moisture is within the validated range. In such a scenario, cake appearance may not matter.

6.5.4 "Intelligent" Formulation and Process Design

Through molecular modeling, we can design molecules (more well behaved from the perspective of viscosity, less aggregation prone, etc.), which can be matched with most effective stabilizers and other components to design "intelligent" or "lyo-friendly" formulations. In silico modeling, similar to the published approach [160], can be used as a first step of molecule design. While there is limited literature on the use of modeling to understand the interactions between proteins, carbohydrates, and other excipients during freezing and drying [161–163] and there are no robust models to date for protein–excipient interaction, one can employ best practices in formulation design for lyophilized products [1, 2, 11, 164] to identify combinations of excipients and compositions that provide optimal stabilization [51, 54, 129]. Low frequency Raman scattering and hydrogen–deuterium exchange MS (HDX-MS)-based methods have been utilized to rank-order formulations during initial formulation screening and have demonstrated the potential to predict long-term stability. Low frequency Raman scattering is not available as a routine screening tool yet, but will be available for formulation scientists in the recent future [118]. HDX-MS-based characterization (described earlier) has been utilized extensively within both academic and industry settings and shows great promise for inclusion into routine formulation screening and analytical toolboxes. Once an optimal formulation targeting the highest glass transition temperature (T'_g, using the Fox equation) has been identified, the currently available primary drying model [96] coupled with best practices in the development of freezing and secondary drying steps [15] can be utilized to design an efficient process cycle, which can be confirmed experimentally. In silico tools, best practices in formulation and process development, and modeling should be utilized in modern formulation and process design. The lessons learned in the formulation development of proteins such as mAbs, ADCs, and fusion and PEGylated proteins could be extended to newer modalities (cell and gene therapy), but may need additional formulation development efforts coupled with the use of alternate technologies (such as spray freeze drying, foam drying, and other methods described in the subsequent chapters of this book).

6.5.5 How Could Alternate Drying Technologies and Freeze Drying Coexist?

6.5.5.1 Alternatives to the Current Batch-Based Vial Drying

Continuous Vial Freeze Drying Given the heterogeneity of the current batch vial freeze-drying process (in the absence of annealing or controlled ice nucleation), continuous vial freeze drying could provide a reasonable alternative offering shorter drying cycles per unit (vial) and, possibly, smaller equipment footprint. Currently, two concepts of continuous processing are available: spin freezing rotary drying [165] and suspended vial drying [166].

During spin freezing, the vial is rotated at about 3000 rpm and quickly cooled by nitrogen flow, forming a thin layer (less than 2 mm) of product [165]. IR radiators provide uniform energy input to the product by rotating the vials during drying. NIR is used to confirm the end of the drying process. The drying time is $\approx$1 hour even for low collapse temperature products. While visual inspection of the vial with product (the product is a shell along the walls and bottom of the vial as opposed to a conventional cake/cylinder) could be challenging, NIR confirms that residual moisture is around the target. This method could be used for products that require very fast freezing (>5 °C/min).

In the second concept based on drying of suspended vials [166], ice nucleation occurs at a high temperature (ensuring low degree of supercooling) by induction of vacuum such that the nucleation temperature is the same for all vials. Then, the vials are transferred to the drying chamber and transported inside the chamber in a continuous manner while remaining suspended. The heat is supplied by radiation and convection, evenly for each vial. By induction of controlled nucleation and elimination of the edge effect, the drying time could be reduced by factor of 3.

To date, there is no commercial continuous manufacture of biologics in vials. In the opinion of the authors, continuous vial freeze drying has the potential to replace traditional freeze dryers, especially when a small footprint is needed and lot size is relatively small.

Spray Freeze Drying Another alternative to vial drying is spray freeze drying (atmospheric spray freezing followed by vacuum drying in either rotating drum or on vibrating shelfs), which could produce relatively large particles (≈0.3–1 mm). These particles (pellets) are still mechanically strong resulting in excellent flowability, but are small enough to allow almost 40X faster drying when compared with vial-based drying [167, 168]. Production of dry pellets provides flexibility in manufacturing of pharmaceutical products by powder filling of targeted doses using previously dried bulk. Spray freeze drying can also be conducted in continuous mode [169].

6.6 Summary

There have been significant efforts in the use and development of rational formulation and process design of biologics when compared with trial-and-error approaches utilized as recently as 10–15 years ago. The emphasis on moving away from empirical strategies for freeze drying has been coupled with the advances in frozen and dried product characterization, equipment design and characterization, process control, monitoring, and characterization approaches and container-closure options for lyophilization. The range of therapeutic biologic compounds requiring removal of water for long-term stabilization has also expanded to cover mAbs, fusion proteins, ADCs and other conjugated proteins, bispecific compounds, vaccines, and cell and gene therapy modalities. In several cases, the advances in alternate drying technologies (discussed in the subsequent chapters of this book) have presented options to stabilize compounds without the need to formulate to counter the damaging effects of ice formation and the accompanying changes in the environment of the protein. In spite of the limitations associated with freeze drying either from the challenges presented by ice formation or equipment costs and maintenance or process inefficiency, lyophilization will continue to serve as the gold standard to which other drying methods will be compared. The challenges presented by newer modalities will provide opportunities for freeze drying (vial- and non-vial-based) and other drying technologies to continue to develop innovative strategies for stabilization and manufacture of biologics and meet the needs of the patients and the healthcare industry.

Acknowledgments

The authors would like to thank Steve Nail and Evgenyi Shalaev for their valuable comments.

Tributes

Dr. Michael (Mike) Pikal (1939–2018)

Michael J. Pikal, Professor Emeritus in the Department of Pharmaceutical Sciences at the University of Connecticut (UConn) and the world's leading expert in pharmaceutical freeze drying, passed away in 2018. A collaborator of Dr. Pikal, the late Felix Franks had aptly described Dr. Pikal as the undisputed "King of Pharmaceutical Freeze Drying."

A physical chemist by training, Dr. Pikal began his career in the pharmaceutical industry as a scientist at Lilly Research Laboratories in the early 1970s after undergraduate work at St. John's University (Minnesota), graduate work at Iowa State University, postdoctoral fellowship at Lawrence Livermore Laboratory, and an assistant professor stint at the University of Tennessee in Knoxville. At Lilly, he began his groundbreaking research in the science of freeze drying after having been introduced to the technology by Alan MacKenzie. Over the next four decades, he published several key papers on lyophilization formulation and process design/characterization (including principles governing heat and mass transfer and models for primary and secondary drying) and stability of pharmaceuticals. While at Lilly, he was also selected as a Fellow of the American Association of Pharmaceutical Scientists (AAPS) and was a recipient of the Ebert Prize for a manuscript published in the *Journal of Pharmaceutical Sciences*.

After a distinguished career at Lilly, Dr. Pikal joined the Department of Pharmaceutical Sciences at UConn in 1996 where he went on to build a world-class program in lyophilization. He mentored more than 40 PhD students, postdoctoral fellows, and visiting scholars, who engaged in finding answers to more fundamental scientific questions as well as resolving practical challenges. Dr. Pikal emphasized the need for utilizing systematic approaches to solving formulation, processing, and stability challenges instead of "throwing a patch on them and hoping they'll go away." While at UConn, another feather was added to his cap following his appointment as the first Pfizer Distinguished Endowed Chair in Pharmaceutical Technology in 2005. He was the driving force and a critical contributor in establishing research consortia such as the Center for Pharmaceutical Processing Research (CPPR), the National Institute for Pharmaceutical Technology and Education (NIPTE), and the National Institute for Innovation in Manufacturing Biopharmaceuticals (NIIMBL). Dr. Pikal was also instrumental in the development of a technology roadmap for lyophilization within the LyoHub consortium to survey the current state, develop the vision for the future, identify the critical gaps in practices and barriers in implementation, and define the goals for the development of new lyophilization methods. In 2009, he was the recipient of the AAPS Distinguished Pharmaceutical Scientist Award, recognizing his achievements that have made a lasting impact on freeze drying and pharmaceutical sciences. In recognition of his contributions, the *Journal of Pharmaceutical Sciences* published a special issue highlighting his key scientific accomplishments in pharmaceutical sciences. While the scientific community will sorely miss Dr. Pikal, we also celebrate his contributions and accomplishments to freeze drying.

Dr. Alan MacKenzie (1932–2018)

Dr. Alan Mackenzie, who was one of the pioneers in the field of lyophilization, also passed away in 2018 after over five decades of stellar contributions to freeze drying. His undergraduate work and doctoral work in chemistry were completed at the Imperial College in London, and he subsequently moved to the United States on a King George VI Memorial Scholarship. While in the United States, he held appointments at the American Foundation for Biological Research, the University of Wisconsin, and the University of Washington and also served as the past president of the Society for Cryobiology. He was a contemporary and collaborator of J. D. Davis, Samuel Goldblith, Basile Luyet, Harold Meryman, Don Rasmussen, Louis Rey, W. W. Rothmayr, and Terence Rowe. The collaborations led to the publication of over 60 manuscripts, including seminal work on freezing and freeze drying of aqueous solutions, foods, pharmaceuticals, cells, and tissues. We note that the current design of the freeze-drying microscope in many of our laboratories is credited to Dr. MacKenzie's efforts to improve the first-generation microscope designed by Dr. Louis Rey and documented in publications in the early 1960s.

Dr. MacKenzie's seminar on freeze drying at Eli Lilly became Dr. Mike Pikal's first introduction to lyophilization, who in turn went on to become the world's foremost expert in the science and technology of freeze drying. Dr. MacKenzie along with Dr. Mike Pikal and Dr. Felix Franks (from Cambridge University) were a powerhouse within the field of freeze drying. Their collaborations with peers such as Dr. Steven Nail (from Upjohn Laboratories and now at Baxter Biopharma) led to a number of innovations in freeze drying. Dr. Mike Pikal paid a tribute to Dr. Mackenzie in an email to Graham MacKenzie shortly before his passing: "Alan was a friend for about 40 years and was the one who got me interested in freeze drying. He has made great contributions to the science of freeze drying, and all of us who knew him will miss him greatly." While his passing is a tremendous loss, we believe that his outstanding contributions to freeze-drying science will continue to inspire the current and future generations of researchers.

References

1 Pikal, M.J. (2006). Freeze drying. In: *Encyclopedia of Pharmaceutical Technology* (ed. J. Swarbick), 1807–1833. New York: Informa Healthcare USA, Inc.

2 Bhatnagar, B.S., Tchessalov, S., Lewis, L.M., and Johnson, R.E. (2013). Freeze drying of biologics. In: *Encyclopedia of Pharmaceutical Science and Technology* (ed. J. Swarbrick), 1673–1722. New York: Taylor and Francis.

3 Flosdorf, E.W. and Mudd, S. (1935). Procedure and apparatus for preservation in "lyophile" form of serum and other biological substances. *Journal of Immunology* 29: 389–425.

4 Flosdorf, E.W., Stokes, F.J., and Mudd, S. (1940). The desivac process for drying from the frozen state. *Journal of the American Medical Association* 115: 1095–1097.

5 Greaves, R.I. (1941). The freezing of human serum and plasma in medical research council transfusion bottles, before drying by sublimation from the frozen state. *The Journal of Hygiene* 41 (5–6): 489–495.

6 Greaves, R.I. (1956). The preservation of bacteria. *Canadian Journal of Microbiology* 2 (3): 365–371.

7 Greaves, R.I. (1960). Preservation of living cells by freeze-drying. *Annals of the New York Academy of Sciences* 85: 723–728.

8 Greaves, R.I. (1965). Preservation of antigens and antibodies. *Federation Proceedings* 24: S263–S266.

9 Greaves, R.I. and Adair, M.E. (1936). A simple method for the preservation of sera by desiccation in the frozen state without the use of refrigerants. *The Journal of Hygiene* 36 (4): 507–513.

10 Greaves, R.I. and Adair, M.E. (1939). High-vacuum condensation drying of proteins from the frozen state. *Journal of Hygiene* 39: 413–445.

11 Carpenter, J.F., Pikal, M.J., Chang, B.S., and Randolph, T.W. (1997). Rational design of stable lyophilized protein formulations: some practical advice. *Pharmaceutical Research* 14 (8): 969–975.

12 Pikal, M.J. (1990). Freeze-drying of proteins. Part II: formulation selection. *BioPharm* 3 (9): 26–30.

13 Pikal, M.J. (1990). Freeze-drying of proteins. Part I: process design. *BioPharm* 3 (8):18–20, 22–14, 26–18.

14 Pikal, M.J. (2010). Mechanisms of protein stabilization during freeze-drying storage: the relative importance of thermodynamic stabilization and glassy state relaxation dynamics. In: *Freeze Drying/Lyophilization of Pharmaceutical and Biological Products*, Drugs and the Pharmaceutical and Sciences, vol. 206 (eds. L. Rey and J.C. May), 198–232. New York: Marcel Dekker.

15 Tang, X. and Pikal, M.J. (2004). Design of freeze-drying processes for pharmaceuticals: practical advice. *Pharmaceutical Research* 21 (2): 191–200.

16 Long, G. (2017). The Biopharmaceutical Pipeline: Innovative Therapies in Clinical Development. Analysis group inc., Pharmaceutical Research and Manufacturers of America, Boston, MA.

17 Bhatnagar, B.S., Pikal, M.J., and Bogner, R.H. (2008). Study of the individual contributions of ice formation and freeze-concentration on isothermal stability of lactate dehydrogenase during freezing. *Journal of Pharmaceutical Sciences* 97 (2): 798–814.

18 Bhatnagar, B.S., Bogner, R.H., and Pikal, M.J. (2007). Protein stability during freezing: separation of stresses and mechanisms of protein stabilization. *Pharmaceutical Development and Technology* 12 (5): 505–523.

19 Luthra, S., Obert, J.-P., Kalonia Devendra, S., and Pikal, M.J. (2007). Investigation of drying stresses on proteins during lyophilization: differentiation between primary and secondary-drying stresses on lactate dehydrogenase using a humidity controlled mini freeze-dryer. *Journal of Pharmaceutical Sciences* 96 (1): 61–70.

20 Luthra, S., Obert, J.-P., Kalonia, D.S., and Pikal, M.J. (2007). Impact of critical process and formulation parameters affecting in-process stability of

lactate dehydrogenase during the secondary drying stage of lyophilization: a mini freeze dryer study. *Journal of Pharmaceutical Sciences* 96 (9): 2242–2250.

21 Greiff, D. and Kelly, R.T. (1966). Cryotolerance of enzymes. I. Freezing of lactic dehydrogenase. *Cryobiology* 2 (6): 335–341.

22 Lazar, K.L., Patapoff, T.W., and Sharma, V.K. (2010). Cold denaturation of monoclonal antibodies. *MAbs* 2 (1): 42–52.

23 Privalov, P.L. (1990). Cold denaturation of proteins. *Critical Reviews in Biochemistry and Molecular Biology* 25 (4): 281–305.

24 Rosa, M., Lopes, C., Melo, E.P. et al. (2013). Measuring and modeling hemoglobin aggregation below the freezing temperature. *The Journal of Physical Chemistry B* 117 (30): 8939–8946.

25 Rosa, M., Roberts, C.J., and Rodrigues, M.A. (2017). Connecting high-temperature and low-temperature protein stability and aggregation. *PLoS ONE* 12 (5): e0176748/0176741–e0176748/0176712.

26 Heller, M.C., Carpenter, J.F., and Randolph, T.W. (1996). Effects of phase separating systems on lyophilized hemoglobin. *Journal of Pharmaceutical Sciences* 85 (12): 1358–1362.

27 Padilla, A.M., Chou, S.G., Luthra, S., and Pikal, M.J. (2011). The study of amorphous phase separation in a model polymer phase-separating system using raman microscopy and a low-temperature stage: effect of cooling rate and nucleation temperature. *Journal of Pharmaceutical Sciences* 100 (4): 1362–1376.

28 Chatterjee, K., Shalaev, E.Y., and Suryanarayanan, R. (2005). Raffinose crystallization during freeze-drying and its impact on recovery of protein activity. *Pharmaceutical Research* 22 (2): 303–309.

29 Izutsu, K.-I., Yoshioka, S., and Kojima, S. (1997). Phase separation and crystallization of components in frozen solutions: effect of molecular compatibility between solutes. In: *Therapeutic Protein and Peptide Formulation and Delivery*, ACS Symposium Series, vol. 675, 109–118.

30 Pyne, A., Surana, R., and Suryanarayanan, R. (2002). Crystallization of mannitol below T_g' during freeze-drying in binary and ternary aqueous systems. *Pharmaceutical Research* 19 (6): 901–908.

31 Pyne, A. and Suryanarayanan, R. (2001). Phase transitions of glycine in frozen aqueous solutions and during freeze-drying. *Pharmaceutical Research* 18 (10): 1448–1454.

32 Gomez, G., Pikal, M.J., and Rodriguez-Hornedo, N. (2001). Effect of initial buffer composition on pH changes during far-from-equilibrium freezing of sodium phosphate buffer solutions. *Pharmaceutical Research* 18 (1): 90–97.

33 Pikal-Cleland, K.A. and Carpenter, J.F. (2001). Lyophilization-induced protein denaturation in phosphate buffer systems: monomeric and tetrameric β-galactosidase. *Journal of Pharmaceutical Sciences* 90 (9): 1255–1268.

34 Szkudlarek, B.A. (1997). *Selective Crystallization of Phosphate Buffer Components and pH Changes During Freezing: Implications to Protein Stability*, 188. Ann Arbor, MI: University of Michigan.

35 Connolly, B.D., Le, L., Patapoff, T.W. et al. (2015). Protein aggregation in frozen trehalose formulations: effects of composition, cooling rate, and storage temperature. *Journal of Pharmaceutical Sciences* 104 (12): 4170–4184.
36 Singh, S.K., Kolhe, P., Mehta, A.P. et al. (2011). Frozen state storage instability of a monoclonal antibody: aggregation as a consequence of trehalose crystallization and protein unfolding. *Pharmaceutical Research* 28 (4): 873–885.
37 Gabellieri, E. and Strambini, G.B. (2003). Perturbation of protein tertiary structure in frozen solutions revealed by 1-anilino-8-naphthalene sulfonate fluorescence. *Biophysical Journal* 85 (5): 3214–3220.
38 Strambini, G.B. and Gabellieri, E. (1996). Proteins in frozen solutions: evidence of ice-induced partial unfolding. *Biophysical Journal* 70 (2): 971–976.
39 Rambhatla, S., Ramot, R., Bhugra, C., and Pikal Michael, J. (2004). Heat and mass transfer scale-up issues during freeze drying: II. Control and characterization of the degree of supercooling. *AAPS PharmSciTech* 5 (4): e58.
40 Bhatnagar, B., Zakharov, B., Fisyuk, A. et al. (2019). Protein/ice interaction: high-resolution synchrotron x-ray diffraction differentiates pharmaceutical proteins from lysozyme. *The Journal of Physical Chemistry B* 123 (27): 5690–5699.
41 Varshney, D.B., Elliott, J.A., Gatlin, L.A. et al. (2009). Synchrotron x-ray diffraction investigation of the anomalous behavior of ice during freezing of aqueous systems. *The Journal of Physical Chemistry B* 113 (18): 6177–6182.
42 Shalaev, E.Y., Wang, W., and Gatlin, L.A. (2008). Rational choice of excipients for use in lyophilized formulations. In: *Protein Formulation and Delivery*, 2e (eds. E.J. McNally and J.E. Hastedt), 197–217. Boca Raton, FL: CRC Press.
43 Shalaev, E.Y. (2005). The impact of buffer on processing and stability of freeze-dried dosage forms, part 1: solution freezing behavior. *American Pharmaceutical Review* 8, 80 (5): 82–87.
44 Shalaev, E.Y. and Gatlin, L.A. (2010). The impact of buffer on solid-state properties and stability of freeze-dried dosage forms. In: *Formulation and Process Development Strategies for Manufacturing Biopharmaceuticals* (eds. F. Jameel and S. Hershenson), 507–519. New York: Wiley.
45 Lam, X.M., Costantino, H.R., Overcashier, D.E. et al. (1996). Replacing succinate with glycolate buffer improves the stability of lyophilized interferon-γ. *International Journal of Pharmaceutics* 142 (1): 85–95.
46 Sundaramurthi, P., Shalaev, E., and Suryanarayanan, R. (2010). Calorimetric and diffractometric evidence for sequential crystallization of buffer components and consequential pH swing in frozen solutions. *The Journal of Physical Chemistry B* 114 (14): 4915–4923.
47 Piedmonte, D.M., Hair, A., Baker, P. et al. (2015). Sorbitol crystallization-induced aggregation in frozen mab formulations. *Journal of Pharmaceutical Sciences* 104 (2): 686–697.
48 Piedmonte, D.M., Summers, C., Mcauley, A. et al. (2007). Sorbitol crystallization can lead to protein aggregation in frozen protein formulations. *Pharmaceutical Research* 24 (1): 136–146.

49 Arakawa, T., Prestrelski, S.J., Kenney, W.C., and Carpenter, J.F. (1993). Factors affecting short-term and long-term stabilities of proteins. *Advanced Drug Delivery Reviews* 10 (1): 1–28.

50 Wang, B., Tchessalov, S., Cicerone, M.T. et al. (2009). Impact of sucrose level on storage stability of proteins in freeze-dried solids: II. Correlation of aggregation rate with protein structure and molecular mobility. *Journal of Pharmaceutical Sciences* 98 (9): 3145–3166.

51 Wang, B., Tchessalov, S., Warne, N.W., and Pikal, M.J. (2009). Impact of sucrose level on storage stability of proteins in freeze-dried solids: I. Correlation of protein-sugar interaction with native structure preservation. *Journal of Pharmaceutical Sciences* 98 (9): 3131–3144.

52 Pikal, M.J., Rigsbee, D., Roy, M.L. et al. (2008). Solid state chemistry of proteins: II. The correlation of storage stability of freeze-dried human growth hormone (hGH) with structure and dynamics in the glassy solid. *Journal of Pharmaceutical Sciences* 97 (12): 5106–5121.

53 Cicerone, M.T. and Soles, C.L. (2004). Fast dynamics and stabilization of proteins: binary glasses of trehalose and glycerol. *Biophysical Journal* 86 (6): 3836–3845.

54 Chang, L., Shepherd, D., Sun, J. et al. (2005). Mechanism of protein stabilization by sugars during freeze-drying and storage: native structure preservation, specific interaction, and/or immobilization in a glassy matrix? *Journal of Pharmaceutical Sciences* 94 (7): 1427–1444.

55 Hu, Y., Arora, J., Joshi, S.B. et al. (2019). Characterization of excipient effects on reversible self-association, backbone flexibility, and solution properties of an igg1 monoclonal antibody at high concentrations: part 1. *Journal of Pharmaceutical Sciences* pii: S0022-3549(19)30373-9.

56 Inoue, N., Takai, E., Arakawa, T., and Shiraki, K. (2014). Specific decrease in solution viscosity of antibodies by arginine for therapeutic formulations. *Molecular Pharmaceutics* 11 (6): 1889–1896.

57 Staertzel, P., Gieseler, H., Gieseler, M. et al. (2015). Freeze-drying of l-arginine/sucrose-based protein formulations, part 2: optimization of formulation design and freeze-drying process conditions for an l-arginine chloride-based protein formulation system. *Journal of Pharmaceutical Sciences* 104 (12): 4241–4256.

58 Staertzel, P., Gieseler, H., Gieseler, M. et al. (2016). Mannitol/l-arginine-based formulation systems for freeze drying of protein pharmaceuticals: effect of the l-arginine counter ion and formulation composition on the formulation properties and the physical state of mannitol. *Journal of Pharmaceutical Sciences* 105 (10): 3123–3135.

59 Kerwin, B.A. (2008). Polysorbates 20 and 80 used in the formulation of protein biotherapeutics: structure and degradation pathways. *Journal of Pharmaceutical Sciences* 97 (8): 2924–2935.

60 Jones, M.T., Mahler, H.-C., Koulov, A. et al. (2018). Considerations for the use of polysorbates in biopharmaceuticals. *Pharmaceutical Research* 35 (8): 148.

61 Mahler, H-C and Ravuri, K. (2010). Understanding polysorbates in protein formulation. Abstracts of Papers, 239th ACS National Meeting, San Francisco, CA, 21–25 March 2010, BIOT-169.

62 Mahler, H.-C. and Allmendinger, A. (2017). Stability, formulation, and delivery of biopharmaceuticals. In: *Protein Therapeutics*, Methods and Principles in Medicinal Chemistry, vol. 71 (eds. T. Vaughan, J. Osbourn and B. Jallal), 469–491. Weinheim, Germany: Wiley-VCH.

63 Searles, J.A., Carpenter, J.F., and Randolph, T.W. (2001). Annealing to optimize the primary drying rate, reduce freezing-induced drying rate heterogeneity, and determine T_g' in pharmaceutical lyophilization. *Journal of Pharmaceutical Sciences* 90 (7): 872–887.

64 Searles, J.A., Carpenter, J.F., and Randolph, T.W. (2001). The ice nucleation temperature determines the primary drying rate of lyophilization for samples frozen on a temperature-controlled shelf. *Journal of Pharmaceutical Sciences* 90 (7): 860–871.

65 Chatterjee, K., Shalaev, E.Y., and Suryanarayanan, R. (2005). Partially crystalline systems in lyophilization: II. Withstanding collapse at high primary drying temperatures and impact on protein activity recovery. *Journal of Pharmaceutical Sciences* 94 (4): 809–820.

66 Heller, M.C., Carpenter, J.F., and Randolph, T.W. (1999). Protein formulation and lyophilization cycle design: prevention of damage due to freeze-concentration induced phase separation. *Biotechnology and Bioengineering* 63 (2): 166–174.

67 Chakravarty, P., Lee, R., Demarco, F., and Renzi, E. (2012). Ice fog as a means to induce uniform ice nucleation during lyophilization. *BioPharm International* 25 (1): 33–38.

68 Patel, S.M., Bhugra, C., and Pikal, M.J. (2009). Reduced pressure ice fog technique for controlled ice nucleation during freeze-drying. *AAPS PharmSciTech* 10 (4): 1406–1411.

69 Rowe, T.D. (1990). A technique for the nucleation of ice. *International Symposium on Biological Product Freeze-Drying and Formulation*. Geneva, Switzerland (26 October 1990).

70 Konstantinidis, A.K., Kuu, W., Otten, L. et al. (2011). Controlled nucleation in freeze-drying: effects on pore size in the dried product layer, mass transfer resistance, and primary drying rate. *Journal of Pharmaceutical Sciences* 100 (8): 3453–3470.

71 Kramer, M., Sennhenn, B., and Lee, G. (2002). Freeze-drying using vacuum-induced surface freezing. *Journal of Pharmaceutical Sciences* 91 (2): 433–443.

72 Liu, J., Viverette, T., Virgin, M. et al. (2005). A study of the impact of freezing on the lyophilization of a concentrated formulation with a high fill depth. *Pharmaceutical Development and Technology* 10 (2): 261–272.

73 Hottot, A., Nakagawa, K., and Andrieu, J. (2008). Effect of ultrasound-controlled nucleation on structural and morphological properties of freeze-dried mannitol solutions. *Chemical Engineering Research and Design* 86 (2): 193–200.

74 Nakagawa, K., Hottot, A., Vessot, S., and Andrieu, J. (2006). Influence of controlled nucleation by ultrasounds on ice morphology of frozen formulations for pharmaceutical proteins freeze-drying. *Chemical Engineering and Processing* 45 (9): 783–791.

75 Saclier, M., Peczalski, R., and Andrieu, J. (2009). A theoretical model for ice primary nucleation induced by acoustic cavitation. *Ultrasonics Sonochemistry* 17 (1): 98–105.

76 Saclier, M., Peczalski, R., and Andrieu, J. (2010). Effect of ultrasonically induced nucleation on ice crystals' size and shape during freezing in vials. *Chemical Engineering Science* 65 (10): 3064–3071.

77 Daoussi, R. and Weber, F.H. (2018). Lyophilization methods that provide stably dehydrated protozoans for use as potent live vaccines. Application WO WO 2018/067647 A1, Zoetis Services LLC, USA, p. 31pp.

78 Colandene, J.D., Maldonado, L.M., Creagh, A.T. et al. (2007). Lyophilization cycle development for a high-concentration monoclonal antibody formulation lacking a crystalline bulking agent. *Journal of Pharmaceutical Sciences* 96 (6): 1598–1608.

79 Nail, S., Tchessalov, S., Shalaev, E. et al. (2017). Recommended best practices for process monitoring instrumentation in pharmaceutical freeze drying-2017. *AAPS PharmSciTech* 18 (7): 2379–2393.

80 Milton, N., Pikal, M.J., Roy, M.L., and Nail, S.L. (1997). Evaluation of manometric temperature measurement as a method of monitoring product temperature during lyophilization. *PDA Journal of Pharmaceutical Science and Technology* 51 (1): 7–16.

81 Tang, X., Nail, S.L., and Pikal, M.J. (2005). Freeze-drying process design by manometric temperature measurement: design of a smart freeze-dryer. *Pharmaceutical Research* 22 (4): 685–700.

82 Gieseler, H., Kramer, T., and Pikal, M.J. (2007). Use of manometric temperature measurement (MTM) and smart freeze dryer technology for development of an optimized freeze-drying cycle. *Journal of Pharmaceutical Sciences* 96 (12): 3402–3418.

83 Patel, S.M., Doen, T., and Pikal, M.J. (2010). Determination of end point of primary drying in freeze-drying process control. *AAPS PharmSciTech* 11 (1): 73–84.

84 Connelly, J.P. and Welch, J.V. (1993). Monitor lyophilization with mass spectrometer gas analysis. *Journal of Parenteral Science and Technology* 47 (2): 70–75.

85 Ganguly, A., Stewart, J., Rhoden, A. et al. (2018). Mass spectrometry in freeze-drying: motivations for using a bespoke pat for laboratory and production environment. *European Journal of Pharmaceutics and Biopharmaceutics* 127: 298–308.

86 Wang, Q. and Shalaev, E. (2018). Process analytical technology in freeze-drying: detection of the secondary solute + water crystallization with heat flux sensors. *AAPS PharmSciTech* 19 (3): 1477–1482.

87 Pisano, R., Fissore, D., and Barresi, A.A. (2014). A new method based on the regression of step response data for monitoring a freeze-drying cycle. *Journal of Pharmaceutical Sciences* 103 (6): 1756–1765.

88 Gieseler, H., Kessler, W.J., Finson, M. et al. (2007). Evaluation of tunable diode laser absorption spectroscopy for in-process water vapor mass flux measurements during freeze drying. *Journal of Pharmaceutical Sciences* 96 (7): 1776–1793.

89 Schneid, S.C., Gieseler, H., Kessler, W.J., and Pikal, M.J. (2009). Non-invasive product temperature determination during primary drying using tunable diode laser absorption spectroscopy. *Journal of Pharmaceutical Sciences* 98 (9): 3406–3418.

90 Kuu, W.Y., Nail, S.L., and Sacha, G. (2009). Rapid determination of vial heat transfer parameters using tunable diode laser absorption spectroscopy (TDLAS) in response to step-changes in pressure set-point during freeze-drying. *Journal of Pharmaceutical Sciences* 98 (3): 1136–1154.

91 Kuu, W.Y., O'bryan, K.R., Hardwick, L.M., and Paul, T.W. (2011). Product mass transfer resistance directly determined during freeze-drying cycle runs using tunable diode laser absorption spectroscopy (TDLAS) and pore diffusion model. *Pharmaceutical Development and Technology* 16 (4): 343–357.

92 De Beer, T.R.M., Alleso, M., Goethals, F. et al. (2007). Implementation of a process analytical technology system in a freeze-drying process using Raman spectroscopy for in-line process monitoring. *Analytical Chemistry* 79 (21): 7992–8003.

93 De Beer, T.R.M., Vercruysse, P., Burggraeve, A. et al. (2009). In-line and real-time process monitoring of a freeze drying process using Raman and NIR spectroscopy as complementary process analytical technology (PAT) tools. *Journal of Pharmaceutical Sciences* 98 (9): 3430–3446.

94 Emteborg, H., Zeleny, R., Charoud-Got, J. et al. (2014). Infrared thermography for monitoring of freeze-drying processes: instrumental developments and preliminary results. *Journal of Pharmaceutical Sciences* 103 (7): 2088–2097.

95 Colucci, D., Maniaci, R., and Fissore, D. (2019). Monitoring of the freezing stage in a freeze-drying process using ir thermography. *International Journal of Pharmaceutics* 566: 488–499.

96 Tchessalov, S., Nulu, S., Latshaw, D.,.I.I., and Dassu, D. (2017). An industry perspective on the application of modeling to lyophilization process scale up and transfer. *American Pharmaceutical Review* 20 (2): 52–58.

97 Sahni, E.K. and Pikal, M.J. (2017). Modeling the secondary drying stage of freeze drying: development and validation of an excel-based model. *Journal of Pharmaceutical Sciences* 106 (3): 779–791.

98 Stotz, C.E., Winslow, S.L., Houchin, M.L. et al. (2004). Degradation pathways for lyophilized peptides and proteins. In: *Lyophilization of Biopharmaceuticals*, Biotechnology: Pharmaceutical Aspects, vol. 2 (eds. H.R. Costantino and M.J. Pikal), 443–479. Arlington: American Association of Pharmaceutical Scientists.

99 Carpenter, J.F., Prestrelski, S.J., and Dong, A. (1998). Application of infrared spectroscopy to development of stable lyophilized protein formulations. *European Journal of Pharmaceutics and Biopharmaceutics* 45: 231–238.

100 Krishnan, S., Cao, W., and Phillips, J. (2009). Applying raman spectroscopy to design of lyophilization cycles for protein formulation development. *American Pharmaceutical Review* 12 (6):44–48, 50–51, 53.
101 Pieters, S., Roger, J.-M., De Beer, T. et al. (2014). Raman model development for the protein conformational state classification in different freeze-dried formulations. *Analytica Chimica Acta* 825: 42–50.
102 Sane, S.U. (1999). Secondary structure characterization of proteins using amide I band raman spectroscopy: methods development and applications to bioprocessing. Troy, NY: Rensselaer Polytechnic Institute, p. 178.
103 Li, Y., Williams, T.D., Schowen, R.L., and Topp, E.M. (2007). Characterizing protein structure in amorphous solids using hydrogen/deuterium exchange with mass spectrometry. *Analytical Biochemistry* 366 (1): 18–28.
104 Moorthy, B.S., Iyer, L.K., and Topp, E.M. (2015). Mass spectrometric approaches to study protein structure and interactions in lyophilized powders. *Journal of Visualized Experiments* 98: e52503/52501–e52503/52512.
105 Moorthy, B.S., Zarraga, I.E., Kumar, L. et al. (2018). Solid-state hydrogen-deuterium exchange mass spectrometry: correlation of deuterium uptake and long-term stability of lyophilized monoclonal antibody formulations. *Molecular Pharmaceutics* 15 (1): 1–11.
106 Liu, J. (2006). Physical characterization of pharmaceutical formulations in frozen and freeze-dried solid states: techniques and applications in freeze-drying development. *Pharmaceutical Development and Technology* 11 (1): 3–28.
107 Izutsu, K.-I., Yonemochi, E., Yomota, C. et al. (2014). Studying the morphology of lyophilized protein solids using x-ray micro-CT: effect of post-freeze annealing and controlled nucleation. *AAPS PharmSciTech* 15 (5): 1181–1188.
108 Haeuser, C., Goldbach, P., Huwyler, J. et al. (2018). Imaging techniques to characterize cake appearance of freeze-dried products. *Journal of Pharmaceutical Sciences* 107 (11): 2810–2822.
109 Abdul-Fattah, A.M., Truong-Le, V., Yee, L. et al. (2007). Drying-induced variations in physico-chemical properties of amorphous pharmaceuticals and their impact on stability (i): Stability of a monoclonal antibody. *Journal of Pharmaceutical Sciences* 96 (8): 1983–2008.
110 Xu, Y., Grobelny, P., Von Allmen, A. et al. (2014). Protein quantity on the air-solid interface determines degradation rates of human growth hormone in lyophilized samples. *Journal of Pharmaceutical Sciences* 103 (5): 1356–1366.
111 Cicerone, M.T., Pikal, M.J., and Qian, K.K. (2015). Stabilization of proteins in solid form. *Advanced Drug Delivery Reviews* 93: 14–24.
112 Cicerone, M.T. and Douglas, J.F. (2012). Β-relaxation governs protein stability in sugar-glass matrices. *Soft Matter* 8 (10): 2983–2991.
113 Shamblin, S.L., Tang, X., Chang, L. et al. (1999). Characterization of the time scales of molecular motion in pharmaceutically important glasses. *The Journal of Physical Chemistry B* 103 (20): 4113–4121.
114 Chang, L. and Pikal, M.J. (2009). Mechanisms of protein stabilization in the solid state. *Journal of Pharmaceutical Sciences* 98 (9): 2886–2908.

115 Cicerone, M.T., Soles, C.L., Chowdhuri, Z. et al. (2005). Fast dynamics as a diagnostic for excipients in preservation of dried proteins. *American Pharmaceutical Review* 8 (6):22, 24–27.

116 Yoshioka, S., Aso, Y., and Kojima, S. (2002). Different molecular motions in lyophilized protein formulations as determined by laboratory and rotating frame spin-lattice relaxation times. *Journal of Pharmaceutical Sciences* 91 (10): 2203–2210.

117 Yoshioka, S., Miyazaki, T., Aso, Y., and Kawanishi, T. (2007). Significance of local mobility in aggregation of β-galactosidase lyophilized with trehalose, sucrose or stachyose. *Pharmaceutical Research* 24 (9): 1660–1667.

118 Cicerone, M.T. (2019). Measuring and using terahertz timescale dynamics to predict solid state protein stability. *International Society of Lyophilization-Freeze Drying, Midwest Chapter Conference*. Chicago, IL (11 April 2019).

119 Padilla, A.M., Ivanisevic, I., Yang, Y. et al. (2011). The study of phase separation in amorphous freeze-dried systems. Part I: raman mapping and computational analysis of XRPD data in model polymer systems. *Journal of Pharmaceutical Sciences* 100 (1): 206–222.

120 Padilla, A.M. and Pikal, M.J. (2011). The study of phase separation in amorphous freeze-dried systems, part 2: investigation of raman mapping as a tool for studying amorphous phase separation in freeze-dried protein formulations. *Journal of Pharmaceutical Sciences* 100 (4): 1467–1474.

121 Govindarajan, R., Chatterjee, K., Gatlin, L. et al. (2006). Impact of freeze-drying on ionization of sulfonephthalein probe molecules in trehalose-citrate systems. *Journal of Pharmaceutical Sciences* 95 (7): 1498–1510.

122 Lu, E., Ewing, S., Gatlin, L. et al. (2009). The effect of bulking agents on the chemical stability of acid-sensitive compounds in freeze-dried formulations: sucrose inversion study. *Journal of Pharmaceutical Sciences* 98 (9): 3387–3396.

123 Abdul-Fattah, A.M., Truong-Le, V., Yee, L. et al. (2007). Drying-induced variations in physico-chemical properties of amorphous pharmaceuticals and their impact on stability II: Stability of a vaccine. *Pharmaceutical Research* 24 (4): 715–727.

124 Cook, I.A. and Ward, K.R. (2011). Applications of headspace moisture analysis for investigating the water dynamics within a sealed vial containing freeze-dried material. *PDA Journal of Pharmaceutical Science and Technology* 65 (1): 2–11.

125 Hede, J.O., Fosbol, P.L., Berg, S.W., and Dahl, S. (2019). Container closure integrity testing-method development for freeze-dried products using laser-based headspace oxygen analysis. *PDA Journal of Pharmaceutical Science and Technology* 73 (2): 170–180.

126 Salnikova, M., Varshney, D., and Shalaev, E. (2015). Heterogeneity of protein environments in frozen solutions and in the dried state. In: *Lyophilized Biologics and Vaccines* (eds. D. Varshney and M. Singh), 11–24. New York: Springer.

127 Arakawa, T., Kita, Y., and Carpenter, J.F. (1991). Protein-solvent interactions in pharmaceutical formulations. *Pharmaceutical Research* 8 (3): 285–291.
128 Arakawa, T. and Timasheff, S.N. (1982). Stabilization of protein structure by sugars. *Biochemistry* 21 (25): 6536–6544.
129 Cleland, J.L., Lam, X., Kendrick, B. et al. (2001). A specific molar ratio of stabilizer to protein is required for storage stability of a lyophilized monoclonal antibody. *Journal of Pharmaceutical Sciences* 90 (3): 310–321.
130 Mensink, M.A., Frijlink, H.W., Van Der Voort Maarschalk, K., and Hinrichs, W.L.J. (2017). How sugars protect proteins in the solid state and during drying (review): mechanisms of stabilization in relation to stress conditions. *European Journal of Pharmaceutics and Biopharmaceutics* 114: 288–295.
131 Johnson, R.E. and Lewis, L.M. (2011). Freeze-drying protein formulations above their collapse temperatures: possible issues and concerns. *American Pharmaceutical Review* 14 (3): 50–54.
132 Schersch, K., Betz, O., Garidel, P. et al. (2010). Systematic investigation of the effect of lyophilizate collapse on pharmaceutically relevant proteins i: stability after freeze-drying. *Journal of Pharmaceutical Sciences* 99 (5): 2256–2278.
133 Tchessalov, S., Dixon, D., and Warne, N. (2010). Lyophilization of pharmaceuticals above collapse temperature. Application: WO 9884019, p. 58pp, Wyeth, John, and Brother Ltd., Philadelphia, PA, filed 5 August 2009 and issued 6 Febraury 2018.
134 Wang, D.Q., Hey, J.M., and Nail, S.L. (2004). Effect of collapse on the stability of freeze-dried recombinant factor VIII and α-amylase. *Journal of Pharmaceutical Sciences* 93 (5): 1253–1263.
135 Abdul-Fattah, A.M., Oeschger, R., Roehl, H. et al. (2013). Investigating factors leading to fogging of glass vials in lyophilized drug products. *European Journal of Pharmaceutics and Biopharmaceutics* 85 (2): 314–326.
136 Huang, M., Childs, E., Roffi, K. et al. (2019). Investigation of fogging behavior in a lyophilized drug product. *Journal of Pharmaceutical Sciences* 108 (3): 1101–1109.
137 Williams, N.A. and Dean, T. (1991). Vial breakage by frozen mannitol solutions: correlation with thermal characteristics and effect of stereoisomerism, additives, and vial configuration. *Journal of Parenteral Science and Technology* 45 (2): 94–100.
138 Williams, N.A. and Guglielmo, J. (1993). Thermal mechanical analysis of frozen solutions of mannitol and some related stereoisomers: evidence of expansion during warming and correlation with vial breakage during lyophilization. *Journal of Parenteral Science and Technology* 47 (3): 119–123.
139 Williams, N.A., Lee, Y., Polli, G.P., and Jennings, T.A. (1986). The effects of cooling rate on solid phase transitions and associated vial breakage occurring in frozen mannitol solutions. *Journal of Parenteral Science and Technology* 40 (4): 135–141.
140 Milton, N., Gopalrathnam, G., Craig, G.D. et al. (2007). Vial breakage during freeze-drying: crystallization of sodium chloride in sodium chloride-sucrose frozen aqueous solutions. *Journal of Pharmaceutical Sciences* 96 (7): 1848–1853.

141 Hirakura, Y., Kojima, S., Okada, A. et al. (2004). The improved dissolution and prevention of ampoule breakage attained by the introduction of pretreatment into the production process of the lyophilized formulation of recombinant human interleukin-11 (RHIL-11). *International Journal of Pharmaceutics* 286 (1–2): 53–67.
142 Bhambhani, A. and Medi, B.M. (2010). Selection of containers/closures for use in lyophilization applications: possibilities and limitations. *American Pharmaceutical Review* 13 (4): 86–91.
143 Degrazio, F. (2007). Considerations for packaging and delivery systems for biopharmaceutical products. *Bioprocessing Journal* 6 (4): 39–40.
144 Rambhatla, S. and Pikal, M.J. (2003). Heat and mass transfer scale-up issues during freeze-drying, I: atypical radiation and the edge vial effect. *AAPS PharmSciTech* 4 (2): E14.
145 Alexeenko, A., Ganguly, A., and Nail, S.L. (2010). Modeling and simulation of vapor and ice dynamics in pharmaceutical freeze-drying. *Freeze Drying of Pharmaceuticals and Biologicals*. Garmisch-Partenkirchen, Germany.
146 Goldman, J.M., Chen, X., Register, J.T. et al. (2019). Representative scale-down lyophilization cycle development using a seven-vial freeze-dryer (microfd). *Journal of Pharmaceutical Sciences* 108 (4): 1486–1495.
147 Tchessalov, S. (2011). Methodology of lyophilizers characterization to enable modeling of process parameters during cycle scale up. *International Society of Lyophilization-Freeze Drying, Midwest Chapter Conference*. Chicago, IL (15 April 2011).
148 Tchessalov, S. (2012). Specifics of heat and mass transfer during freeze-drying above collapse temperature. *International Society of Lyophilization-Freeze Drying, Midwest Chapter Conference*. Chicago, IL (12 April 2012).
149 Kuu, W.Y., Hardwick, L.M., and Akers, M.J. (2005). Correlation of laboratory and production freeze drying cycles. *International Journal of Pharmaceutics* 302 (1–2): 56–67.
150 Kobayashi, M. (1984). Development of new refrigeration system and optimum geometry of the vapor condenser for pharmaceutical freeze dryers. In: *Fourth International Drying Symposium*, vol. 2 (eds. R. Toei and A. Mujumdar), 464–471. Kyoto, Japan: Kyoto International Conference Hall.
151 Ganguly, A., Venkattraman, A., and Alexeenko, A.A. (2011). Simulations of vapor/ice dynamics in a freeze-dryer condenser. *AIP Conference Proceedings* 1333(Pt. 1, 27th International Symposium on Rarefied Gas Dynamics, 2010: 254–259.
152 Ganguly, A., Alexeenko, A.A., Schultz, S.G., and Kim, S.G. (2013). Freeze-drying simulation framework coupling product attributes and equipment capability: toward accelerating process by equipment modifications. *European Journal of Pharmaceutics and Biopharmaceutics* 85 (2): 223–235.
153 Alexeenko, A.A., Ganguly, A., and Nail, S.L. (2009). Computational analysis of fluid dynamics in pharmaceutical freeze-drying. *Journal of Pharmaceutical Sciences* 98 (9): 3483–3494.
154 Kshirsagar, V., Tchessalov, S., Kanka, F. et al. (2019). Determining maximum sublimation rate for a production lyophilizer: computational modeling and

comparison with ice slab tests. *Journal of Pharmaceutical Sciences* 108 (1): 382–390.

155 Patel, S.M., Chaudhuri, S., and Pikal, M.J. (2010). Choked flow and importance of Mach I in freeze-drying process design. *Chemical Engineering Science* 65 (21): 5716–5727.

156 Tchessalov, S. and Warne, N. (2008). Lyophilization: cycle robustness and process tolerances, transfer, and scale up. *European Pharmaceutical Review* 3: 76–83.

157 Schersch, K., Betz, O., Garidel, P. et al. (2012). Systematic investigation of the effect of lyophilizate collapse on pharmaceutically relevant proteins, part 2: stability during storage at elevated temperatures. *Journal of Pharmaceutical Sciences* 101 (7): 2288–2306.

158 Schersch, K., Betz, O., Garidel, P. et al. (2013). Systematic investigation of the effect of lyophilizate collapse on pharmaceutically relevant proteins III: collapse during storage at elevated temperatures. *European Journal of Pharmaceutics and Biopharmaceutics* 85 (2): 240–252.

159 Patel, S.M., Nail, S.L., Pikal, M.J. et al. (2017). Lyophilized drug product cake appearance: what is acceptable? *Journal of Pharmaceutical Sciences* 106 (7): 1706–1721.

160 Rawat, P., Kumar, S., and Michael Gromiha, M. (2018). An in-silico method for identifying aggregation rate enhancer and mitigator mutations in proteins. *International Journal of Biological Macromolecules* 118 (Part_A): 1157–1167.

161 Arsiccio, A., Mccarty, J., Pisano, R., and Shea, J.-E. (2018). Effect of surfactants on surface-induced denaturation of proteins: evidence of an orientation-dependent mechanism. *The Journal of Physical Chemistry B* 122 (49): 11390–11399.

162 Arsiccio, A. and Pisano, R. (2018). Clarifying the role of cryo- and lyo-protectants in the biopreservation of proteins. *Physical Chemistry Chemical Physics* 20 (12): 8267–8277.

163 Arsiccio, A., Paladini, A., Pattarino, F., and Pisano, R. (2019). Designing the optimal formulation for biopharmaceuticals: a new approach combining molecular dynamics and experiments. *Journal of Pharmaceutical Sciences* 108 (1): 431–438.

164 Costantino, H.R. (2004). Excipients for use in lyophilized pharmaceutical peptide, protein, and other bioproducts. *Biotechnology: Pharmaceutical Aspects* 2(Lyophilization of Biopharmaceuticals): 139–228.

165 Van Bockstal, P.-J., De Meyer, L., Corver, J. et al. (2017). Noncontact infrared-mediated heat transfer during continuous freeze-drying of unit doses. *Journal of Pharmaceutical Sciences* 106 (1): 71–82.

166 Capozzi, L.C., Trout, B.L., and Pisano, R. (2019). From batch to continuous: freeze-drying of suspended vials for pharmaceuticals in unit-doses. *Industrial & Engineering Chemistry Research* 58 (4): 1635–1649.

167 MERIDION Technologies (2017). MERIDION technologies: processes from lab to productions scale. http://meridion-technologies.de/en/produkte.php#lab (accessed 15 May 2019).

168 Tchessalov S. (2018). Exploring new opportunities beyond vial freeze-drying: aseptic spray freeze-drying and foam drying of complex biologicals. *Freeze Drying of Pharmaceuticals and Biologicals*. Garmisch-Partenkirchen, Germany.

169 IMA Group. (2019) Continuous manufacturing. https://ima.it/pharma/lynfinity/ (accessed 15 May 2019).

7

Spray Drying

Reinhard Vehring[1], *Herm Snyder*[2], *and David Lechuga-Ballesteros*[3]

[1] *University of Alberta, Department of Mechanical Engineering, 5-1G Mechanical Engineering Building, Edmonton, AB T6G 2G8, Canada*
[2] *PARSEC Solutions LLC, Purdue Technology Center, 1281 Win Hentschel Blvd., West Lafayette, IN 47906, USA*
[3] *AstraZeneca Pharmaceuticals LP, Pharmaceutical Technology and Development, 121 Oyster Point Boulevard, South San Francisco, CA 94080, USA*

7.1 Background

The spray drying of biotherapeutics is a well-established technology to enable stabilization as well as functionality for drug delivery applications. The current range of active pharmaceutical ingredients (APIs) that can be successfully spray-dried include the traditional small molecules to biologics, spanning peptides to high molecular weight proteins and further into complex vaccine structures. Materials previously thought not suitable for spray drying, such as temperature and mechanical shear-sensitive compounds, have been successfully processed with appropriate formulation and process design. In addition, the process is well suited for continuous manufacturing scenarios with the properly designed equipment and process conditions. The technology has proven to be both robust and scalable in the pharmaceutical development and current good manufacturing process (cGMP) manufacturing environments with an increasing number of toll manufacturing options available.

Conversion of liquid feedstock containing a biologic into a stable, flowable, dried powder using spray evaporative drying processes is a long-established technology in the food processing industry. A patent issued in 1865 describes spray-drying eggs to improve shelf life [1]. Another one issued in 1872 outlines the basic spray-drying process for producing dried starch and gelatin [2]. In addition, heat-sensitive proteins such as milk products were spray-dried prior to World War II at equipment scales capable of processing tons per day of dry powder.

Spray evaporation processes have been utilized to isolate small molecule active ingredient removing volatile solvents from the mother liquor following a crystallization step. In this example, the evaporation process has little impact on the key particle properties such as size, density, surface morphology, or product's solid-state form. The purpose is simply to remove solvent and yield a powder with low residual solvent level.

Drying Technologies for Biotechnology and Pharmaceutical Applications, First Edition.
Edited by Satoshi Ohtake, Ken-ichi Izutsu, and David Lechuga-Ballesteros.

More recently pharmaceutical spray drying has become a valuable tool in the general formulation toolbox known as "particle engineering" in which the API can be co-sprayed with excipients to enable precise control of the particle size, density, surface energy, solid-state form, and residual solvents. This level of particle property precision is unrivaled among pharmaceutical powder production technologies and enables particle attributes designed for the demands of the API and selected drug delivery method. Product performance enhancements are possible in the fields of inhalation drug delivery (oral/nasal), controlled release capsules/tablets, and room-temperature stabilized biologics using spray-drying technologies.

7.1.1 Spray-Drying Fundamentals

Spray drying is a one-step process transforming a prepared liquid feedstock to solid powder in a conceptually simple manner. The fundamental subprocesses involved in spray drying are conceptually illustrated in Figure 7.1. A spray plume of liquid droplets is generated from a prepared feedstock using a spray atomizer. The individual droplets contain solid components that interact with a heated gas stream that promotes the rapid evaporative mass transfer of the liquid volatile component from the droplet into the process gas. When sufficient liquid mass has been transformed to vapor, the remaining solid material from the droplet forms an individual dried particle, which is then separated from the process stream with an inertial separation or a filtration step.

Spray drying typically produces near-spherical particles with favorable flow characteristics conducive to subsequent downstream handling and packaging. The concept has been implemented over a range of equipment scales from bench units to large multistory commercial drying towers. Powder production rates for a typical bench spray dryer are on the order of grams per hour, while the commercial pharmaceutical systems process tons per year, as shown in Figure 7.2.

7.1.2 Feedstock Preparation

A broad range of feedstock rheological properties can be utilized in spray drying: low viscosity solutions, emulsions, and suspensions to high viscosity slurries.

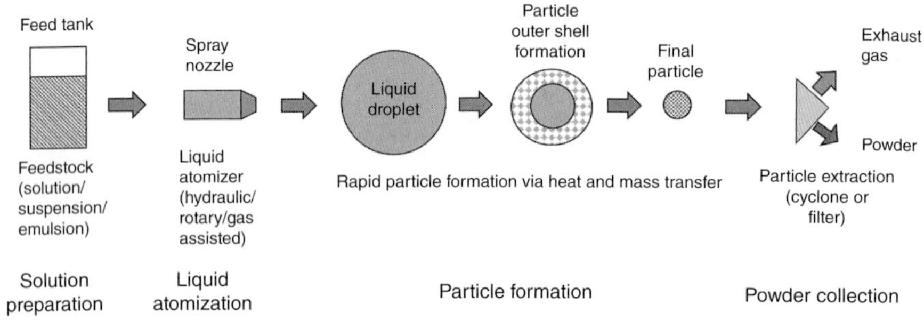

Figure 7.1 Key elements of the spray-drying process.

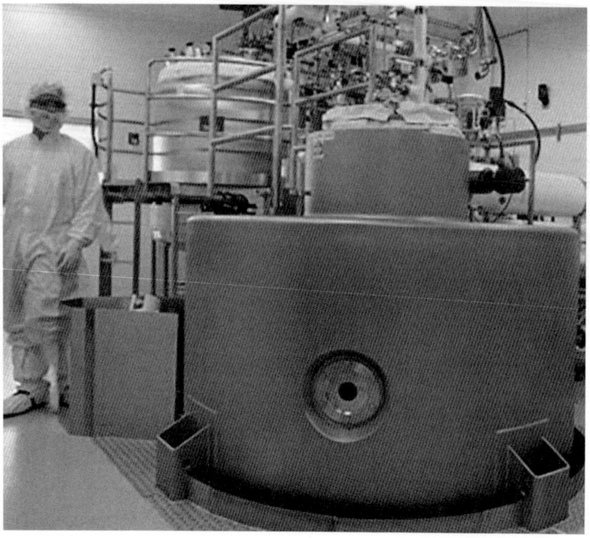

Figure 7.2 Example of a cGMP commercial spray-drying system.

The main limitation is the ability to pump the feedstock and produce suitable atomized droplets inside the drying chamber. The design of the feedstock is driven by target product characteristics, formulation, API solubility, and liquid stability considerations. Both aqueous and organic solvent systems are used in commercially spray-dried pharmaceutical powders, along with emulsions and suspension preparations that have additional feedstock physical stability challenges compared with solutions. The greater the tendency for component separation in the delivery tank due to component density differences, the higher the chance for dryer operational issues (pump pulsations/nozzle blockage) and variable product quality.

Emulsion or suspension feedstock systems can be effectively processed when the dispersed phase component of emulsion droplets or suspended particles is significantly smaller than the atomizer nozzle restricting orifices to avoid clogging and assure for stable dryer operation. In addition, the dispersed phase components should be approximately one order of magnitude smaller in size compared with the atomized droplet size in order to assure consistent composition across the final spray-dried particle population.

Biopharmaceutical spray-drying processes typically utilize aqueous-based formulations with low shear-inducing solution preparation equipment and various methods of solution thermal control to minimize stresses imposed on the feedstock. Given the often-extended time required for solution preparation and hold, which can take minutes to hours, compared with the actual spray-drying event, which is over in seconds, the opportunity for damage to large biomolecules during preparation should not be ignored.

7.1.3 Spray-Drying Equipment

Spray dryers typically used in pharmaceutical applications are considered "co-flow" designs [3] in which the drying gas interacts initially with the spray plume and both are introduced to the drying chamber in the same direction. This is in contrast to counterflow design dryers commonly used for processing metals and ceramics in which the spray is injected opposite the drying gas and at some axial distance such that the freshly formed particle, not the droplet, is impinged by the drying gas. The co-flow dryer, when properly designed and implemented, will buffer the drug compound within the liquid droplets from direct exposure to the high dryer inlet temperature due to evaporative cooling. The rapid mixing between the drying gas and spray plume acts to localize the majority of the solvent mass transfer process to the upper region of the drying chamber. As the droplet solvent mass transfer rate declines and the protective evaporative cooling is reduced, the particle has transitioned into the lower region of the dryer and experiences the significantly lower outlet temperature. In addition, at this point in the process, the particle is largely formed with the solidification acting to limit protein mobility and potential denaturation. These two processing factors coupled with stabilizing formulation excipients have enabled the production of a stable spray-dried powder from a liquid feedstock containing a labile biopharmaceutical such as a protein or an antibody.

Pharmaceutical spray-drying systems can be configured for single-pass, open-loop operation using air as the process gas to dry aqueous-based formulations, such as biologic compounds. When organic solvents are required for the formulation, a closed-loop dryer system is used, typically with nitrogen as the processing gas. The process stream exhaust is directed through condenser hardware to recover the majority of the solvent, and this reduced partial vapor pressure stream is fed back into the dryer inlet. Such a closed system will produce powder with an elevated residual solvent level in comparison with an open-loop system due to the residual solvent level present in the recycle stream.

The mixing process inside a spray dryer can be examined using three-dimensional computational fluid dynamics (CFD) modeling tools. Figure 7.3 illustrates the output from the model of a clinical-scale spray dryer, drying an aqueous formulation. Figure 7.3 (left panel) illustrates the gas velocity magnitude contours in the dryer center-plane region. Note the velocity scale is logarithmic and in units of meters per second. The gas-assisted atomizer creates a narrow angle gas jet, which penetrates into the lower region of the drying chamber. Figure 7.3 (right panel) shows the static temperature profile, in degrees celsius, at this center plane, indicating rapid near-nozzle mixing with the lower half of the chamber, creating a gas field close to the dryer outlet temperature

Typical droplet lifetimes, and hence particle formation rates, can occur over a range of time from milliseconds to many seconds. This time is controlled by both the initial liquid droplet size and evaporation rate. The latter is dictated by the heat transfer to the droplet, mass transfer of the vapor away from the droplet into the process stream, and the specific formulation chemistry and particle shell formation rate. The rate of particle formation is a key parameter that dictates the minimum required size of the drying chamber and hence the scale of equipment required to produce a desired particle size at the target production rate. Bench-scale spray dryers typically produce particles in the 1–15 μm particle size range, while large multistory, single-pass dryers can produce particles up to 100 μm in diameter or greater if configured to produce particle agglomerates.

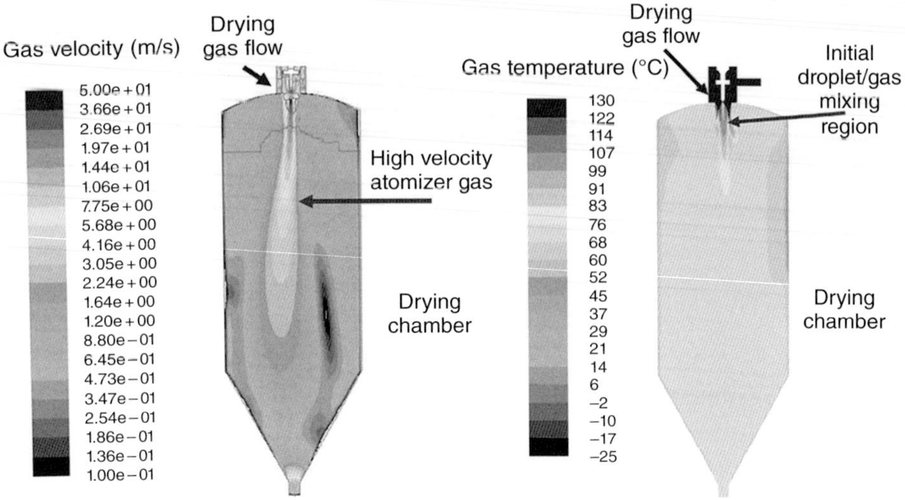

Figure 7.3 Computational fluid dynamics modeling results showing dryer center-plane gas velocity (left) and temperature contours (right).

The final non-agglomerated product particle size can be estimated for the initial liquid droplet size and solution feedstock by equating the mass of dissolved solids to the mass of the dried particle yielding the following:

$$d_{\text{particle}} = \sqrt[3]{\left(\frac{C\,\rho_{\text{solution}}}{\rho_{\text{particle}}}\right)} d_{\text{droplet}} \tag{7.1}$$

where d_{particle} is the particle diameter, d_{droplet} is the droplet diameter, C is the solution concentration (total solids %wt) ρ_{particle} is the particle density, and ρ_{solution} is the solution density.

Hence the final product particle size is controlled predominantly by the initial liquid droplet size and to a lesser degree by the feedstock concentration, along with the feed solution to particle density ratio. Therefore, understanding the spray atomizer design options and performance limitations is essential for controlling the product primary particle size from the dryer.

7.1.4 Atomization

Effective spray atomization of the formulated feedstock is a key aspect required for any successful spray-drying process. Selection of the appropriate nozzle design is driven by the target liquid flow rate required and the resulting liquid droplet size distribution. Both the mean and width parameters of the size distribution play a role in determining final product particle size as well as process yield. Ideally a narrow droplet size distribution, with a geometric standard deviation below 2, should be targeted to enable a more uniform drying event and prevent product loss to the dryer sidewalls due to incomplete drying of the larger droplets. Controlling the droplet size distribution is essential for precise control of the spray-dried particles required for certain applications such as inhalation drug delivery and a critical control parameter for a successful scale-up. This process must start with the appropriate nozzle design selection and be completed with an appropriate development process for setting nozzle operating parameters.

Clinical and commercial-scale pharmaceutical spray dryers to date have utilized one of the following design approaches for spray atomization: twin-fluid (gas-assisted) nozzle, pressure (hydraulic) nozzle, or rotary (spinning disk or cup) atomizer.

7.1.4.1 Twin-Fluid or Gas (Air)-Assisted Atomizer

Twin-fluid nozzles utilize a low pressure liquid delivery system such as a peristaltic pump and extract energy for atomization from a high-speed gas stream brought into intimate contact with the liquid, typically in the shape of a jet or a sheet, which drives droplet production. One example of this concept is shown in Figure 7.4, which generates a narrow spray angle, sub-10 μm droplet size spray.

In comparison with the pressure and rotary atomizers, the twin-fluid atomizer generates smaller liquid droplet sizes, and droplet size performance is less sensitive to changes in feedstock rheology such as viscosity. The twin-fluid atomizer is capable to operate over a wider range of liquid feed flows and can tune the shape and mean values of the droplet sizes produced by altering the mass flow ratio of atomization gas to liquid at the nozzle. Due to the existence of a localized reduced

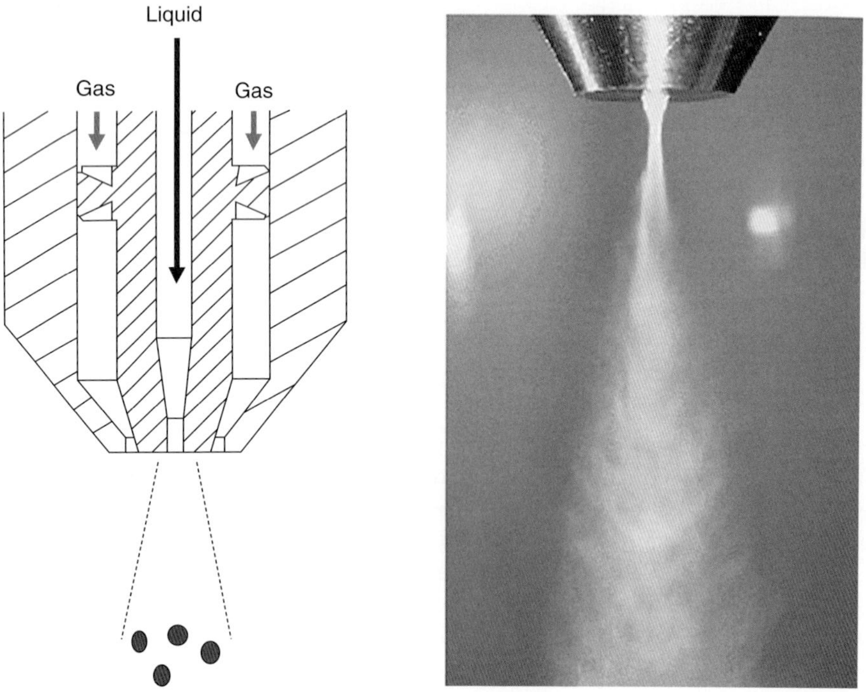

Figure 7.4 Example of a twin-fluid/gas-assisted atomizer.

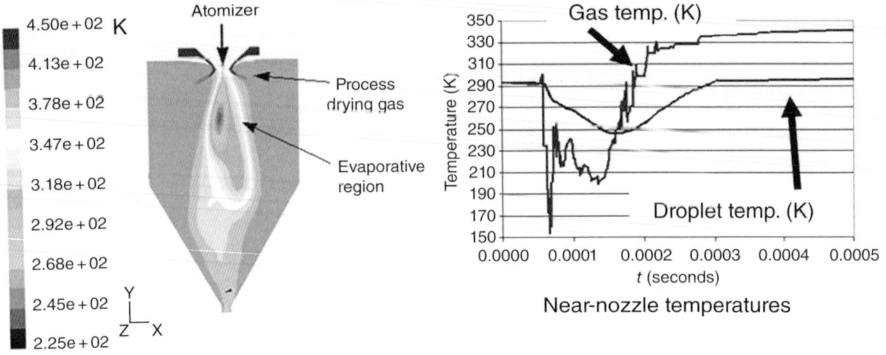

Figure 7.5 Computational fluid dynamics modeling results in a clinical scale spray dryer showing temperature distribution in drying chamber (left) and gas and droplet temperatures near the nozzle exit.

temperature region near the nozzle, twin-fluid atomizers can briefly buffer the drug compound containing droplets from the high-temperature drying gas.

These attributes make the twin-fluid nozzles well suited for spray drying from the small benchtop systems to multistory commercial dryers. The ability to generate small droplet sizes favors the use of these nozzles in small-scale drying systems with limited droplet drying residence time available. Large droplets will tend to be lost to the sidewall of bench units due to incomplete drying. The concept can be scaled to large dryers as well, but does require a suitable high pressure gas source, which can impact system capital and operating expenses at very large scale.

The combination of small droplet size, the ability to modulate the size distribution, and the localized buffering effect on heat transfer in the near-nozzle region make the twin-fluid atomizer the preferred choice for specialized drug delivery applications such as inhalation drug delivery of biomolecules. The micron-level precision control of droplet size translates to exceedingly small and narrow final particle size distributions required to efficiently deliver 1–3 μm-sized particles into the respiratory tract. The added buffering from the cold atomization gas flow benefits the processing of thermally labile compounds by reducing thermal shock to the drug in the near-nozzle region while still in the liquid droplet form. Figure 7.5 displays CFD results of a cGMP spray-drying process illustrating a central evaporation zone with a near-nozzle calculated droplet temperature profile indicating a rapid decrease in liquid droplet temperature due to the gas expansion cooling of the surrounding atomization gas stream.

Design variations of the twin-fluid atomizer concept have successfully been implemented in a range of validated cGMP pharmaceutical spray-drying processes, including aseptic spray-drying systems.

7.1.4.2 Pressure or Hydraulic Nozzle

Pressure or hydraulic atomization nozzles do not use a supplemental gas stream to create droplets but rely upon the pressure from the liquid feedstock delivery system to create a high-speed liquid exit velocity and induce droplet production. This principle has broad spray applications across many different industries such

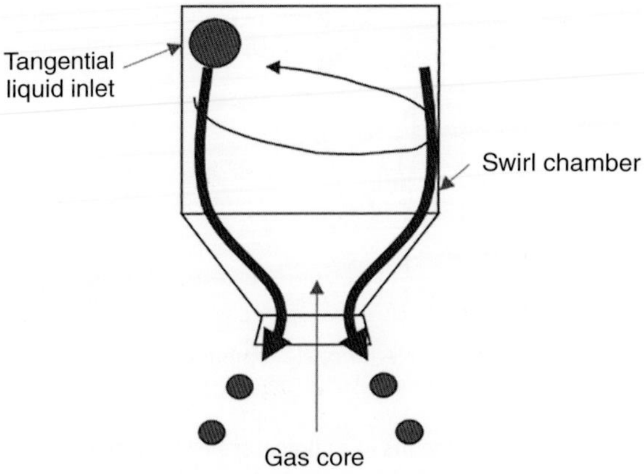

Figure 7.6 Pressure-swirl atomizer concept.

a painting (fan spray) and automotive engine fuel injection (plain orifice) but for pharmaceutical spray drying has been applied mostly in larger spray dryers producing particles in the 20–60 μm size range. The preferred pressure nozzle version for this application is called a pressure-swirl design and generates a hollow cone spray plume by introducing the liquid into a swirl chamber within the nozzle, just prior to the exit opening with sufficient tangential velocity to create an expanding liquid cone structure, as illustrated in Figure 7.6.

Any pressure atomizer will require elevated liquid feed delivery pressure (40–200 bar) compared with a twin-fluid nozzle design (0.5 bar), which necessitates the use of one or more high pressure gear pumps in series to drive the atomizer. This type of feed system will impose elevated mechanical stress on the feedstock compared to a peristaltic pump typically used for a twin-fluid nozzle, which could be detrimental to shear-sensitive biomolecules.

The gear pump systems generally require careful cleaning and maintenance procedures to operate consistently in a cGMP production environment. In addition, by the nature of the operating physics for pressure nozzles, the flow rate and droplet sizes are inherently coupled. Therefore, it is common to change nozzle hardware when performing process development activities in order to accommodate a range of feed rates while maintaining suitable atomization performance to prevent incomplete product drying and poor process yield.

Despite these limitations, pressure nozzles have found acceptance in some large-scale commercial spray dryers because they do not require a supplemental high pressure gas supply system, required for a twin-fluid nozzle. For closed-loop dryer systems, the lack of additional atomization gas flow into the process stream allows for a simplified control and pressure bleed systems.

For spray-drying applications in which relatively large particles (2–60 μm) are produced using a formulation capable of withstanding high mechanical shear and thermal stresses, the pressure nozzle can be effectively implemented in a commercial cGMP environment.

7.1.4.3 Rotary Atomizer

Rotary atomizers operate by flinging the liquid from a high-speed rotating disk or wheel directly into the drying environment. The motive force can be derived from a high pressure pneumatic source for the smaller units or electric motor-driven unit for large-scale production. A range of atomizer rotating wheels and spinning cup designs exist [4]. The radial nature of this type of droplet production creates a wide spray angle near the atomizer as the droplet trajectories form a two-dimensional sheet radiating outward from the wheel. Once the droplets have escaped the near wheel region, they are susceptible to the aerodynamic forces imposed by the drying gas flow, and their trajectories will be altered, or they will impact a sidewall causing potential loss of product yield. The impact of this spray geometry difference imposes different design constraints on the dryer body shape and airflow pattern when compared with the twin-fluid nozzle. For both cases the droplets need sufficient drying time prior to contacting the chamber sidewalls in order to assure complete particle formation and minimize film deposition losses to the chamber.

Rotary atomizer produce larger, more uniform droplet spray fields in comparison with the twin-fluid nozzle. The atomization energy is provided by the rotation speed of the wheel, and the droplet size will decrease with increased wheel rotation. For pharmaceutical applications, cleaning validation can be a challenge as the moving mechanical parts require seals that require suitable cleaning method development.

The previous section outlines several atomizer design and performance parameters that should be considered when developing a spray-drying process for a target set of powder properties. The impact of nozzle selection propagates into the drying environment by dictating the initial droplet size and trajectory. These initial conditions set the stage for the evaporation process within the drying chamber.

7.1.5 Drying Chamber

Conversion of the atomized spray droplets into fine particles involves multiple steps as the droplets are exposed to the drying gas medium. First, the droplet must adjust to the temperature of the near-nozzle environment. During this period, the type of atomizer will play a role in the local droplet environment and hence impact the early droplet temperature as previously discussed. The second stage occurs when the liquid droplet has established equilibrium evaporation of the carrier solvent into the gas surroundings. The evaporation process can be modeled as it will be discussed below. During the second stage of drying, the liquid droplet will experience a temperature close to the thermodynamic wet bulb value, which will be significantly below the surrounding gas temperature. For example, the liquid droplet experiences only 40 °C under steady-state evaporation when the internal dryer chamber contains hot air at 80 °C and 10% relative humidity (RH). Increased RH in the process stream acts to slow the mass transfer into the gas phase, decreasing the particle formation rate and reducing the evaporative cooling of the droplet and elevating the equilibrium droplet temperature. The relative humidity in the spray-drying chamber is defined as the partial vapor pressure of water divided by the saturation vapor pressure at a target temperature [5]. For particles in mass transfer equilibrium with the process gas stream, the dryer exit humidity will control the final product moisture level, which can be calculated using the relative humidity value and the product specific sorption isotherms. For products in which low particle moisture is key, the outlet RH will effectively limit the powder production rate for a given dryer outlet temperature. The relationship between dryer outlet temperature and RH is nonlinear with an increase of a few degrees enabling a significant feed rate and hence powder throughput increase for moisture-limited drying processes.

The third stage of particle formation occurs after a portion of the solvent carrier has been evaporated and the solid content within the droplet influences the evaporation rate into the gas medium. Typically, this reduces the mass transfer rate for the remaining solvent; hence this stage is commonly referred to as the "falling rate period" [6]. At this point in time, the droplet surface has started to solidify, forming a viscous shell. This creates an internal droplet diffusion-controlled [7] mass transfer process slowing the rate of solvent escape from the inner core to the surface prior to evaporation into the gas medium. For solution-based feedstock with dissolved solids, the particle morphology is set in this third drying stage. The particle formation kinetics, controlled by the evaporation rate in conjunction with the rising droplet viscosity, imposes stresses on the forming surface, which control the final shape and surface roughness of the spray-dried product.

The detailed physics of the entire droplet to particle formation process is highly complex and dependent upon the coupled interplay between the initial droplet size, evaporation rate, feedstock concentration, formulation chemistry, and solid mechanics. Certain aspects of this process can be simulated using computational simulation tools. The impact of fluid mechanics on the drying and particle formation process is further illustrated by the range of calculated droplet pathways generated in the simulation shown in Figure 7.7. Significantly different particle pathways inside the drying chamber can occur, impacting the particle residence time in the chamber and the resulting thermal exposure. The particle formed near the spray centerline will directly exit the drying chamber and experience a

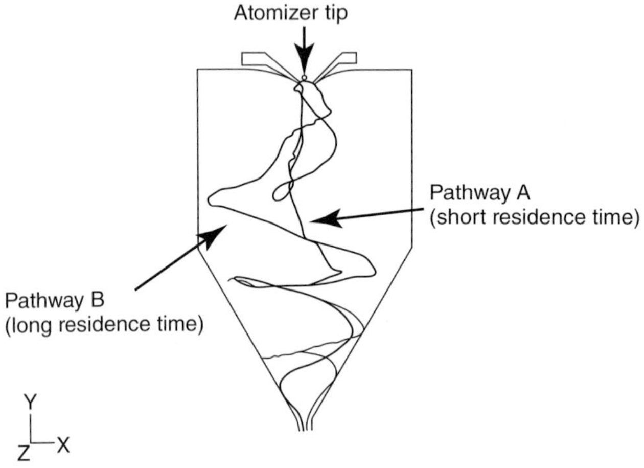

Figure 7.7 Calculated particle trajectories in a clinical-scale spray dryer.

residence time of approximately 42 ms. The particles that get entrained within a recirculation eddy will experience much greater residence times and expose thermally sensitive biomolecules particles to the inlet drying gas temperature, without the protective shield of evaporation to insulate the compound.

7.1.6 Particle Collection

Pharmaceutical spray dryers create a dispersed particulate aerosol in which a high-value solid material must be recovered from the process stream. One of two different technologies is typically used for product capture in such a process: inertial cyclone separation or baghouse filtration. Both approaches have evolved out of the dust pollution control and chemical processing industries in which particle abatement was the primary goal, not particulate recovery. As a result, some design modification of these established technologies is required to assure product quality and maximum product yield.

Cyclones have the following advantages for particle collection in a pharmaceutical spray-drying process: mechanically simple, with no moving parts; can be designed for high recovery efficiency; and amenable to being cleaned in place. Disadvantages can include both hardware scale and particle size-dependent capture efficiency, which must be addressed during process transfer and scale-up.

Refinements to the traditional reverse-flow Stairmand cyclone design [8] for use in therapeutic protein spray drying have focused on thermal control around the particles during collection for improved product moisture control, enabling effective clean-in-place (CIP) methodology and minimizing particle attrition during inertial separation while maximizing product recovery from the bottom collector region. Such designs have been implemented in commercial validated manufacturing systems for spray-dried inhalation powders with high efficiency product recovery performance above >90% for a mean particle size of 2 μm.

Figure 7.8 displays the results from a simulation of a high efficiency cyclone. The particle-laden stream is fed tangentially into the top of the unit, creating a hybrid vortex flow inside the cyclone. Along the outer wall, the particle-laden gas flow spirals downward, both accelerating and decelerating until the particles disengage from the gas flow in the final product collector region. The gas flow turns back upward via a high tangential velocity central vortex and exhausts through the top of the cyclone. For applications requiring high collection efficiency of <5 μm diameter particles, understanding the impact of cyclone design and operating conditions is crucial for the obtainment of high process yields.

7.2 Particle Engineering

Particle engineering provides the mechanistic understanding that is necessary to design advanced microparticles with an interior structure that can determine or enhance the functionality of products that are based on these particles. Inhalation products that rely on such structured particles have entered the

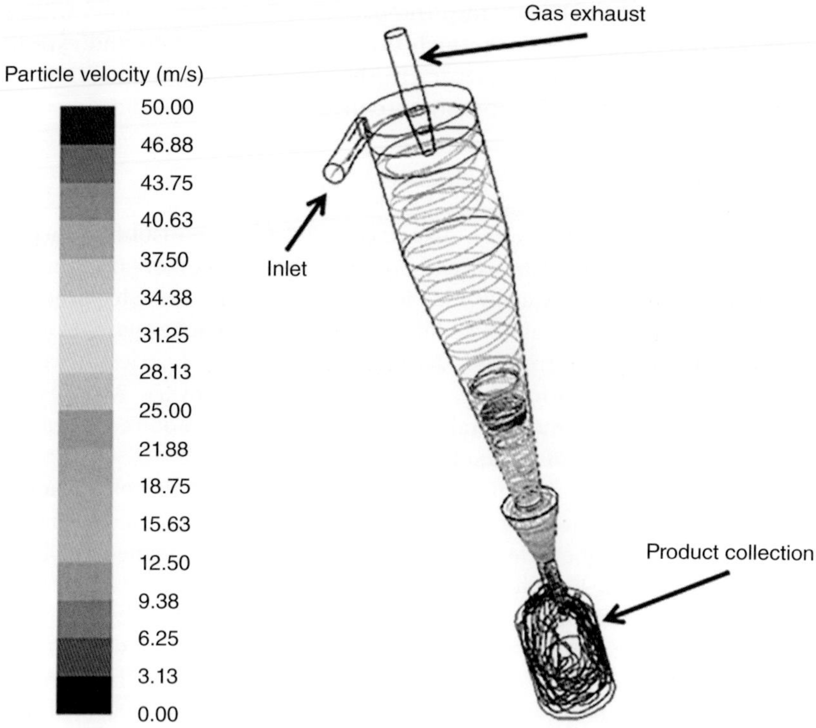

Figure 7.8 Computational fluid dynamics modeling results of a clinical scale spray dryer shown in temperature distribution in drying chamber (left) and gas and droplet temperatures near the nozzle exit.

marketplace in recent years. Pioneering for the field of biologics was the work on inhaled insulin Exubera® [9–11] and more recently Afrezza® [12]. Structured lipid porous particle-based products have been successful as inhaled antibiotic such as TOBI® Podhaler™ [13] and in a metered dose inhaler format for chronic obstructive pulmonary disease (Bevespi Aerosphere™) [14]. In all of these products, the particle morphology contributes to the functionality of the dosage form. Typical targets for particle design are increased dispersibility or powder flowability, increased dosing uniformity, improved delivery efficiency, and, particularly important for biologics, physical, chemical, and biological stabilization of the product during shipping, storage, and patient use. These targets can be achieved by particle features such as low particle density, layers and shells for encapsulation, and favorable surface properties, e.g. low surface energy or high surface roughness, in combination with careful control of the particle's solid phase. The design targets are too diverse and too complex to be attainable on practical time scales with an empirical approach. Hence mechanistic understanding and the predictive tools that follow from it are the keys to successful particle design.

The complete particle formation process from atomization to powder collection is rather complex. Therefore, it is helpful to separately discuss four stages of the process. Each stage is dominated by different physicochemical processes.

7.2.1 Particle Formation: Evaporation Stage

During the *evaporation stage*, the drying process is controlled by coupled heat and mass transfer between the liquid phase, i.e. the atomized droplets, and the gas phase, i.e. the drying gas. Immediately after atomization, the droplets will assume a spherical shape and reach thermal equilibrium, determined by the evaporation rate. For typical droplet diameters, this equilibration process is fast compared with the time it takes to evaporate the solvent. The equilibration phase is often neglected in particle formation models, because it is thought to have little influence on the particle morphology. Once in equilibrium the evaporation of one or more solvents proceeds. The evaporation rate, κ, is primarily determined by the heat transfer from the drying gas to the droplets and can be calculated without much difficulty for many cases. A common simplification for single solvent systems such as aqueous solution droplets is the constant rate assumption, also known as the d^2-law. It states that the surface area of the evaporating droplet with diameter, d, decreases linearly with time, t [15]:

$$d^2(t) = d_0^2 - \kappa t \tag{7.2}$$

Here, d_0 is the initial diameter of the atomized droplets. The constant rate assumption is not realistic for drying in an actual spray dryer because the evaporation rate depends on the drying gas temperature, which is spatially heterogeneous in an actual spray dryer, as shown in Figure 7.3. Furthermore, the evaporation rate will change over time in systems with more than one solvent and also in the later stages of evaporation when highly concentrated solutes start to affect the partial pressure of the solvent on the droplet surface. This assumption is nevertheless popular, because it allows a semi-analytical solution for the mass transport in the interior of the droplet. From a perspective of particle engineering, describing the mass transport inside of the droplet is quite important, because by this mechanism multicomponent solutions may de-mix, e.g. one component may become enriched on the surface. This may be a desirable particle design target, e.g. in encapsulation applications. Mass transport inside of the droplet is caused by the receding droplet surface. Solutes become concentrated at the droplet surface due to solvent loss, and the resulting concentration gradient causes diffusion of the solutes toward the droplet center. For small microdroplets, convective transport within the droplet is usually neglected, and diffusion is the only transport mechanism considered, e.g. via Fick's second law of diffusion, which links the concentration field with the change of concentration, c, over time:

$$\frac{\partial c}{\partial t} = \nabla \bullet (D \nabla c) \tag{7.3}$$

This general form permits the diffusion coefficient of a solute, D, to vary spatially and temporally, but has no analytical solution. With the assumption of a constant diffusion coefficient, however, this equation can be fully normalized and expressed as a function of a single dimensionless number, the Péclet number, Pe. In one-dimensional spherical coordinates, it takes the form [16]

$$\frac{\partial c}{\partial \tau} = \frac{1}{2Pe(1-\tau)} \left[\frac{\partial^2 c}{\partial R^2} + \frac{2}{R} \frac{\partial c}{\partial R} \right] - \frac{R}{2(1-\tau)} \frac{\partial c}{\partial R} \tag{7.4}$$

Here R is the radial coordinate normalized by the droplet radius. Normalized time, τ, is the ratio of time and droplet lifetime, τ_D, which is the time at which Eq. (7.2) predicts a droplet radius of zero:

$$\tau_D = \frac{d_0^2}{\kappa} \tag{7.5}$$

The droplet lifetime is a useful approximation for the time required to dry a droplet in a spray dryer, which can be compared to the results of residence time calculations, as shown in Figure 7.7. In this theoretical framework, the Péclet number is defined as

$$Pe = \frac{\kappa}{8D} \tag{7.6}$$

The Péclet number describes the relative importance of the rate of surface recession and the rate of diffusion for dissolved or suspended components in the droplet. The utility of Eq. (7.4) for particle design lies in the fact that in this simplified form, a semi-analytical solution exists, which yields the equilibrium radial concentration profile, including the surface concentration, $c_{S,j}$, for each component, j, in the droplet. If the surface concentration is normalized by the average concentration, $c_{m,j}$, simple expressions [7] for the surface enrichment, E, can be fitted to the semi-analytical solution of the partial differential equation (7.4):

$$E_j = \frac{c_{S,j}}{c_{m,j}} = 1 + \frac{Pe_j}{5} + \frac{Pe_j^2}{100} - \frac{Pe_j^3}{4000} \quad \text{for } Pe < 20 \tag{7.7}$$

Equation (7.7) is a good approximation for small Péclet numbers, which are often encountered in evaporation of aqueous small molecule solution droplets. However, biologics are often large molecules or even nanoparticles that can diffuse only very slowly, leading to very large Péclet number. In these cases,

$$E_j = \frac{Pe_j}{3} + 0.363 \quad \text{for } Pe > 20 \tag{7.8}$$

is a better approximation [17]. The steady-state solutions described in Eqs. (7.7) and (7.8) may not be reached in cases with relatively short droplet lifetime or for very large Péclet numbers. In these cases the development of the surface enrichment over time can be approximated by [17]

$$E_j(\tau) = \frac{1}{32}\left[(15Pe_j - 4) - (15Pe_j - 36)\exp\left(-\frac{5}{4}\tau\right)\right] \tag{7.9}$$

In summary, the internal redistribution of components in the droplets during the evaporation phase is the key feature for the sake of particle design. In general, the spatial component distribution as a function of time can only be provided by a full numerical model, referred to as the Vehring, Foss, Lechuga (VFL) model [15]. However, under the assumption of constant evaporation rate and constant material properties, useful and much easier-to-use approximations for the surface enrichment of components can be found. These approximations are only dependent on a single dimensionless parameter, the Péclet number, which is rather straightforward to estimate in most practical cases.

7.2.2 Particle Formation: Solidification Stage

During the second stage of the drying process, the *solidification stage*, the liquid droplets transition into a solid particle. Depending on the nature of the feedstock, different processes may occur during this stage. Some solutes are difficult or impossible to crystallize during the droplet lifetime, for example, if their solubility in the solvent is high, supersaturation levels will remain low, leading to slower nucleation or crystal growth rates compared with the evaporation rate. The particles dried from these solutes have an amorphous solid phase. The solutes will reach a state of supersaturation due to solvent removal at some time during the evaporation process, but crystallization does not commence before the droplet is dried. In this case, the viscosity of the solutions increases continuously during the solidification phase, and the solution transitions into an amorphous glass. The theoretical description of the evaporation phase can be used to find an approximation for the timing of this phase transition. Once the local density at the surface of the droplet is predicted to be equal to the true density of the amorphous solid, the transition to an amorphous shell has occurred there. The time, $\tau_{t,j}$, it takes for a solute, j, to reach the true density, ρ_t, of its dry solid can be derived by inserting an expression for the average concentration as a function of time into Eq. (7.7) [7]:

$$\tau_{t,j} = \tau_D \left(1 - \left(\frac{c_{o,j}}{\rho_{t,j}} E_j \right)^{\frac{2}{3}} \right) \tag{7.10}$$

In cases with little surface enrichment, the resulting particles likely have a low void fraction, with a particle density close to the true density of the solute. An example is shown in Figure 7.9, which shows the spatial and temporal distribution of trehalose in a case with a low surface enrichment of 1.22. The insert show a fractured dried particle without evidence of internal voids. The particle density of the dried particles was within 10% of the true density of trehalose.

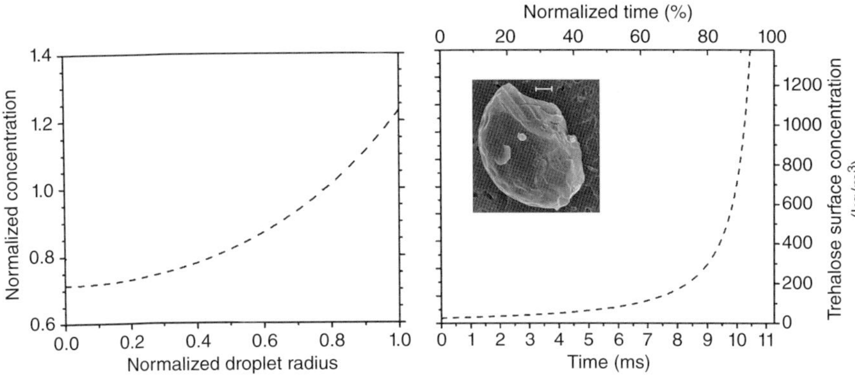

Figure 7.9 The left panel shows the steady state radial concentration profile for a trehalose solution droplet drying with a Péclet number of 1.05. The concentration is normalized by the average concentration. The right panel shows the evolution of the surface concentration as a function of time and time normalized by the droplet lifetime of 11.4 ms. The insert depicts an electromicrograph of a resulting particle that was cryo-fractured. The scale bar denotes 1 μm.

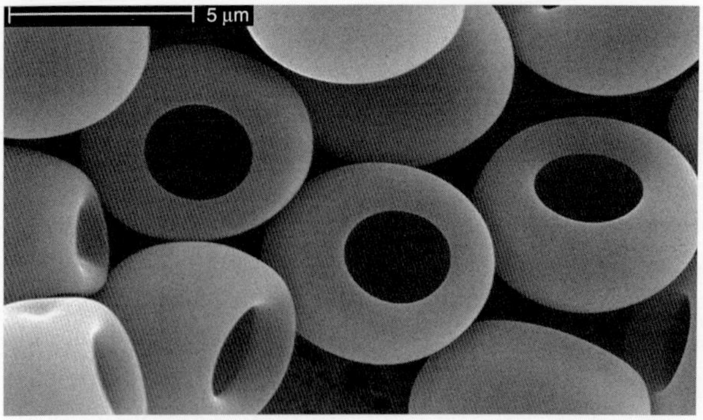

Figure 7.10 Electromicrograph of amorphous protein particles dried at a drying gas temperature of 125 °C, leading to a sixfold surface enrichment.

In cases with high surface enrichment, on the other hand, it is likely that hollow particles with large void volume are formed, because the surface of the droplet changes into a solid much earlier than the interior. Figure 7.10 shows hollow protein particles that were dried under conditions corresponding to a Péclet number of 16.8, which leads to a steady-state surface enrichment of 6. These particles have a large central void and a low particle density of 0.1 g/cm^3. It is possible to predict the particle density using Eq. (7.10) in combination with a mass balance, but it requires the assumption that the particle does not shrink after true density is reached at the surface [16]. This assumption may not hold in many cases, but the result is still useful to demonstrate the potential effect of the Péclet number on the particle density of the dried particles:

$$\rho_\mathrm{P} = \frac{c_0}{(1-\tau_\mathrm{t})^{\frac{3}{2}}} \tag{7.11}$$

Equation (7.11) shows that a low particle density is achieved if true density is reached on the surface of the droplet early in the evaporation process. According to Eq. (7.10), this happens for large Péclet numbers, i.e. large surface enrichment. Equation (7.11) also shows that the particle density cannot be lower than the initial concentration of the solute in the droplet.

7.2.3 Particle Formation: Solidification Stage for Crystallizing Excipients

The solidification stage for crystallizing excipients is dominated by different mechanisms, which are depicted in the cartoon in Figure 7.11. The evaporation process starts with a dilute solution. Once critical supersaturation is reached at the droplet surface, nucleation and crystal growth commence. The growing crystals remain or accumulate on the surface, because their mobility is insufficient to diffuse to the droplet center. Once the crystals form a closed shell, further droplet shrinkage may be arrested. In this case the remaining solvent evaporates through pores in the shell, leaving a hollow interior. The resulting particle will be mostly or completely crystalline.

This type of particle formation has recently been studied in detail using a sodium nitrate model system [17]. This study concluded that not only the timing of the onset of crystallization but also the time that is available for crystal growth

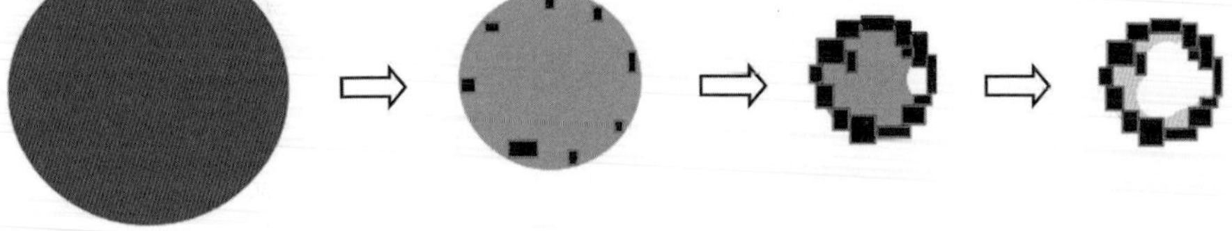

Figure 7.11 Schematic representation of the particle formation process for a single-component crystallizing solute.

is important for the morphology of the particles. Assuming that nucleation and crystal growth commence when a critical supersaturation, c_c, is reached and that it cannot proceed beyond the droplet lifetime, the time available for crystallization, Δt_c, can be approximated by

$$\Delta t_c = \frac{d_0^2}{\kappa}\left(\frac{c_{0,j}}{c_{c,j}}E_j\right)^{\frac{2}{3}} \tag{7.12}$$

The effect of decreasing the time available for crystallization is shown in Figure 7.12. If more than 200 ms is available for crystallization, large crystals with curved faces form a closed, smooth particle surface. At around 100 ms, individual crystals are visible. With decreasing Δt_c, the crystal size decreases, transitioning to nanocrystals. If Δt_c is reduced by another order of magnitude, crystals are no longer detectable, and Raman spectroscopic analysis [18] indicates a predominantly amorphous solid phase. Maintaining a consistent crystal size in particles that are composed of individual crystals is very important, because crystal size affects surface roughness, which in turn has a strong influence on particle cohesion [19]. It can be concluded that all formulation and process parameters that can influence Eq. (7.12) can be critical for the performance of a product based on such particles. Therefore these parameters need to be controlled carefully, e.g. during scale-up.

In the case of multicomponent solutions, a shell can potentially be formed by any of the components, either via accumulation on the surface, as shown in Figure 7.12, or via crystallization. The question arises whether it is possible to design the formulation and the drying process in a way that a specific excipient occupies the surface, e.g. for encapsulation or dispersibility enhancement

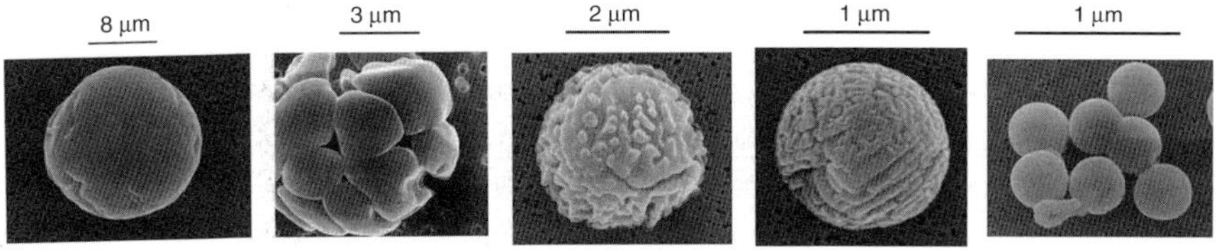

Figure 7.12 Effect of decreasing the available time for crystallization, Δtc, of evaporating sodium nitrate solution droplets on the morphology of the resulting particles. Δtc from left to right: 221 ± 6 ms, 119 ± 18 ms, 117 ± 2 ms, 101 ± 3 ms, 18 ± 2 ms. Initial solution concentration from left to right: 5 mg/ml, 0.5 mg/ml, 50 µg/ml, 5 µg/ml, 0.05 µg/ml. Drying gas temperature from left to right: 75 °C, 100 °C, 75 °C, 75 °C, 125 °C.

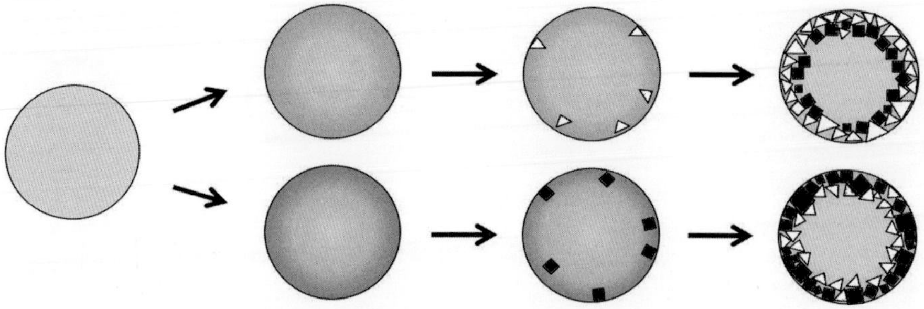

Figure 7.13 Schematic representation of the particle formation process for a particle with two crystallizing components. In the top row, the crystallization process for the component color coded in white begins first. The bottom row shows the reverse sequence.

purposes. Figure 7.13 shows two hypothetical options for the particle formation of a binary solution with two crystallizing solutes, one color-coded in white and the other in black. In the option shown on top, the white component reaches critical supersaturation earlier than the black component. Hence, this component crystallizes first and the black component second. Assuming similar crystal growth rates, a composite shell with the white component predominantly on the surface is created. In the option shown on the bottom, the black component reaches critical supersaturation first, and both the crystallization sequence and the radial composition of the resulting shell are reversed. The times at which each solute reaches critical supersaturation, $\tau_{c,j}$, can be estimated using a modified version of Eq. (7.10):

$$\tau_{c,j} = \tau_D \left(1 - \left(\frac{c_{o,j}}{c_{c,j}} E_j\right)^{\frac{2}{3}}\right) \tag{7.13}$$

It is apparent that the initial concentration of the solutes in relation to their critical supersaturation is the primary determinant of the crystallization sequence.

This hypothesis was tested in a binary solution of sodium nitrate and potassium nitrate as a model system [20]. Figure 7.14 shows the key result from this study. The first three panels show that the surface concentration of the component that reaches its critical supersaturation first is indeed enriched relative to its nominal concentration. In the leftmost case, potassium nitrate has a head start of nearly 300 ms over sodium nitrate. Hence, mostly potassium nitrate crystals form the surface of the particle. Reversing sodium to potassium ratio gives sodium nitrate about 100 ms advantage in the onset of crystallization, which leads to a surface rich in sodium nitrate, in agreement with the hypothesis described above.

The rightmost case in Figure 7.6 is instructive because it shows that the surface composition is not exclusively determined by the formulation composition. This case also has a 7 : 3 Na/K molar ratio, as the one immediately left of it. However, its surface is not enriched in sodium. The model predicts that potassium retains about 100 ms advantage in this case, a result that is due to a difference in the temperature dependence of the critical supersaturation for sodium and potassium nitrate. This case represents a higher drying gas temperature that led to a higher droplet temperature. This example shows the importance of model calculations

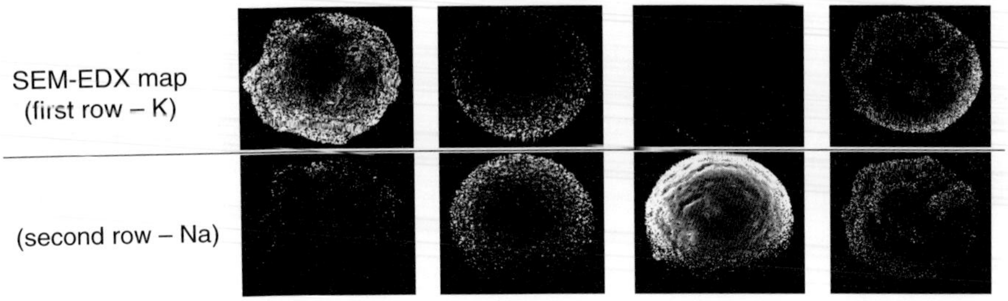

Na/K ratio nominal	3:7	1:1	7:3	7:3
Na/K ratio EDX	12/88	50/50	93/7	47:53
$\tau_{c,Na} - \tau_{c,K}$	+273 ms	+9 ms	–86 ms	+95 ms

Figure 7.14 The effect of crystallization sequence on the surface composition of binary sodium nitrate–potassium nitrate particles. The particles were dried from an aqueous solution with a total solution concentration of 10 mg/ml at drying temperatures of 50 °C (left three panels) or 100 °C (right panel). The first two rows show an intensity-coded representation of the near-surface composition measured by low overvoltage scanning electron microscopy equipped with energy-dispersive X-ray spectroscopy. The third row shows the nominal molar ratios in the solution. The fourth row reports the actual near-surface composition measured by energy-dispersive X-ray spectroscopy. The bottom row shows the time difference between sodium and potassium nitrate reaching critical supersaturation. Positive values indicate that potassium nitrate reaches critical supersaturation first.

in the interpretation of counterintuitive results and provides further evidence for the presented hypothesis.

7.2.4 Particle Formation: Deformation Stage

During the third stage of the drying process, the *deformation stage*, particles that are partially solid may deform. During this phase, surface tension may cause stress in the newly formed shell, and this may lead to shell buckling, folding, or hole formation. The cartoon in Figure 7.15 shows as an example a possible mechanism for the creation of the particle morphology depicted in Figure 7.10.

Once a shell is thick and rigid enough to impede droplet shrinkage, further loss of solvent will lead to an inward bending stress on the shell. The shell is

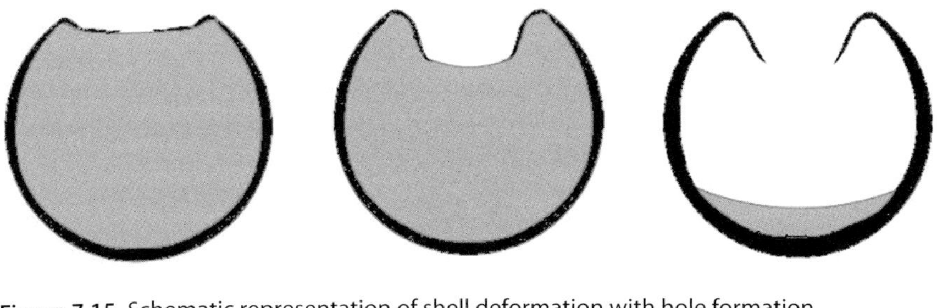

Figure 7.15 Schematic representation of shell deformation with hole formation.

likely to deform where it is thinnest. This may cause the shell to tear open and the liquid meniscus that spans the hole in the shell will then continue to pull the shell edges inward. At some point the liquid meniscus may detach, and the remaining solvent evaporates through the hole. This mechanism explains why many spray-dried microparticles have holes that have been interpreted before as "blowholes" created by solvent vapor expansion. However, these holes generally have edges that are folded inward and also occur in particles dried well below the boiling temperature of the solvent. This indicates that the mechanism proposed here is more likely.

In some cases the deformation of the particles leads to unexpected results. In a recent study on polymer particles [7], higher Péclet number conditions during drying lead to an increase in particle density, contrary to what Eqs. (7.10) and (7.11) would predict. Ion beam sectioned particles showed a reduction in shell thickness with increasing Péclet number, as expected. However, the particles with thin, pliable shells were folded very tightly, removing nearly all void volume, whereas the particles with thicker shells retained more void space due to incomplete folding. This example shows that the deformation phase can be critical for the final morphology of the particles.

Of particular interest for biologics is the drying behavior of suspensions, because virus particles or bacteria will be suspended in the feedstock, similar to nanoparticle suspensions. While a general theory of folding or buckling of composite shells made of nanoparticles has not been developed to date, some key parameters controlling the process have been identified and reviewed [21]. It is generally agreed that nanoparticles accumulate at the droplet surface during drying, because their Péclet number would be very large. The distance between nanoparticles at the surface decreases as the droplet shrinks and aggregation of the particles may occur. Once a closed nanoparticle shell is formed, capillary forces can lead to buckling as described in Figure 7.6. Whether this particle formation mechanism occurs depends strongly on the nature of the colloidal interactions between the particles. Hence, it may be possible to affect the morphology of such particles by adding a surfactant to modify repulsive or attractive forces between the nanoparticles.

7.2.5 Particle Formation: Equilibration Phase

The last phase of the drying phase can be described as *equilibration phase*. In a spray dryer, the particles are separated from the gas phase, e.g. by a cyclone, and then collected in a collection container. This container may be thermostated to provide a controlled environment for the collected powder. In the collector the residual solvent content in the powder equilibrates with the gas phase conditions, for example, RH and temperature. Understanding of the equilibration phase is important for amorphous systems that are designed to provide glass stabilization of the active ingredient. It has been proposed that the design of such products can be assisted by a combination of a supplemented phase diagram with the output from a spry-drying process model [22]. An example is shown in Figure 7.16.

Figure 7.16 illustrates spray drying of aqueous binary solutions of trehalose, a glass stabilizer, and a model pharmaceutical active. The supplemented phase diagram does not contain solidus or liquidus lines. They are not relevant because

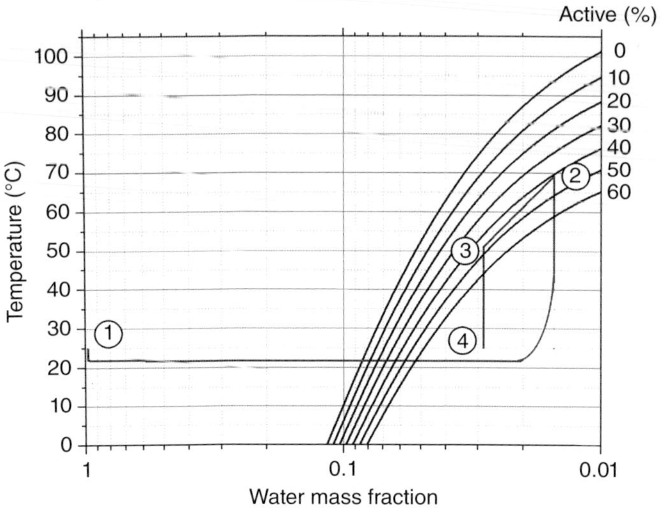

Figure 7.16 Process model output in gray (process conditions: drying gas inlet temperature, 75 °C; feedstock flow rate, 1 mg/ml; feedstock temperature, 25 °C) superimposed on a simulated phase diagram showing the plasticization curves for binary amorphous mixtures of trehalose (T_g = 117 °C) and a pharmaceutical active (T_g = 57 °C) for different mass fractions of active in the formulation. Position 1: atomizer. Position 2: cyclone. Position 3: collector. Position 4: storage.

the drying process remains above freezing and crystallization does not occur in this system. Instead plasticization curves for different ratios of active to glass stabilizer (mass fractions 0–60%) in the binary amorphous mixture are shown. The plasticization curves describe the depression of the glass transition temperature, T_g, of the amorphous mixture by water. Plasticization curves for unknown amorphous mixtures would need to be determined experimentally. However, a first approximation for product design purposes can be achieved by first calculating the dry glass transition of the mixture using the Fox equation [23], which relates the mixture glass transition temperature to the mass fractions, Y_j, and glass transition temperatures of the pure components, $T_{g,j}$. For binary systems it has the form

$$T_{\mathbf{g,mix}} = \frac{1}{\frac{Y_1}{T_{G,1}} + \frac{Y_2}{T_{G,2}}} \tag{7.14}$$

Subsequently the Gordon–Taylor equation [23] can be utilized to account for the plasticization effect assuming a T_g of −137 °C for solid amorphous water.

Superimposing particle conditions during the drying process onto the phase diagram can assist in predicting stability during manufacture and on storage. In Figure 7.3, the process begins with an atomized feedstock droplet at room temperature, 25 °C. The much higher drying gas temperature (75 °C) causes rapid droplet evaporation, during which the droplet temperature decreases slightly due to evaporative cooling. Position (2) in Figure 7.7 denotes the end of the evaporation process when solid particles with a temperature equal to the outlet drying gas temperature exit the drying chamber and enter the cyclone. Toward the end of the drying process, the particle temperature increases, because evaporative cooling is no longer effective. The model assumes that at this point the moisture content reaches the value given by the moisture sorption isotherm of trehalose at the drying gas relative humidity. The particles then transition from the cyclone to the collector (position 3), and in this particular case, it is assumed that the collector temperature is lower than the gas temperature in the cyclone. This leads to an increase in relative humidity and causes reuptake of moisture in the particles. Finally, the powder is removed from the collector and stored at room temperature (position 4). Storage relative humidity is assumed to be unchanged from collector relative humidity.

To ensure physical stability during manufacturing and physical and biochemical stability during storage, a certain temperature differential to the glass transition must be maintained for each position shown in Figure 7.7. The required temperature difference can be based on published mobility data [24] or experience with similar systems. For the example shown in Figure 7.3, instability is likely when the active mass fraction in the formulation exceeds 15 %. For higher mass fractions, process positions (2) and (3) are predicted to be too close to the glass transition temperatures, which would likely lead to particle aggregation and fusing.

7.3 Current Status

Much progress has been achieved since the first published reviews on the use of spray drying for pharmaceutical applications [25]. Several reviews have reported on the subject of biotherapeutics stabilization via spray drying [7, 26–30].

Many comparative studies show that spray drying is equivalent to other drying technologies used to stabilize biotherapeutics [31–35]. There are also many studies demonstrating that the observed protein aggregation during spray drying is not due to shearing or temperature stress during particle formation but more a consequence of adsorption at the air–liquid interface of the atomized spray [28] as well as exposure to temperatures in excess of the glass transition during collection of the dry powder [36]. The effect of shear forces during atomization or drying temperature on stability of spray-dried particles is well understood [22, 28, 37]. Drying air temperature is unlikely to cause degradation since, as pointed above, the drying liquid droplet will experience a temperature close to the thermodynamic wet bulb temperatures, which is significantly below the surrounding gas temperature (e.g. 40 °C under steady-state evaporation when the drying hot air is at 80 °C and 10% relative humidity). Protein unfolding requires large shear rates, and studies have shown that shear forces alone are not a major cause of denaturation when compared against air–liquid interfacial adsorption [38].

Successful formulation approaches have been used to overcome the effect of atomization of the liquid feedstock and temperature of the drying gas, which also determines the temperature at which the powder is collected. During atomization the liquid feedstock is broken into small droplets, thereby exponentially increasing the air–liquid interface where adsorption of proteins is often followed by denaturation or conformational changes. The use of surface active excipients has been shown to aid in stabilization by minimizing the protein surface enrichment during drying [39]. Other excipients that can minimize the surface concentration of proteins are excipients with high molecular weight, such as polymers, which slowly move with the receding liquid front during drying, and excipients with low solubility in the liquid feedstock, which tend to precipitate early in the drying process, enriching the surface and thus reducing the protein concentration at the air–liquid interface [40–42].

Most notably leucine [43–49] and trileucine [39] have been extensively used as ideal excipients to provide stabilization during atomization due to their surface activity and their low aqueous solubility that promote surface enrichment during particle formation. Leucine is a crystallizing excipient and trileucine forms an amorphous phase with high glass transition, which both furnish a hydrophobic particle coating that aids in flowability and enables aerosolization even in humid environments [50].

As explained above, even for crystallizing excipients, rapid drying usually leads to the formation of an amorphous solid matrix, which is desirable when spray-drying biotherapeutics since the biomolecule is dispersed in the amorphous matrix; thus in addition to surface activity to protect the air–liquid interface, an excipient is needed to maintain a glass transition temperature higher than the drying and collector's temperature to afford stabilization during processing and long-term stability during storage (see Figure 7.16).

The use of stabilizers, such as nonreducing disaccharides and amino acids, to preserve bioactivity during spray drying and also on subsequent storage of the dried product is also abundantly described. In addition, sound mechanisms of biotherapeutics stabilization via spray drying have been proposed, and the field has made a great deal of progress since the design of spray-dried formulations of therapeutic proteins was described as a "fortuitous affair" [28]. Numerous examples exist describing the use of spray drying to achieve the stabilization of therapeutic peptides [51] and proteins [9], enzymes [35], antibodies [33], bacteriophages [45, 52, 53], and vaccines [34, 54, 55].

The selection of appropriate glass-forming excipients with a high glass transition is also a requirement to providing long-term stability without the need for refrigeration. Nonreducing sugars such as sucrose, trehalose, and raffinose and other polysaccharides such as cyclodextrin, dextrin, and inulin have been the preferred glass-forming excipients that provide an amorphous matrix with a high glass transition. It is also recognized that the use of plasticizers as stabilizers such as glycerol and sorbitol may improve the stabilization in cases where the use of a high glass transition excipient alone is not sufficient. Addition of small amounts of plasticizer excipients reduces the overall glass transition temperature of the desiccated formulation, which may be thought of as counterproductive, but the free volume the amorphous matrix formed during the drying process is also reduced, thereby decreasing the overall molecular mobility, which may result in increased stabilization [56, 57].

As in any desiccated formulation, residual water content in spray-dried powders needs to be controlled in order to ensure long-term stability. It is generally accepted that keeping the residual water content below the "hydration limit" ensures long-term chemical and physical stability. The hydration limit is the maximum amount of water that can be hydrogen bound by the amorphous matrix, and additional water molecules in excess of the hydration limit will interact with bound water molecules, eventually forming domains within the amorphous matrix containing water molecules as reactive as liquid water that dissolve the amorphous solid, accelerating chemical degradation. Understanding the temperature dependence of the hydration limit offers a straightforward way to visualize the complex relation between water content, glass transition, and stability [58–60].

As noted above, comparative studies demonstrate spray drying is as good as freeze drying to provide stabilization; however, spray drying has been shown to have advantages to freeze or foam drying when the use of engineered particles is required. For example, spray drying has been extensively used to produce dry powders for inhalation with controlled size, morphology, density, and surface composition. Spray-dried powders for inhalation perfectly illustrate the evolution of spray drying from a research laboratory-scale operation to now be fully adopted as a contemporary pharmaceutical unit operation. Representative examples of spray-dried biotherapeutics for inhalation that demonstrate the breath of the production scale from grams per hour to 15 kg/d that have been tested in early clinical trials or commercialized are shown in Table 7.1. Many other examples have been described in the literature [66].

Spray drying has also been extensively proven to be a viable process for vaccine stabilization. The need to develop a technology to break the cold chain needed for vaccine stockpiling and distribution has been addressed using spray drying with the purpose of achieving vaccine thermostabilization [47, 67–70].

One of the first patents described spray drying as method to obtain thermostable vaccines [71], protecting against pathogens such as influenza virus, parainfluenza virus, respiratory syncytial virus, herpes simplex virus, SARS virus, cytomegalovirus, coronavirus family members, human metapneumovirus,

Table 7.1 Spray-dried inhaled biotherapeutics that have been commercialized or tested in clinical trials.

Biotherapeutic	Indication	Stage of development	Reference
Tobramycin	Cystic fibrosis (CF) lung infection	Commercial	[13]
Insulin (Pfizer/Nektar)	Diabetes	Commercial	[11]
Leuprolide (Nektar)	Endometriosis	Phase 2	[61]
Calcitonin (Nektar)	Osteoporosis	Phase 2	[62]
Human growth hormone (Lilly/advance inhalation research (AIR))	Growth hormone deficiency	Phase 2	[63]
Pitrakinra (Aerovance)	Asthma	Phase 2	[64]
VR942 antibody (union chimique belge (UCB) therapeutics/Vectura)	Asthma	Phase 2	[65]

Table 7.2 Investigational spray-dried vaccine formulations.

Vaccine	Shelf life	Route of administration/ composition	Reference
Anthrax Recombinant protective antigen (rPA) of *Bacillus anthracis* bacterium	20 °C; >1 mo 40 °C; >1 mo	Nasal/trehalose	[72]
Cholera Inactivated *Vibrio cholerae* bacterium	Not reported	Oral/microparticles with enteric coating Eudragit® L 30 D-55 and FS 30 D	[73]
Hepatitis B Recombinant hepatitis B surface antigen	37 °C; >2 y	Intramuscular/trehalose, mannitol	[74]
Hepatitis B virus (HBV) Recombinant hepatitis B surface antigen	Not reported	Pulmonary/nanoparticle aggregate, poly(lactic acid) and poly(lactic-co-glycolic acid), L-leucine	[75]
Human papillomavirus (HPV) Bacteriophage virus-like particle against human papillomavirus	37 °C; > 1 y	Oral, intramuscular/mannitol, trehalose, dextran, and L-leucine	[76]
Influenza Influenza antigen	Not reported	Pulmonary, subcutaneous/trehalose and L-leucine	[77]
Influenza Subunit vaccine	20 °C; >3 y	Pulmonary/inulin	[78]
Influenza Live attenuated virus	25 °C; 6 mo	Pulmonary, subcutaneous, nasal/sucrose, trehalose, Pluronic F68, methionine, arginine, ethylenediamine tetraacetic acid (EDTA), citrate	[71]
Influenza Live attenuated virus	4 °C; 30 wk 25 °C; 1 wk	Pulmonary, subcutaneous, nasal/sucrose, Pluronic F68	[34]
Influenza/tetanus/ diphtheria/pertussis *Haemophilus influenzae* type b conjugate, diphtheria toxoid, tetanus toxoid, and pertussis toxin	Not reported	Subcutaneous/poly(lactic acid) and poly(lactic-co-glycolic acid), trehalose microspheres	[79]
Measles Live attenuated virus	Not reported	Buccal/bovine serum albumin particles dispersed in orally dissolving film Lycoat RS 720®, Neosorb P 60W®, and Tween 80	[80]
Measles Live attenuated virus	Not reported	Pulmonary/specific immunity was induced after dry powder vaccination although levels induced were lower than injection and nebulization	[81]
Meningitis group A Protein–polysaccharide conjugate vaccine	40 °C; ≥20 wk 60 °C; ≥2 wk	Intramuscular/trehalose $AlPO_4$ adjuvant	[74]

(*continued*)

Table 7.2 (Continued)

Vaccine	Shelf life	Route of administration/ composition	Reference
Pneumonia Pneumococcal surface protein A	Not reported	Pulmonary/antigen-loaded polyvinyl alcohol (PVA) nanoparticles embedded in L-leucine microparticles	[82]
Tularemia Recombinant live attenuated bacteria *Listeria monocytogenes* expressing *Francisella tularensis* immune protective antigen pathogenicity island protein IglC	Room temperature (~23 °C); >1 y 40 °C; >180 d	Pulmonary/mannitol, trehalose, dextran, L-leucine, and inositol	[83]
Tuberculosis Live attenuated adenovirus vector	25 °C; >12 mo 37 °C; >5 wk	Pulmonary/mannitol, trehalose cyclodextrin, dextran	[84]
Tuberculosis Recombinant antigen 85B expressed in *Escherichia coli*	Not reported	Pulmonary/poly(lactic-co-glycolic acid) microparticles	[85] [86]
Tuberculosis Live attenuated *Bacillus* Calmette–Guérin	5 °C; >9 mo 25 °C; 30 d	Pulmonary/L-leucine	[87], [88], [89]

and Epstein–Barr virus. The formulation described consisted of a polyol (e.g. trehalose, sucrose, raffinose, lactose, glycerol, mannitol, or sorbitol), a polymer (e.g. polyvinylpyrrolidone, hydroxyethyl starch, serum albumin, or gelatin), and a surfactant (e.g. polyethylene glycol, sorbitan monolaurate, block copolymers, polyethylene, polypropylene glycol, or polyoxyethylenesorbitan monooleate), and an amino acid (e.g. arginine, lysine, methionine, histidine, or glutamic acid).

Ever since, several examples describing investigational spray-dried vaccine formulations have been published (see Table 7.2). A cursory analysis of such examples demonstrates the applicability of spray-dried formulations to stabilize antigens, which are usually proteins and polysaccharides and less frequently lipids (anthrax, hepatitis B, influenza, tetanus, diphtheria, meningitis, pertussis, pneumonia, tuberculosis), live attenuated viruses (influenza, rotavirus, measles, human papillomavirus, live attenuated virus vector for tuberculosis), and live attenuated bacteria (anthrax, cholera, tuberculosis, tularemia). Vaccine thermostability is achieved in all instances, and the formulation complexity increases from stabilizing an antigen to stabilizing a virus to stabilizing a bacterium. The formulations described for all the reported examples are combination variations of a polyol, polymer, surfactant, and an amino acid.

Encouraging results can be highlighted, for example, a flu vaccine stable for at least six months at 25 °C [71] stability defined as the vaccine losing less than 1 log potency titer in focus-forming units per milliliter. Or a spray-dried measles vaccine that can remain stable for at least eight weeks at 37 °C [55] or even achieving one month at 25 °C for a live attenuated bacteria tuberculosis vaccine would make a difference in the field of mass vaccination.

In addition to thermostability, particle engineering via spray drying has enabled pulmonary delivery of influenza subunit vaccine [90], measles vaccine [81], or tuberculosis [88]. Another notable example of the use of particle engineering of spray-dried particles to enable novel dosage forms is the formulation of spray-dried rotavirus vaccine particles into an oral quick dissolve strip [91]. In this application a rotavirus vaccine is stabilized in a dry powder to enable room-temperature stability, and the spray-dried powder is so stable that it can be dispersed into an organic solvent containing a dissolved polymer, which is made into a film. More recently a similar application has been reported for a buccal measles vaccine [80].

7.4 Future Direction: Aseptic Spray Drying

The application of spray drying within an aseptic pharmaceutical process can be traced back to at least 1975 [92] yet is still considered a new technology in many ways as the first biologic product utilizing this technology was approved by the FDA in 2015 [93]. During this 40-year span, patents and studies were published supporting the viability of aseptic spray-drying equipment and processes [94–97] for the production of dried pharmaceutical and biological entities. Spray-dried biologics such as monoclonal antibodies have been shown to maintain viability and in some cases demonstrate superior dried product stability compared with the lyophilized product [98].

While freeze drying is an established technology for aseptic processing of biologics, spray-drying equipment vendors are now providing hardware and support for good manufacturing process (GMP) aseptic installations over a range of processing scales from benchtop to pilot to commercial production levels [99, 100]. One example of a large-scale commercial aseptic system is shown in Figure 7.17. In addition to the availability of commercial aseptic spray-drying equipment, at least one contract manufacturing organization (CMO) has made this technology available [101] on a toll basis, enabling more groups to explore this alternative form of dry powder production while deferring large capital outlays to bring the technology in-house.

The advantages of aseptic spray drying include the ability to implement particle engineering techniques within an aseptic process to create the desired product attributes such as particle size, density, surface composition and energy, etc. These properties drive product performance characteristics such as surface composition, powder flowability, wetting, and rehydration. Controlling properties at the particle level is not available to the product designer utilizing standard lyophilization technology, which creates a packed "cake" product. The solid form requires subsequent milling to generate a flowable powder, should this be required for subsequent downstream processing or to aliquot unit dose below a full vial volume. Milling creates new surface areas from the solid interior; hence for a multicomponent solid, control of the surface composition of the final powder is not possible. While sub-vial unit dosing can be conducted from a vial at the point of use via rehydration, the product stability of any remaining vial material becomes limited to that of the liquid state.

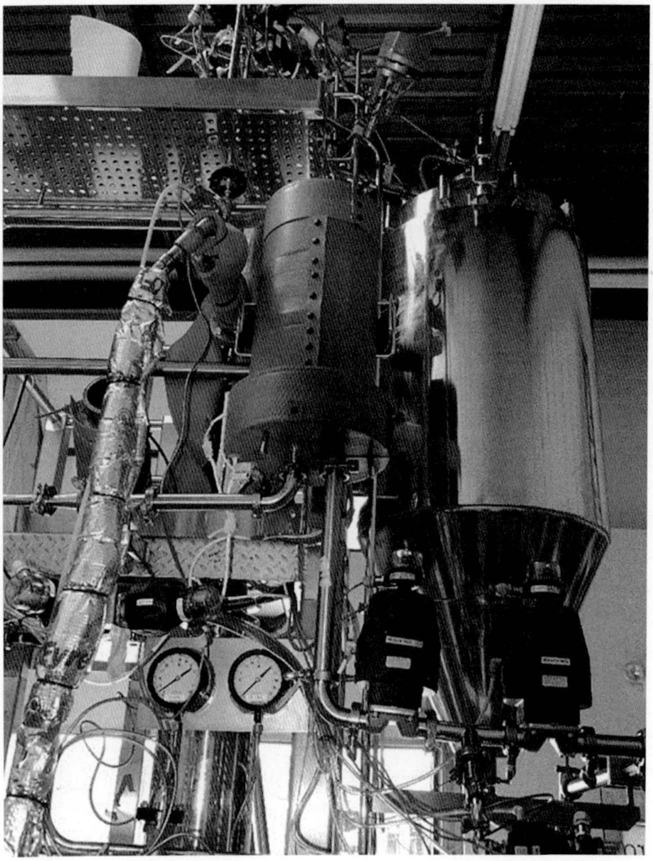

Figure 7.17 Commercial-scale aseptic spray-drying system. Source: Image courtesy of SPX Flow Inc.

In comparison, bulk free-flowing spray-dried powder can be blended and filled into many desired product formats through implementation of appropriate aseptic powder handing and filling processes while maintaining the enhanced stability of the dried solid product. The continuous flow nature of the spray-drying process provides an inherent process throughput advantage over lyophilization when coupled with aseptic powder filling technology. The powder is created in a matter of seconds, with potential powder production rates in the kilogram per hours range. The bulk powder can then be aseptically filled into a variety of product formats. In comparison, the cycle times for lyophilization can require multiple days to produce a dried powder, and the product format is limited to those compatible with the freeze-drying process, typically vials or bags.

System losses with aseptic spray drying and powder filling are dependent upon particle sizes produced during the drying operation. Existing spray-drying technology producing mean particle sizes above 30 μm routinely recover in excess of 95% of the spray dried product in commercial operations with kilogram-scale batch sizes. The dryer yield will decline as the particle diameter decreases with spray-dried inhalation products targeting sub-5 μm mean diameters. Custom-developed cyclone separator technologies have demonstrated 85–91% recovery of inhalation particles in commercial processes with future improvements possible through the use of multiple inertial separators in convert with filtration capture designs.

For processes involving a separate aseptic dried powder filling operation, additional material loss of 10–15% can be expected, with the higher loss attributed to smaller mean particle sizes that tend to aerosolize during filling. Continuing advancements in this field have been reported [102] with the application of ultrasonic vibration to improve the powder filling efficiency of small-diameter cohesive powders and small fill weights.

Most spray-drying systems designed for processing API under validated cGMP conditions utilize a sealed system with high efficiency particulate air (HEPA)-level filtered inputs and the unit operating in a clean room environment, typically class 10K or 100K (ISO 7 or 8). Such systems routinely produce "low-bioburden" dried powder products, but not necessarily aseptic (free from microbial pathogens) and therefore not considered sterile, the absence of all microorganisms.

Conversion of a low-bioburden spray dryer to an aseptic one involves adherence to aseptic processing guidance documents [103, 104] through modified dryer hardware and additional engineered environmental controls to address areas of potential microbial contamination. Spray-dryer specific areas for attention involve three fundamental functions [105].

7.4.1 Initial System Sterilization of Product Contact Surfaces

For small powder production requirements (<1 kg/h) applications, such as clinical development batches, small-scale spray dryers can be disassembled, cleaned, and autoclaved at the component level and reassembled inside a class 100 (ISO 5) isolator system. This would require appropriate facilities to handle the sterilized components as well as sterilize the interior of the glovebox isolator system inside the cGMP suite environment.

For larger-scale and commercial processing systems where disassembly is not feasible, both appropriate CIP and sterilization systems are required. Assembled system sterilization can be performed with a number of methods such as:

(a) Clean steam (steam in place [SIP]).
(b) Dry heat.
(c) Chemical vapor phase disinfection, such as ethylene oxide or hydrogen peroxide.

The standard for in-process sterilization is considered to be the SIP approach for sterilizing direct product contact surfaces. This process exposes the equipment to lower temperatures, but elevated pressure for a shorter period of time compared with the dry heat approach. A system pressure check is required, and the SIP system approach requires appropriate equipment accommodations such as condensate traps and thermal insulation strategy, but does not introduce the complications involved with handling sterilizing vapor compounds.

Design modifications of the spray-drying hardware itself may also be required to aid in validation of the CIP and SIP steps, for example, the elimination of any mechanical threads potentially exposed to the process stream. While it is common practice for non-aseptic cGMP spray-dryer systems to have atomizer designs with replaceable nozzle tips utilizing internal thread connections, these parts are traditionally cleaned out of place with the potential product contact surfaces fully exposed for cleaning and validation. For aseptic operation with CIP and SIP, the assembled system is sterilized prior to processing start-up, and crevices that act to shelter the microorganisms from the sanitization process should be eliminated. In addition, appropriate drainage of condensate should be addressed with a suitable aseptic atomizer design.

7.4.2 Maintaining a Sterile Environment over the Course of the Spray-Dried Batch

Once the system is considered sterilized and ready for start-up, maintaining sterility for a continuous flow-through spray-drying process is controlled by the appropriate design and implementation of a sterile barrier filtration strategy. Validated filter integrity testing (FDA Guidance [103]) procedures assure that the dryer input streams and any potential backflow into the product stream are controlled to maintain the sterile environment from the initial contact point with the filtered liquid feed through to the collection point of the dried particles, typically occurring in a product recovery cyclone separator.

Additional process monitoring points can be implemented during operation, such a filter differential pressure measurements along with pre/post-run integrity testing. Aseptic spray drying should be conducted under mildly elevated drying chamber pressure conditions above ambient (<1 psig or 0.069 bar) to assure that no ambient air can be ingested into the process.

7.4.3 Aseptic Extraction and Handling the Dried Powder Product from the Dryer System

Pharmaceutical spray-dried product collection typically occurs downstream of the drying chamber in a cyclone separation system, as shown in Figure 7.2. The powder is captured at the bottom of the cyclone in a collection vessel, sealed within the process stream. For standard, non-aseptic systems, the collector is removed on a regular basis throughout the drying run with the interval based upon the collector size, cyclone efficiency, and powder production rate. The dryer continues to operate during this "change-out" period with the collector being isolated from the process stream, typically by utilizing a "butterfly"-type valve arrangement. Implementation of a split plate design enables both the lower cyclone exit and collector entrance to be sealed upon collector removal. This enables the drying process to continue and the product to not be exposed to the local environment. When closed, these valves must form an effective gas seal across the lower cyclone outlet diameter, which vary from 2 to 6 in., during the collector change-out process. However, when the valve is opened and powder is filling the collection vessel, the mechanism must not create a disruption in the cyclone outlet flow pattern, which could reduce product recovery yield. Loss of yield can be a major driver for process economics when spray-drying high-value biologics.

For aseptic systems, the need for CIP and SIP sterilization requirements can present additional implementation challenges for collector valve isolation during operation. These valves can be difficult to clean and sterilize in place due the exposed crevices in which powder can migrate and the thermal mass of the valve body. Continued development of robust valve hardware design approaches would be beneficial to allow multiple powder extraction events to occur during extended spray drying while still meeting the requirements for aseptic processing and high product yield.

One effective approach is to eliminate the isolation valve all together and size the collector to enable extended run times, with appropriate vessel thermal control. The dryer flow would be momentarily interrupted, and the collector removed from the cyclone inside a sterilized glovebox isolator. A replacement sterilized collection vessel would be connected to the cyclone and the flow reinitiated. The amount of production time lost during this process will depend upon the thermal stabilization time of the spray dryer as equilibrium conditions will be interrupted.

Future demand for stabilized dry powder biologic products suitable for parenteral or alternate delivery platforms could benefit from the ability to engineer powder properties at the particle level while utilizing a rapid, scalable, high throughput, continuous production process. All characteristics embodied in aseptic spray-drying technology.

References

1 La Mont, C.A. (1865). Improvement in preserving eggs. US Patent 51,263A. issued 28 November 28 1965.

2 Peroy, S. (1872). Improvement in drying and concentrating liquid substances by atomizing. US Patent 125406 A., filed 9 April 1872

3 Masters, K. (1979). Applications of spray drying. In: *Spray Drying Handbook* (ed. E.J. Crosby), 481–516. New York: Halsted Press.

4 Lefebvre, A.H. (1989). *Atomization and Sprays*. New York: Hemisphere Publishing Corporation.

5 Sonntag, R.E. and Van Wylen, G.V. (1982). *Introduction to Thermodynamics, Classical and Statistical*, 2e. New York: Wiley.

6 Crowe, C., Sommerfeld, M., and Tsuji, Y. (1998). *Multiphase Flows with Droplets and Particles*. Boca Raton, FL: CRC Press.

7 Vehring, R. (2008). Expert review: pharmaceutical particle engineering via spray drying. *Pharmaceutical Research* 25: 999–1022.

8 Heumann, W.L. (1997). *Industrial Air Pollution Control Systems*. New York: McGraw-Hill.

9 Sadrzadeh, N., Miller, D.P., Lechuga-Ballesteros, D. et al. (2010). Solid-state stability of spray-dried insulin powder for inhalation: chemical kinetics and structural relaxation modeling of EXUBERA above and below the glass

transition temperature. *Journal of Pharmaceutical Sciences* 99: 3698–3710. Selected for special issue dedicated to Professor Stephen R. Byrn.

10 Stevenson, C.L. and Bennett, D.B. (2014). Development of the EXUBERA insulin pulmonary delivery system. In: *Mucosal Delivery of Biopharmaceuticals* (eds. J. das Neves and B. Sarmento), 461–481. New York: Springer.

11 White, S., Bennett, D.B., Cheu, S. et al. (2005). EXUBERA®: Pharmaceutical development of a novel product for pulmonary delivery of insulin. *Diabetes Technology & Therapeutics* 7: 896–906.

12 Kling, J. (2014). Sanofi to propel inhalable insulin Afrezza into market. *Nature Biotechnology* 32: 851–852.

13 Geller, D.E., Weers, J.G., and Heuerding, S. (2011). Development of an inhaled dry-powder formulation of tobramycin using PulmoSphere™ technology. *Journal of Aerosol Medicine and Pulmonary Drug Delivery* 24: 175–182.

14 Vehring, R., Lechuga-Ballesteros, D., Joshi, V. et al. (2012). Cosuspensions of microcrystals and engineered microparticles for uniform and efficient delivery of respiratory therapeutics from pressurized metered dose inhalers. *Langmuir* 28: 15015–15023.

15 Vehring, R., Foss, W.R., and Lechuga-Ballesteros, D. (2007). Particle formation in spray drying. *Journal of Aerosol Science* 38: 728–746.

16 Boraey, M.A. and Vehring, R. (2014). Diffusion controlled formation of microparticles. *Journal of Aerosol Science* 67: 131–143.

17 Baldelli, A., Boraey, M.A., Nobes, D.S., and Vehring, R. (2015). Analysis of the particle formation process of structured microparticles. *Molecular Pharmaceutics* 12: 2562–2573.

18 Baldelli, A., Power, R.M., Miles, R.E.H. et al. (2016). Effect of crystallization kinetics on the properties of spray dried microparticles. *Aerosol Science and Technology* 50: 693–704.

19 Baldelli, A. and Vehring, R. (2016a). Analysis of cohesion forces between monodisperse microparticles with rough surfaces. *Colloids and Surfaces A: Physicochemical and Engineering Aspects* 506: 176–189.

20 Baldelli, A. and Vehring, R. (2016b). Control of the radial distribution of chemical components in spray-dried crystalline microparticles. *Aerosol Science and Technology* 50: 1130–1142.

21 Lintingre, E., Lequeux, F., Talini, L., and Tsapis, N. (2016). Control of particle morphology in the spray drying of colloidal suspensions. *Soft Matter* 12: 7435–7444.

22 Hoe, S., Boraey, M.A., Ivey, J.M. et al. (2014). Manufacturing and device options for the delivery of biotherapeutics. *Journal of Aerosol Medicine and Pulmonary Drug Delivery* 27: 315–328.

23 Katkov, I. and Levine, F. (2004). Prediction of the glass transition temperature of water solutions: Comparison of different models. *Cryobiology* 49: 62–82.

24 Hancock, B.C., Shamblin, S.L., and Zografi, G. (1995). Molecular mobility of amorphous pharmaceutical solids below their glass transition temperatures. *Pharmaceutical Research* 12: 799–806.

25 Broadhead, J., Rouan, S.K.E., and Rhodes, C.T. (1992). The spray drying of pharmaceuticals. *Drug Development and Industrial Pharmacy* 18: 1169–1206.

26 Ameri, M. and Maa, Y.-F. (2006). Spray drying of biopharmaceuticals: stability and process considerations. *Drying Technology* 24: 763–768.

27 Krzysztof, S. and Krzysztof, C. (2010). Spray drying technique: II. Current applications in pharmaceutical technology. *Journal of Pharmaceutical Sciences* 99: 587–597.

28 Lee, G. (2002). Spray drying of proteins. In: *Rational Design of Stable Protein Formulations* (eds. J.F. Carpenter and M.C. Manning), 135–158. New York: Kluwer Academic/Plenum.

29 Maa, Y.-F. and Prestrelski, S.J. (2000). Biopharmaceutical powders: particle formation and formulation considerations. *Current Pharmaceutical Biotechnology* 1: 283–302.

30 Snyder, H.E. and Lechuga-Ballesteros, D. (2008). Spray drying: theory and pharmaceutical applications. In: *Pharmaceutical Dosage Forms: Tablets* (eds. L.L. Augsburger and S.W. Hoag). New York: Informa Health Care.

31 Abdul-Fattah, A., Kalonia, D.S., and Pikal, M.J. (2007a). The challenge of drying method selection for protein pharmaceuticals: product quality implications. *Journal of Pharmaceutical Sciences* 96: 1886–1916.

32 Abdul-Fattah, A., Lechuga-Ballesteros, D., Kalonia, D., and Pikal, M.J. (2008). The impact of drying method and formulation on the physical properties and stability of methionyl human growth hormone in the amorphous solid state. *Journal of Pharmaceutical Sciences* 1: 163–184.

33 Abdul-Fattah, A., Truong-Le, V., Yee, L. et al. (2007b). Drying-induced variations in physico-chemical properties of amorphous pharmaceuticals and their impact on stability (I): stability of a monoclonal antibody. *Journal of Pharmaceutical Sciences* 96: 1983–2008.

34 Abdul-Fattah, A.M., Truong-Le, V., Yee, L. et al. (2007c). Drying-induced variations in physico-chemical properties of amorphous pharmaceuticals and their impact on stability II: stability of a vaccine. *Pharmaceutical Research* 24: 715–727.

35 de Jesus, S.S. and Maciel Filho, R. (2014). Drying of α-amylase by spray drying and freeze drying: a comparative study. *Brazilian Journal of Chemical Engineering* 31: 625–631.

36 Ståhl, K., Claesson, M., Lilliehorn, P. et al. (2002). The effect of process variables on the degradation and physical properties of spray dried insulin intended for inhalation. *International Journal of Pharmaceutics* 233: 227–237.

37 Maa, Y.-F. and Hsu, C.C. (1997). Protein denaturation by combined effect of shear and air-liquid Interface. *Biotechnology and Bioengineering* 54: 503–512.

38 Hawe, A., Wiggenhorn, M., van de Weert, M. et al. (2012). Forced degradation of therapeutic proteins. *Journal of Pharmaceutical Sciences* 101: 895–913.

39 Lechuga-Ballesteros, D., Charan, C., Stults, C.L.M. et al. (2008). Trileucine improves aerosol performance and stability of spray-dried powders for inhalation. *Journal of Pharmaceutical Sciences* 97: 287–302.

40 Fäldt, P. and Bergenståhl, B. (1994). The surface composition of spray-dried protein—lactose powders. *Colloids and Surfaces A: Physicochemical and Engineering Aspects* 90 (2–3): 183–190.

41 Millqvist-Fureby, A., Malmsten, M., and Bergenstahl, B. (1999). Spray-drying of trypsin: surface characterization and activity preservation. *International Journal of Pharmaceutics* 188: 243–253.

42 Millqvist-Fureby, A., Malmsten, M., and Bergenstahl, B. (1999c). Surface characterization of freeze-dried protein/carbohydrate mixtures. *International Journal of Pharmaceutics* 191: 103–114.

43 Feng, A.L., Boraey, M.A., Gwin, M.A. et al. (2011). Mechanistic models facilitate efficient development of leucine containing microparticles for pulmonary delivery. *International Journal of Pharmaceutics* 409: 155–163.

44 Li, H.-Y., Neill, H., Innocent, R. et al. (2003). Enhanced dispersibility and deposition of spray-dried powders for pulmonary gene therapy. *Journal of Drug Targeting* 11: 425–432.

45 Matinkhoo, S., Lynch, K.H., Dennis, J.J. et al. (2011). Spray-dried respirable powders containing bacteriophages for the treatment of pulmonary infections. *Journal of Pharmaceutical Sciences* 100: 5197–5205.

46 Shur, J., Nevell, T.G., Ewen, R.J. et al. (2008). Cospray-dried unfractionated heparin with L-Leucine as a dry powder inhaler mucolytic for cystic fibrosis therapy. *Journal of Pharmaceutical Sciences* 97: 4857–4868. https://doi.org/10.1002/jps.21362.

47 Sou, T., Forbes, R.T., Gray, J. et al. (2016). Designing a multi-component spray-dried formulation platform for pulmonary delivery of biopharmaceuticals: the use of polyol, disaccharide, polysaccharide and synthetic polymer to modify solid-state properties for glassy stabilisation. *Powder Technology* 287: 248–255.

48 Yamashita, C., Nishibayashi, T., Akashi, S. et al. (1998). A novel formulation of dry powder for inhalation of peptides and proteins. In: *Proceedings of Respiratory Drug Delivery VI* (eds. J. Peart and P.R. Byron), 483–485. Buffalo Grove, IL: Interpharm Press.

49 Yang, B., Lesikar, D., Tan, M.M. et al. (2002). Formulation of human growth hormone for pulmonary delivery. *AAPSPharmSci* 4: Abstract W5073.

50 Li, L., Sun, S., Parumasivam, T. et al. (2016). L-Leucine as an excipient against moisture on in vitro aerosolization performances of highly hygroscopic spray-dried powders. *European Journal of Pharmaceutics and Biopharmaceutics* 102: 132–141.

51 Chan, H.K., Clark, A.R., Feeley, J. et al. (2004). Physical stability of salmon calcitonin spray-dried powders for inhalation. *Journal of Pharmaceutical Sciences* 93: 792–804.

52 Leung, S.S.Y., Parumasivam, T., Gao, F.G. et al. (2016). Production of inhalation phage powders using spray freeze drying and spray drying techniques for treatment of respiratory infections. *Pharmaceutical Research* 33: 1486–1496.

53 Leung, S.S.Y., Parumasivam, T., Gao, F.G. et al. (2017). Effects of storage conditions on the stability of spray dried, inhalable bacteriophage powders. *International Journal of Pharmaceutics* 52: 141–149.

54 Burger, J.L., Cape, S.P., Braun, C.S. et al. (2008). Stabilizing formulations for inhalable powders of live-attenuated measles virus vaccine. *Journal of Aerosol Medicine and Pulmonary Drug Delivery* 21: 25–34.

55 Ohtake, S., Martin, R.A., Yee, L. et al. (2010). Heat-stable measles vaccine produced by spray drying. *Vaccine* 28: 1275–1284.

56 Cicerone, M.T. and Soles, C.L. (2004). Fast dynamics and stabilization of proteins: binary glasses of trehalose and glycerol. *Biophysical Journal* 86: 3836–3845.

57 Maury, M., Murphy, K., Kumar, S. et al. (2005). Spray-drying of proteins: effects of sorbitol and trehalose on aggregation and FT-IR amide I spectrum of an immunoglobulin G. *European Journal of Pharmaceutics and Biopharmaceutics* 59: 251–261.

58 Lechuga-Ballesteros, D. and Miller, D.P. (2005). The hydration limit of amorphous solids and long term stability. In: *Water Properties of Food, Pharmaceutical and Biological Materials* (eds. M.D.P. Buera, J. Welti-Chanes, P.J. Lillford and H.R. Corti), 303–308. Boca Raton, FL: CRC Taylor & Francis.

59 Lechuga-Ballesteros, D., Miller, D.P., and Bakri, A. (2003). Characterization of the interactions of water vapor and amorphous pharmaceutical solids. *Pharmaceutical Research* 20: 308–318.

60 Lechuga-Ballesteros, D., Miller, D.P., and Zhang, J. (2002). Residual water in amorphous solids, measurement and effects on stability. In: *Progress in Amorphous Food and Pharmaceutical Systems* (ed. H. Levine), 275–316. London: The Royal Society of Chemistry.

61 Eldon, M.A. (2003). New developments in inhalation therapy: systemic and local drug treatment. American College of Clinical Pharmacology Annual Meeting, Tampa, Florida. September 21, 2003.

62 Patton, J.S. and Platz, R.M. (1992). (D) Routes of delivery: Case studies: (2) Pulmonary delivery of peptides and proteins for systemic action. *Advanced Drug Delivery Reviews* 8: 179–196.

63 McElroy, M.C., Kirton, C., Gliddon, D., and Wolff, R.K. (2013). Inhaled biopharmaceutical drug development: nonclinical considerations and case studies. *Inhalation Technology* 25: 219–232.

64 Wenzel, S.E., Wilbraham, D., Fuller, R. et al. (2007). Effect of an interleukin-4 variant on late phase asthmatic response to allergen challenge in asthmatic patients: results of two phase 2a studies. *Lancet* 370: 1422–1431.

65 Vectura-Limited. (2015). An evaluation of VR942 in healthy volunteers and patients with mild asthma (NCT02473939). US National Institute of Health, ClinicalTrialsgov, filed 21 December 2016.

66 Weers, J.G., Tarara, T.E., and Clark, A.R. (2007). Design of fine particles for pulmonary drug delivery. *Expert Opinion on Drug Delivery* 4: 297–313.

67 Lu, D. and Hickey, A.J. (2007). Pulmonary vaccine delivery. *Expert Review of Vaccines* 6: 213–226.

68 Sou, T., Meeusen, E.N., Veer, M.D. et al. (2011). New developments in dry powder pulmonary vaccine delivery. *Trends in Biotechnology* 29: 191–198.

69 Tlaxca, J.L., Ellis, S., and Remmele, R.L. Jr., (2015). Live attenuated and inactivated viral vaccine formulation and nasal delivery: potential and challenges. *Advanced Drug Delivery Reviews* 93: 56–78.

70 Truong-Le, V. and Abdul-Fattah, A.M. (2008). Drying process methods for biopharmaceutical products: an overview. In: *Formulation and Process Development Strategies for Manufacturing of a Biopharmaceuticals* (eds. F. Jameel and S. Hershenson). New York: Wiley.
71 Truong-Le, V. and Pham, B. (2007). Preservation of biomaterials by spray drying. US patent 7258873, Medimmune Vaccines, Inc, filed 10 April 2003 and issued 21 August 2007.
72 Jiang, G.E., Joshi, S.B., Peek, L.J. et al. (2006). Anthrax vaccine powder formulations for nasal mucosal delivery. *Journal of Pharmaceutical Sciences* 95: 80–96.
73 Año, G., Esquisabel, A., Pastor, M. et al. (2011). A new oral vaccine candidate based on the microencapsulation by spray-drying of inactivated *Vibrio cholerae*. *Vaccine* 29: 5758–5764.
74 Chen, D., Kapre, S., Goel, A. et al. (2010). Thermostable formulations of a hepatitis B vaccine and a meningitis A polysaccharide conjugate vaccine produced by a spray drying method. *Vaccine* 28: 5093–5099.
75 Muttil, P., Prego, C., García-Contreras, L. et al. (2010). Immunization of guinea pigs with novel hepatitis B antigen as nanoparticle aggregate powders administered by the pulmonary route. *The AAPS Journal* 12: 330–337.
76 Saboo, S., Tumban, E., Peabody, J. et al. (2016). Optimized formulation of a thermostable spray-dried virus-like particle vaccine against human papillomavirus. *Molecular Pharmaceutics* 13: 1646–1655.
77 Sou, T., Morton, D.A.V., Williamson, M. et al. (2015). Spray-dried influenza antigen with trehalose and leucine produces an aerosolizable powder vaccine formulation that induces strong systemic and mucosal immunity after pulmonary administration. *Journal of Aerosol Medicine and Pulmonary Drug Delivery* 28: 361–371.
78 Saluja, V., Amorij, J.-P., Kapteyn, J.C. et al. (2010). A comparison between spray drying and spray freeze drying to produce an influenza subunit vaccine powder for inhalation. *Journal of Controlled Release* 144: 127–133.
79 Boehm, G., Peyre, M., Sesardic, D. et al. (2002). On technological and immunological benefits of multivalent single-injection microsphere vaccines. *Pharmaceutical Research* 19: 1330–1336.
80 Gala, R.P., Popescu, C., Knipp, G.T. et al. (2017). Physicochemical and preclinical evaluation of a novel buccal measles vaccine. *AAPS PharmSciTech* 18: 283–292.
81 de Swart, R.L., LiCalsi, C., Quirk, A.V. et al. (2007). Measles vaccination of macaques by dry powder inhalation. *Vaccine* 25: 1183–1190.
82 Kunda, N.K., Alfagih, I.M., Miyaji, E.N. et al. (2015). Pulmonary dry powder vaccine of pneumococcal antigen loaded nanoparticles. *International Journal of Pharmaceutics* 495: 903–912.
83 Kunda, N.K., Wafula, D., Tram, M. et al. (2016). A stable live bacterial vaccine. *European Journal of Pharmaceutics and Biopharmaceutics* 103: 109–117.
84 Jin, T.H., Tsao, E., Goudsmit, J. et al. (2010). Stabilizing formulations for inhalable powders of an adenovirus 35-vectored tuberculosis (TB) vaccine (AERAS-402). *Vaccine* 28: 4369–4375.

85 Lu, D., García-Contreras, L., Muttil, P. et al. (2010). Pulmonary immunization using antigen 85-B polymeric microparticles to boost tuberculosis immunity. *The AAPS Journal* 12: 338–347.

86 Lu, D., García-Contreras, L., Xu, D. et al. (2007). Poly (lactide-co-glycolide) microspheres in respirable sizes enhance an in vitro T cell response to recombinant Mycobacterium tuberculosis antigen 85B. *Pharmaceutical Research* 24: 1834–1843.

87 Fourie, P.B., Germishuizen, W.A., Wong, Y.L., and Edwards, D.A. (2008). Spray drying TB vaccines for pulmonary administration. *Expert Opinion on Biological Therapeutics* 8: 857–863.

88 García-Contreras, L., Wong, Y.-L., Muttil, P. et al. (2008). Immunization by a bacterial aerosol. *Proceedings of the National Academy of Sciences* 105: 4656–4660.

89 Wong, Y.-L., Sampson, S., Germishuizen, W.A. et al. (2007). Drying a tuberculosis vaccine without freezing. *Proceedings of the National Academy of Sciences of the United States of America* 104: 2591–2595.

90 Amorij, J.P., Saluja, V., Petersen, A.H. et al. (2007). Pulmonary delivery of an insulin-stabilized influenza subunit vaccine prepared by spray-freeze drying induces systemic, mucosal humoral as well as cell-mediated immune responses in BALB/c mice. *Vaccine* 25: 8707–8717.

91 Mao, H.-Q., Ku Yu, C., Truong, V.L., et al. (2008). Quick-dissolving oral thin film for targeted delivery of therapeutic agents. Patent US2008/088300, Johns Hopkins University, USA, filed 1 July 2008 and Publication date 7 January 2010.

92 Masters, K. and Vestergaard, I. (1975). Aseptic and closed cycle spray drying in pharmaceuticals/bio-chemicals manufacture. *Process Biochemistry* 10 (20): 21–23,29.

93 Siew, A. (2016). Exploring the use of aseptic spray drying in the manufacture of biopharmaceutical injectables. *Pharmaceutical Technology* 40: 24–27.

94 Chickering, D.E. (2001). Spray drying apparatus and methods of use. US Patent 6,560,897.

95 Hill, S. (1982). Pharmaceutical composition. US Patent 4,490,383, filed 9 December 9 1982 and issued 25 December 1984.

96 Oftedahl, M. (1979). Polymeric anti-tumor agent and method of preparation. US Patent 4,397,995, filed 29 December 1980 and issued 9 August 1983.

97 Turok, R. (2007). Process gas filtration. US Patent 8,398,732, filed 10 April 2007 and issued 19 March 2013.

98 Bowen, M., Turok, R., and Maa, Y.-F. (2013). Spray drying of monoclonal antibodies: investigating powder-based biologic drug substance bulk storage. *Drying Technology: An International Journal* 31: 1441–1450.

99 GEA. (2017). Aseptic spray dryers: an effective method for sterile solid drug manufacture. http://www.gea.com/zh/binaries/aseptic-spray-dryers-for-sterile-solid-drug-manufacture-brochure-EN_tcm28-24000.pdf (accessed 17 July 2017).

100 SPX Flow. (2013). https://www.spxflow.com/en/literature/articles/efficient-solution-to-pharmaceutical-industry (accessed 7 October 2019).

101 Novalabs. (n.d.). Spray drying solutions for the pharmaceutical industry. https://www.novalabs.co.uk/news-and-events/spray-drying-solutions-for-the-pharmaceutical-industry (accessed 7 July 2017).

102 Naydo, K.A., Parks, D.J., Reich, P. et al. (2014). Powder filling apparatus and methods for their use. US Patent 8,783,305 B2, filed 21 November 2011 and issued 22 July 2014.

103 FDA Guidance. (2004). FDA guidance for industry sterile drug products produced by aseptic processing—current good. Manufacturing Practice, September 2004, Pharmaceutical cGMPs. https://www.fda.gov/downloads/Drugs/Guidances/ucm070342.pdf (accessed 7 July 2017).

104 ISPE. (n.d.). ISPE Baseline® Guide: Sterile Product Manufacturing Facilities (second Edition), September 2011. http://www.ispe.org/publications-guidance-documents/sterile-manufacturing (accessed 7 July 2017).

105 Schwartzbach, H. (2011). Achieving aseptic drying with spray drying technologies. *Pharmaceutical Technology Europe* 23: 90–92.

Part III

Next Generation Drying Technologies

8

Spray Freeze Drying

Bernhard Luy[1] and Howard Stamato[2]

[1] *Meridion Technologies GmbH, Mauchener Str. 14, 79379 Mülheim, Germany*
[2] *Bridgewater, NJ 08807, USA*

8.1 Introduction

Freeze drying is an effective means of preserving the characteristics of temperature- and moisture-sensitive product. The process, referred to as lyophilization in the pharmaceutical industry, removes water by sublimation from the frozen state, leaving a three-dimensional pore network in the resulting solid. These pores enhance reconstitution of the product while the low processing temperatures and low residual water content improve the product stability often allowing storage at room temperature with adequate stability.

The standard practice for lyophilization has evolved from its introduction around 1890 and expansion to industrial applications in the 1950s [1] yet remains a complex process. Typically, the liquid containing dissolved product is filled into vials or in trays. When vials are used, the stopper is loosely put in place to allow escape of vapor during processing. The filled vials or trays are loaded into a vacuum chamber on temperature-controlled shelves used to cycle the product through the desired temperature profile.

There are numerous studies discussing the challenges of heat transfer between the vial and the temperature-controlled shelf due to the shape of the vial, the even distribution of heat or exposure to the desired chamber atmosphere across the geometry of the dryer, the difficulties of measuring product properties during the process, and others [2–5]. These challenges are increased when taken under the conditions of sterile processing. While improved product characteristics are of sufficient value to justify a complex process, there is an opportunity to design an updated system to provide the same advantages in an improved design.

The concept of quality by design (QbD) includes forming a target profile and then designing toward it [6]. In addition to the benefits of low-temperature processing, it would be advantageous to have a homogeneous exposure of the product to the process conditions so that the measurement and control of the process is simplified and the product quality enhanced. The ability to process a larger quantity of product, uniformly, as bulk and then fill into the desired unit doses allows the vials to be filled flexibly, at the desired dose, to

Drying Technologies for Biotechnology and Pharmaceutical Applications, First Edition.
Edited by Satoshi Ohtake, Ken-ichi Izutsu, and David Lechuga-Ballesteros.

meet changing supply chain demands. This forming of a bulk solid requires the formation of mechanically stable, free-flowing solids, with similar reconstitution capabilities to the cake form of lyophilized product. Thus, the requirements of a new process are set out by a simple examination of the product needs.

A process for spray freeze drying has been designed to provide all the desired advantages. The process eliminates the challenges of the vial-on-shelf-in-a-chamber approach, which reduces the development and processing time compared with standard methods. Due to the high sphericity, uniformity, and mechanical properties of the resulting product, the opportunity to provide material efficiently and flexibly from a supply chain standpoint can be achieved. It may also open new applications for lyophilized product in inhalation [7, 8], controlled release formulations [9], or ballistic injection dosage forms [10].

The general operating principle of spray freeze drying is to generate droplets out of a liquid, freeze them under cryogenic conditions, and then remove the solvent from the frozen bulk pellets under freeze-drying conditions. This novel process combines the low-temperature environment, low final moisture content, and porous final product structure of traditional sterile product aseptic lyophilization with favorable aspects of solid dosage form processing. The technology allows for the generation of bulk lyophilized pellets or "bulkware", which is homogeneous and, if required, sterile. By this, it allows application of solid dosage form manufacturing principles for lyophilized products, which to this point was not generally available for formulations that require freeze drying. Therefore, in addition to the product processing and quality improvement aspects, spray freeze drying has the potential for significantly improved efficiency in the supply chain due to increased flexibility of the manufacturing logistics. The technology is currently being introduced by major pharmaceutical companies, and related regulatory aspects are being considered.

8.2 Background

In pharmaceutical process technology, shelf freeze drying is a well-established technology widely used for stabilizing thermosensitive substances or formulations by drying. Solubility enhancement is another reason to use this kind of drying technique [11], in order to increase bioavailability, or for fast disintegrating tablets [12].

8.2.1 Shelf Freeze Drying

Certain limitations are intrinsic to the fact that the freeze drying in shelf-type systems is a static process, except for some process variations, e.g. by introducing rotation of vials in order to increase surface by generating a liquid film along the glass surface [13].

From a process perspective, conventional shelf freeze drying requires the substrate liquid, most often after filling into a vial, to be frozen under static conditions and to be lyophilized under static conditions as well. This prefilled frozen liquid plug limits the heat and mass transfer during drying, because the transfer interface is the cross section of the vial either for heat, at the bottom of the plug through the glass to the shelf, or for mass, at the top of the open vial. As the drying front progresses from the upper end of the frozen liquid where the ice sublimates toward the bottom, the heat to provide sublimation energy must be transferred across the frozen substrate. The heat transfer rate determines the heat energy concentration, which can be applied at the product interface without damaging the product structure. The relevant length scale for water vapor diffusion is on the order of microns. With a typical one centimeter filling height in the vial, the required distance at its maximum is 10 000 μm showing a limitation of the drying process in typical shelf lyophilization.

Finally, the resulting lyo-cake, which remains after sublimation, represents a spongelike structure, which by its nature is not free flowing, even if sectioned into pieces. Due to the geometry of the vial and the processes involved, inhomogeneities may occur, e.g. by circulation and concentration processes during freezing. When lyophilized on shelves, the removal of such lyo-cakes from vials or trays and reduction to particles in a screening mill impose product handling as well as containment and aseptic processing challenges. For product that was lyophilized in a vial or tray and shelf system, this limits the potential use as bulkware.

With respect to manufacturing logistics, the characteristic feature of conventional shelf freeze drying is that with vials being used as primary packaging, the filling is done prior to lyophilization. This has a significant impact on the overall supply chain. In order to fill a liquid, the bulk solution must be available, kept at specific storage conditions and for a limited time prior to processing into the final lyophilized product. In biotechnology processing, the production of the bulk solution is a multistep process that may require weeks prior to lyophilization and in traditional methods will need closely coordinated scheduling.

A freezing of the liquid as bulk with later thawing may be possible, though it carries the risk of loss in activity and furthermore requires cold chain logistics. The shipping containers, the shipping conditions, and any excursions must be specified and qualified for the shipping of the frozen liquid with drug substance if the thawing, drug product formulation, and filling should be done at a different site. Thawing of the bulk solution and any required adjustments for final processing carry risks for inhomogeneity and stability. Once the bulk liquid is filled into a vial, the dosing is fixed, i.e. dose changes or variations in vial numbers require new availability of substrate liquid. This makes the supply chain long, with intrinsic time and cost effects, and at the same time rigid.

8.2.2 Spray Freeze Drying

8.2.2.1 Single Dose vs. Bulk Manufacturing

The concept of solid dosage form technologies is strongly based on availability of pellets, granulation, or powder blend being available for further processing into a variety of forms and strengths of capsules and tablets. Even though there are numerous activities to adopt continuous manufacturing technologies in contrast to batch processing, the general concept of a common intermediate material for further processing remains applicable.

Once the bulk lyophilized pellets are produced, dosing and filling can take place at a different point in time. A combination of products could be as simple as filling pellets of two different types into a capsule due to the limited interaction of components in the solid phase. In contrast, conventional single dose freeze drying in vials puts an end to the bulk status of the substrate, thereby eliminating the degree of flexibility in filling and introducing the possibility of poor stability due to the intimate mixing of components during processing and in the resulting solid.

In comparison with such conventional shelf freeze drying, the most significant difference in logistics is that in spray freeze drying, lyophilization takes place *prior* to filling. The subsequent availability of homogeneous, free-flowing lyophilized bulkware obviously overcomes limitations as described above and is shown in Diagram 8.1.

Bulk intermediate product in general provides a high degree of manufacturing flexibility – for drug product, the filling volume and the number of vials to be filled only depend on the availability of bulk. The filling may take place at any time, independent of the availability of substrate liquid. The primary packaging can take on a variety of forms without constraint by suitability for handling in a shelf-based freeze dryer or for lyophilization processes in general.

Filling on demand, dosing flexibility, small quantity filling, or a single vial aimed at personalized medication are expectations that can be met with lyophilized bulkware. Also, combinatory products can be generated by "compounding on the filling line."

Therefore, bulk availability is a major target when looking at further developments in lyophilization. Advantages and challenges of the two types of lyo-production processing types are described in Table 8.1.

8.2.2.2 Process Considerations

From a product and process point of view, there are several advantages of a droplet/lyophilized sphere conformation compared with a vial with solution/lyophilized cake. For heat and mass transfer, these advantages are driven by geometry. The cake format is bounded on all sides, except the top, by the glass vial. Pellets have an advantage in being exposed on all sides and are easily stirred to homogenize the exposure to a directional heat source.

As an example, the maximum water vapor diffusion distance in a typical lyophilized cake of 1 cm depth is equal to that depth (10 000 μm), while a pellet of typically 0.6 mm diameter will have a maximum diffusion distance equal to the radius (300 μm). Therefore, in vapor diffusion length the pellet form has a threefold advantage.

The surface area available for mass transport is also a factor. The 1 cm diameter cake has only the top surface exposed (78.54 mm^2). The ~6950 (0.6 mm diameter) pellets with equal volume to the lyo-cake (1 cm diameter, 1 cm depth) have a much larger surface area (7854 mm^2). Therefore, in surface area for mass transfer, the pellets have a 100-fold advantage.

Similar advantages exist for heat transfer. The shorter distance and higher surface area to volume ratio for the pellet allow for more efficient heat transfer from

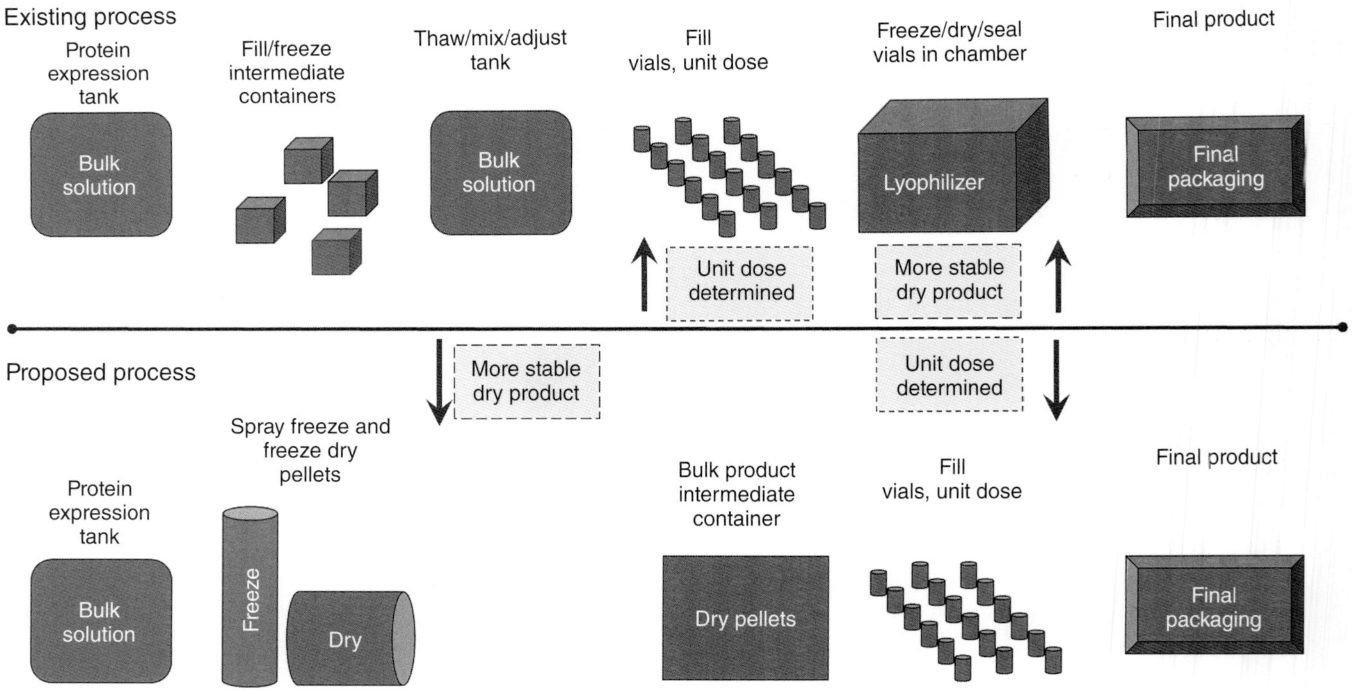

Diagram 8.1 Comparison of process chains for existing and proposed process.

Table 8.1 Process challenges/advantages in lyo-production.

Unit operation	Freeze drying – vial	Spray freeze drying – bulk pellets
Bulk solution	• Batch scheduling and coordination • Storage/shipping of intermediate • Thawing • Mixing/adjustment of bulk liquid • Stability	• Bulk liquid may go directly to more stable bulk solid
Freezing/drying	• Heat transfer • Mass transfer • Cake collapse	• Droplet formation • Attrition
Filling	• Unit dose locked in at viral filling	• Flexible dose and number of units • Alternate delivery modes available
Final package	• Availability dependent on rigid supply chain	• Flexible supply filled as needed

the surface in contact and penetration to more of the product by radiant heating sources compared to the cake format. It depends on the freeze-drying process applied, to which extent this increase in surface is utilized.

Depending on the drying concept used, the drying starts on the surface of each sphere, and the drying front progresses to the core of the particle. This allows more aggressive drying conditions, as the drying energy is applied at a place where the product is already dried, therefore more stable. On the other hand, the heat transfer occurs across the dry product cake, which offers significantly less heat conductivity. Therefore, the method of heat application must take this aspect into account.

8.2.3 Spray-Freeze-Drying Developments

Several approaches have been taken in the past to overcome the limitations of the static nature of conventional shelf freeze drying.

In the 1980s, research was conducted in the area of atmospheric spray freeze drying in fluid-bed processes at Basel University sponsored by the fluid-bed equipment manufacturer Glatt [14, 15]. Specifically, heat and mass transfers were intended to be increased by using a fluidized-bed system, where each single particle exposes the entire surface to the drying process. The process was conducted such that a (heated) nozzle was introduced into a very cold gas stream inside a fluidized-bed apparatus. The droplets generated by the binary nozzle had to be congealed prior to being in contact with each other or with the side walls of the process vessel. In order to provide such conditions, the inlet air had to be reduced to temperatures below −60 °C, with relatively high air velocities in order to prevent any premature contact.

The characteristic feature of this setup was that particle generation and lyophilization (at ambient pressure) took place in one process chamber (single-pot processing). As described by Plitzko [16, 17], the system works in small scale. However, a major limitation is that droplets generated undergo a significant weight reduction, which at high air velocities gives rise to a product accumulation in the upper filter. Thereby, the advantages of fluidization are no longer available to powder on the filters, and recovery of that powder becomes another challenge. Furthermore, for the drying process at ambient pressure, the sublimated vapors must be taken up by the process gas, which at low temperatures has a very low dew point, translating to very low carrying capacity for water vapor. This, in turn, causes the need for gas flow to be very high in order to accommodate the vapor removal rate that may have high operating costs and/or exceed the limit for proper particle motion in the fluidized bed. Therefore, an economically viable and technically feasible process for a sterile pharmaceutical product for parenteral use by using such "single-pot" fluidized-bed process, under atmospheric conditions, turned out to be impractical. The need to separate the freezing and the lyophilization process due to their different processing requirements for optimum conditions was clearly identified.

8.3 Spray Freezing and Dynamic Freeze Drying

For the new technology presented in this chapter, two processes have been developed and adapted for the use in the manufacture of parenteral pharmaceutical formulations [18–20].

In the first process step, frozen microspheres are generated as bulk by dispersing the substrate liquid into single droplets, which fall by gravity through a cooling zone, congealing at ambient pressure, i.e. in a cold gas atmosphere, to frozen spheres.

The second process step is the lyophilization of the frozen bulk material under dynamic conditions with constant gentle mixing in a slowly rotating, temperature-controlled, double wall drum, under typical vacuum conditions, using infrared (IR) radiation as sublimation energy besides the drum surface in contact with the bulk product.

The two processes can be operated in separate units as stand-alone equipment, especially for development purposes. This allows for the parallel development of the frozen droplet and lyophilized pellet steps. For sterile operations, the two process steps are combined to a fully contained, sterilizable process line with product handling by gravity. Configuration options for the process equipment at various scales are shown in Diagram 8.2.

8.3.1 Spray Freezing

A spray freezing in general is often described as a process where liquid droplets that were generated by conventional spray nozzles (binary air nozzles or pressure nozzles) are directed into a cryogenic medium, often liquid nitrogen [21].

Droplet generation technology: The use of conventional spray nozzles (e.g. binary air nozzles or pressure nozzles) allows only limited impact on the droplet size

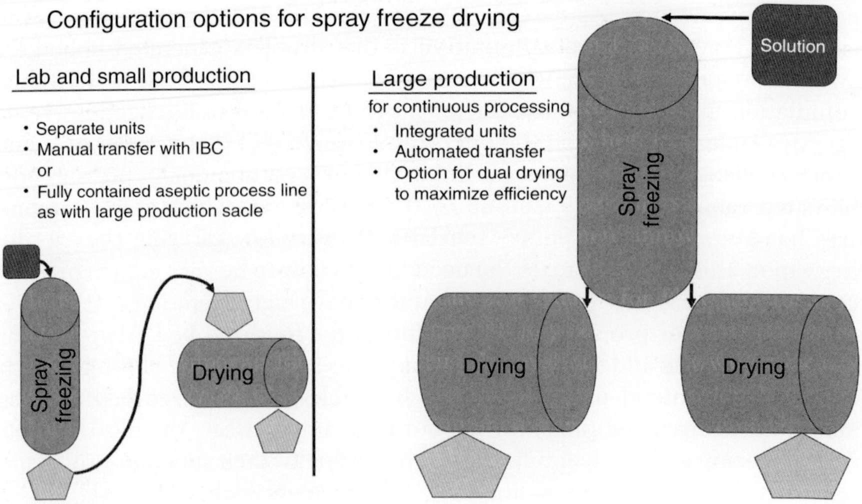

Diagram 8.2 Configuration options for spray freeze drying.

distribution; it will result in a broader particle size range of the frozen bulk, with a significant amount of fines. Also, the impact of spray conditions like high gas velocities and/or pressure conditions with high shear forces must be considered, as a detrimental effect on a sensitive substrate could occur with potential effects on the product potency.

For these reasons, a frequency-driven prilling nozzle is used. It is based on the operating principle of controlled laminar jet breakup. Here, a liquid jet is generated, and a frequency applied to the liquid jet. When at the resonance frequency, the liquid jet disintegrates to sections of similar size, which by surface tension form round droplets of nearly monodisperse size (see Figure 8.1). In this manner about 1000–5000 droplets per second per nozzle can be generated [22]. Once formed, the droplets move by gravity into the cryogenic medium or cryogenic chamber.

Freezing technology: The second part of the initial process step of generating frozen bulk is the freezing of the spherical liquid droplets. For the freezing step, direct contact with liquid nitrogen (LN_2) is avoided. At larger particle sizes, internal mechanical stress may weaken the stability of the frozen particle, when dripping a droplet of several millimeter size into LN_2. For the use in sterile operation, it would furthermore be necessary to use sterile LN_2, which is quite an expensive utility, with challenging validation requirements. On the other hand, it is required to have sufficient transfer of cooling capacity, which is intrinsic to LN_2 (as opposed to gaseous nitrogen [GN_2]).

Furthermore, a directed co- or countercurrent gas flow, similar to that encountered in fluid-bed operations, should be avoided in order to eliminate the need for filters. Such filters can be problematic, especially in sterile and particle-free operations.

Based on these considerations, a new freezing chamber is designed as a cylinder-shaped, double-walled column (see Figure 8.2a). The top lid

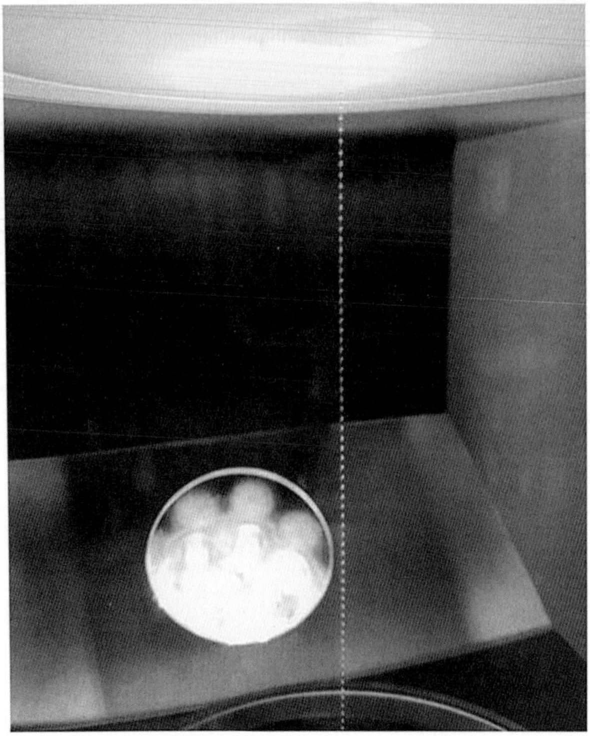

Figure 8.1 Droplet formation by controlled laminar jet breakup: stroboscopic light visualizes single droplets generated with 3500 Hz, i.e. generation of ~3500 droplets/s.

(see Figure 8.2b) carries one or several nozzles for the droplet generation; the lower end is funnel-shaped to guide the frozen spheres to the exit. The double wall is cooled with a mixture of LN_2 and GN_2. As the primary cooling medium is never in direct contact with the substrate, a technical grade LN_2 can be used. The inside of the closed freezing chamber is gas filled with GN_2, if need be sterile, or air as process gas. The heat exchange inside the process chamber is achieved by free convection.

Process considerations for spray freezing: In the droplet generation step, the droplet size depends on several parameters like flow rate, frequency, viscosity (based on formulation and temperature), and orifice diameter. For spray-freeze-drying technology, normally a (selectable) range for the droplets between 300 and 1000 μm is used. Especially for closed sterile operations, an optical monitoring system for the control of droplet generation has been developed as in-process control. The solids content of the substrate liquid can go to 40% for typical bulking agents used in freeze drying, like sucrose or mannitol. The requirements with respect to particle size and size distribution depend also on the accuracy requirements during the filling of the unit dose of the lyophilized bulk.

The freezing step takes place at ambient pressure or at slight overpressure to ensure aseptic processing. The process gas, which can be injected by sterile filtration, is cooled down by the cryogenic atmosphere that is cooled by the chilled walls. Typical operating temperatures for the process gas are in the

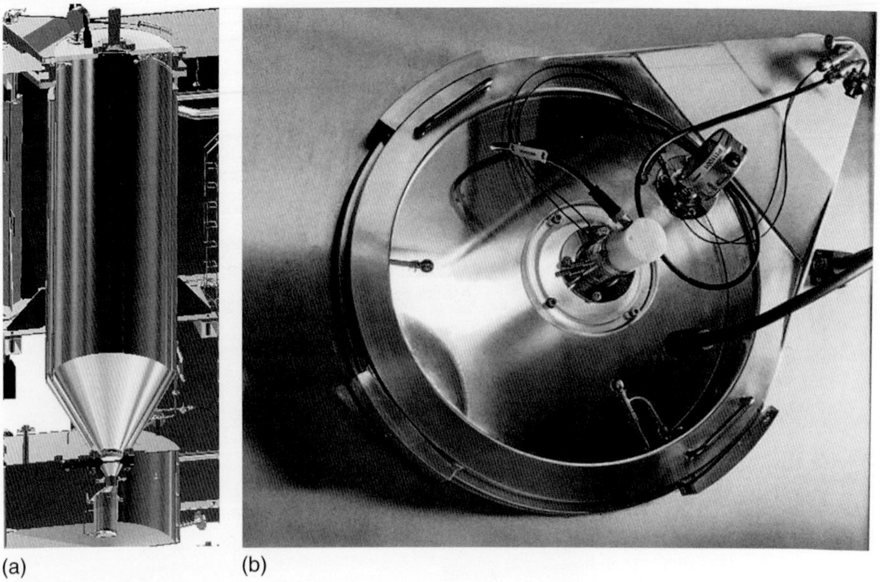

Figure 8.2 (a) Cross-sectional view of spray freezing tower including top lid with nozzle, double wall chamber, and discharge cone (lab scale). (b) Top view of spray freezing tower with lid including frequency nozzle.

range of −80 to −150 °C. In the spray freezing process, a droplet leaving the nozzle falls by gravity through the cold gas atmosphere and congeals into a frozen sphere.

The processing conditions have to ensure that the droplet gets frozen prior to reaching the lower end of the processing chamber. This depends on various parameters like gas temperature, droplet size, formulation (solids content, glass transition temperature), and height of the freezing chamber. The larger the droplets to be frozen, the greater falling height and/or lower gas temperatures required. Spray rates are in the range of 10–35 g/min. For scale-up, multiple nozzles are used.

The height requirement remains unchanged on scale-up, though, as it is determined by the freezing process duration and the droplet falling speed. In the lab environment, height is also to be considered, and a minimum falling distance is required. Typical falling heights for the generation of 300–1000 μm frozen spheres are in the range of 1.5–3.5 m, with traveling times of 1–3 s. As the sinking velocity of droplets may be lower than the velocity of the liquid jet and the droplets that are close to the nozzle orifice, a deflection of the single droplets is recommended to spread out the single line of droplets into a spray cone. This enhances the exposure of the single droplet to the cooling gas and prevents a premature collision of particles, as this could result in coalescence, thereby limiting the control of droplet size.

With respect to bulk volume, there is a volume increase when transforming a liquid into bulkware consisting of frozen pellets. Due to inter- and intraparticle porosity, approximately a doubling of volume can be expected, i.e. 1 l of liquid translates into c. 2 l of frozen bulk.

In a closed setup for aseptic operation, after being sprayed and frozen, the pellets move by gravity down the chamber and through the transfer section to the lyophilization step. In such way, the spray freezing process delivers very homogeneous frozen pellet bulkware, since the liquid that is fed to the nozzle is homogenous, has a rapid heat transfer due to a high surface to volume ratio when formed into a droplet, and with the freezing conditions being controlled results in homogeneous bulkware. Through freezing, the material is transformed from a liquid into a solid bulk, and solid dosage form technology can be applied for further processing.

8.3.2 Dynamic Freeze Drying

Compared with one ice cube or cylinder in a vial or as a thick frozen layer on a shelf, frozen bulk consisting of numerous small spheres have a much larger exposed surface. As used with fluid-bed processing, the large surface of many small frozen particles is a good prerequisite for efficient heat and mass transfer during drying. The dynamic lyophilization process in a rotary freeze dryer provides the process conditions that make use of the large surface area of the pellets. The dynamic freeze-drying process avoids the undesirable aspects of fluid-bed processing, mentioned earlier, and maintains the advantage of high homogeneity of the bulk during drying.

8.3.2.1 Rotary Freeze-Drying Technology

The rotary freeze dryer consists of a cylindrical drum, which is horizontally positioned in a cylindrical vacuum chamber (see Figure 8.3). Adjacent to the chamber are the condenser, vacuum rack, and further installations, comparable with conventional lyophilization. The drum is cantilevered, i.e. there are no support wheels or other moving parts that would cause cleaning or attrition issues. The drum support bearings have a vacuum trap to ensure there is no leakage from the non-clean into the clean area of the process chamber.

The drum itself has front and rear end openings to maximize the cross-sectional area for water vapor flow and is double-walled. Inside the double wall, silicone oil can circulate to cool or heat the inner drum surface. Through the front opening of the drum, one or more IR radiators are introduced that are directing downward. The radiators itself are completely glass covered, and the glass surface is temperature-controlled. The drum rotates around the longitudinal axis, comparable to a tablet coater. Under rotation, the temperature of the bulk, i.e. the product surrounding temperature, is constantly measured, as well as the drum surface temperature.

The drum can be charged with frozen product by gravity. Emptying is achieved by means of integrated discharge scoops that are fully integrated in the drum; by reverse rotation, the bulk product enters the scoops and is conveyed to the rim of the front opening, where it is taken up by a funnel, with further gravity flow downward.

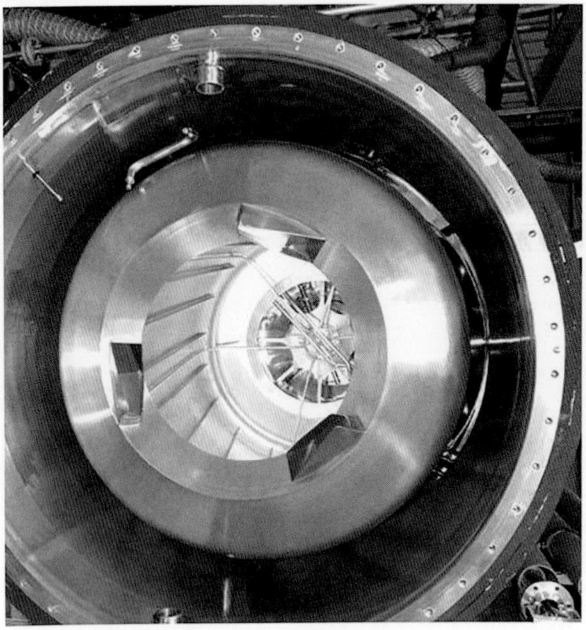

Figure 8.3 Vacuum process chamber housing with rotating double wall drum including three discharge scoops and both rotating and static cleaning nozzles (production size unit with sterilize in place (SIP) and clean in place (CIP), drum diameter c. 1.6 m).

8.3.2.2 Process Considerations

For receiving the frozen bulk, the drum is precooled so that the product stays frozen and free flowing on contact with the drum. In nonsterile development applications, the charging of the drum can be done in open operation. With aseptic process lines, the two process chambers for spray freezing and for rotary freeze drying are connected, with an isolation valve between the spraying chamber and the dryer.

During freezing, the valve is in an open position to allow the frozen pellets to pass into the drying chamber. When the spraying process is completed, the valve is closed to begin drying under vacuum.

For the drying process, the process chamber is evacuated to pressures comparable with conventional freeze drying, e.g. 100 μbar or less, and the drum is put under rotation. By this, the frozen product is under constant movement. The sublimation energy is applied to the product by either IR radiation to the moving surface of the product bed or by conduction via the heated double wall or a combination of both.

Generally speaking, the processing conditions like temperature and pressure, or ramping conditions, are quite similar to the parameters used in conventional freeze drying. Still there are some differences to be noted.

Due to the large surface of the frozen bulk, heat and mass transfer is increased, which allows for generally shorter drying times. In addition, the water vapor diffusion length is significantly reduced. For example, for a 10 mm deep lyo-cake in vial, the maximum diffusion length is 10 000 μm; for a 1 mm diameter microsphere, the maximum diffusion length is 500 μm.

Another improvement of the spray-freeze-drying process is in the heat transfer. In conventional shelf freeze drying, the (contact) heat is transmitted to a limited area across the bottom of the glass vial, and the drying front is moving from the top to the bottom, i.e. the heat transfer takes place across the frozen product. In dynamic freeze drying multiple mechanisms of heat can be used. The heat both from the radiator and the drum surface is transmitted to the surface of a particle. The drying front starts at the surface of the particle and moves from the outside to the center of the microsphere. After an initial phase where a dry outer shell is formed, it is possible to have a high heat flow from the IR radiator. The constantly moving surface of the bulk bed, the high surface area of the pellets, and the high heat flux reduce the drying time.

Both the dynamic conditions inside of the drum and the intended later use of the bulkware as a solid require a minimum mechanical stability of the lyophilized spheres. From a formulation point of view, the overall dissolved solids content of the formulation should be in the range of 5–10% in order to provide a sufficiently strong structure also in the dry state. On the other hand, significantly higher concentrations up to 40% can be processed, still with short processing times, due to the advantageous drying conditions mentioned.

With respect to particle size, the lower end of diameter is in the range of c. 300 μm. From a freezing point of view, even lower sizes are easily feasible. In a dynamic lyophilization process as described, though, specific limitations are given: during drying, a microsphere will typically lose 80–90% of its weight. In combination with high water vapor flow, an entrainment of the mostly dried pellets into the vapor flow is possible, which would cause particle to be carried from the drum, reducing the yield. Higher solids contents reduce the loss in weight reducing the opportunity for particle loss. Electrostatic phenomena can have an influence on particle motion/loss and should also be considered.

Drying times depend on formulation, particle size, scale and load, and process conditions like drum rotation, pressure, temperatures, and heat application rate. There were cases where a several days' process was reduced to less than 24 hours, but this cannot be generalized. Especially with formulations showing low solids content and aiming a larger particle sizes (e.g. 2–3 mm in non-aseptic applications in the food area, generated by dripping into LN_2), the dry shell may act as an insulating barrier that limits heat flux, increasing processing time.

The residual moistures that are achieved are comparable with conventional freeze drying and can be below 1%, if required. The final product that is discharged from the dryer is mostly dust-free, free-flowing, and homogeneous due to constant mixing during drying – the homogeneity that is achieved by the particle generation is maintained during the drying process. It is the homogeneity that allows the use of bulk product filling technologies to create the final packaged product (see Figure 8.4).

8.3.3 Industrial Application: Integration of Process Steps to a Process Line

For sterile operations at manufacturing scale, specific aspects of containment and product handling need to be addressed. As known from solid dosage form processing, a vertical alignment of various process areas can be arranged, which are connected by interfaces and form the entire process line.

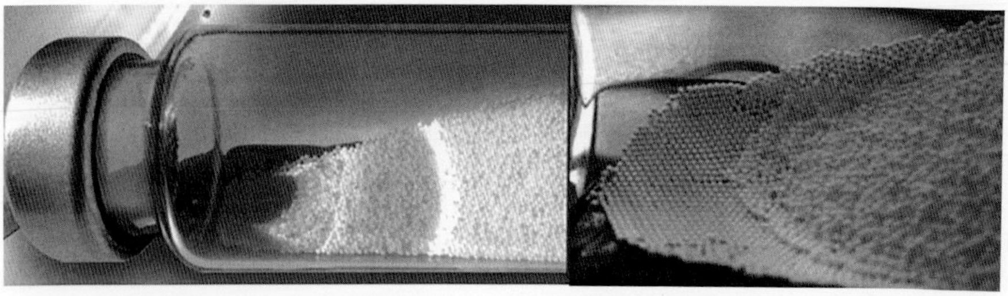

Figure 8.4 Spray-freeze-dried microspheres filled into vial from bulk.

For the industrial application of spray freeze drying, the spray/freeze chamber with a liquid handling area in the upper segment is positioned on top of a rotary freeze dryer (see Figure 8.5). As generally described before, the lower cone of the freezing chamber is connected to a cooled tube that continues into the dryer housing and protrudes into the front opening of the drum. Between freezing chamber and dryer, a flap is installed that can tightly separate both process areas.

In the dryer, the drum that is charged from the top can discharge the product as described by reverse rotation, and the product flows through a funnel that is connected by a tube to an intermediate vessel that receives the product; below this vessel, a docking station or an isolator with sterile docking for intermediate bin containers is located. Due to the round design of all components, the weight of

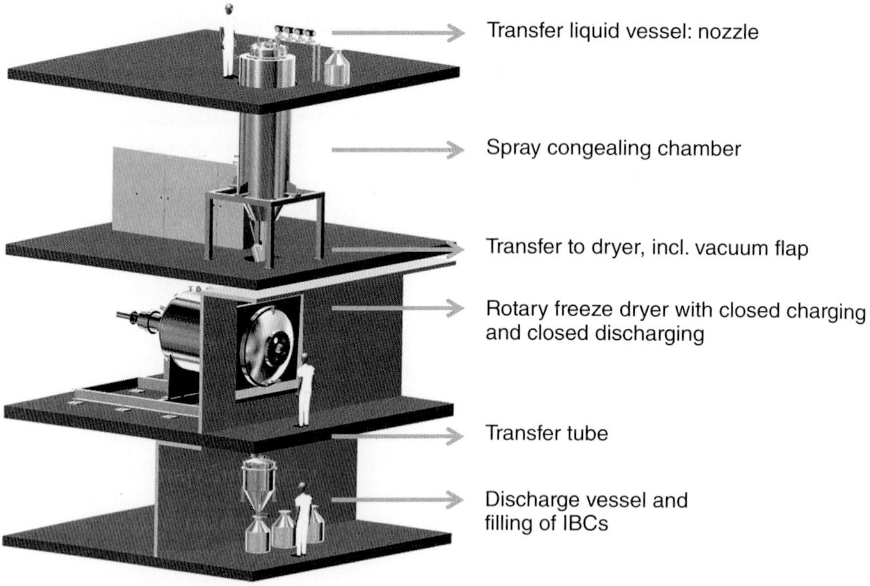

Figure 8.5 Schematic view of a production size contained process line with main components, for aseptic processing.

the entire train is still lower than that for comparable conventional freeze drying, which is relevant for the sterilization step.

By this arrangement, product handling purely by gravity is achieved, and there is no open handling of product or specific loading and unloading systems. The entire process train is executed as fully contained, steam sterilizable line that can be cleaned in place. The building requirements are mainly defined by the height. However, the main room classification does not need to reflect sterile conditions; in the liquid area, tubes are equipped with sterile connectors, the discharge section needs sterile container docking or an isolator.

Processing in such a line is executed consecutively and as batch, i.e. the spray freezing step is performed at ambient pressure until all liquid is frozen to microspheres, which are collected in the cold drum. Then, the separation flap between freezing chamber and dryer closes, the dryer chamber is evacuated, and freeze drying starts. After drying, the product is discharged into the intermediate vessel, the equipment purged to ambient pressure, and discharging into intermediate bulk container (IBC) starts.

In a further arrangement, in order to increase throughput by decreasing idle times, one freezing chamber can be connected to two or more freeze dryers, so the utilization of both process steps is increased, and a quasi-continuous operation is achieved.

A process line as described has been built (see Figure 8.6) and successfully tested for a parenteral pharmaceutical product, designed for a dryer batch size of 100 l (liquid substrate). For a 100 l batch, containing 20% solids, processed in a closed line as shown in Figure 8.6, a processing time of 24 hours for lyophilization can be expected, with an overall yield >97.0%. For frozen bulk generation, typically 10–20 hours is required, dependent on droplet size and spray rate.

Both process technologies are also designed as lab equipment (see Figure 8.7), with a minimum load of 150–200 ml (liquid) and can be arranged as separate stand-alone unit or as a single and continuous process line.

The spray freezing process is intrinsically a continuous process. By combining one spray chamber with one or more freeze dryers, a quasi-continuous operation of a process line can be envisaged – a typical setup of solid dosage form manufacturing technology, where one high shear granulator can serve several fluid-bed dryers.

8.3.4 Product Innovation Potential

Independent of aspects related to the availability of bulkware, the process characteristics and the product appearance open further opportunities for product innovation:

- The possibility to use higher solids contents can reduce the overall processing time.
- Formulations of high viscosity and low collapse temperature can be processed successfully.

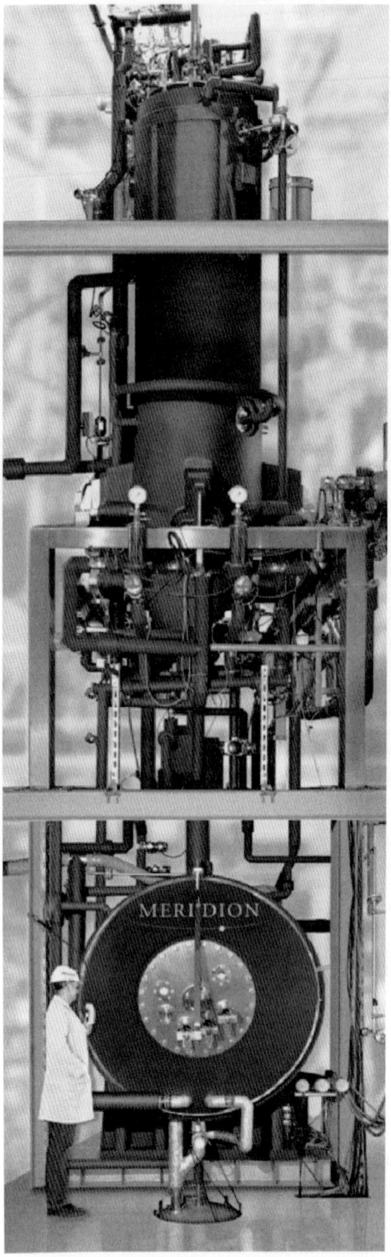

Figure 8.6 Fully contained sterilizable process line in production scale with spray freezing tower, rotary freeze dryer, and discharge container.

- Due to the larger surface, a significant reduction in reconstitution time is possible even with higher concentrated formulations.
- The pellet format is more uniform than a lyo-cake and allows more of the product to be seen during inspection avoiding potential investigations.
- Filling of the pellets can be accomplished in additional types of packages (e.g. syringes) and devices.

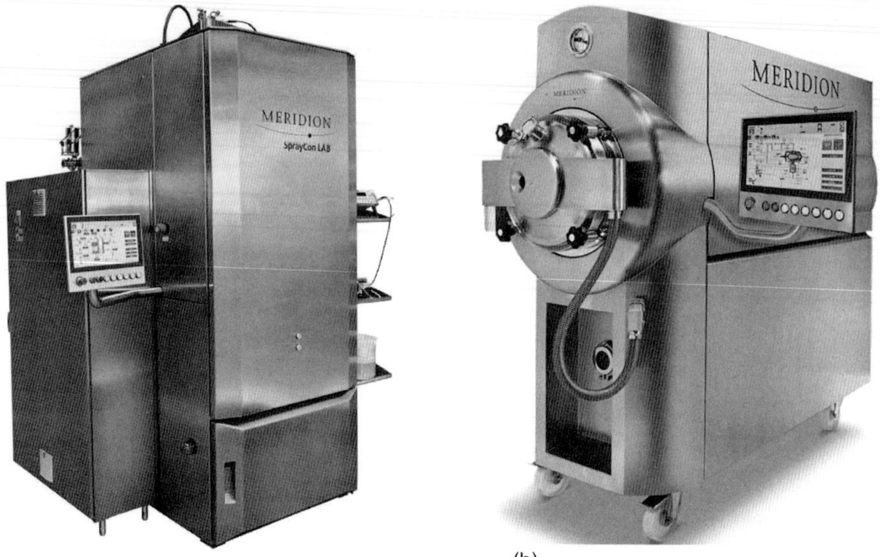

Figure 8.7 (a) Lab-scale freezing chamber. (b) Lab-scale rotary freeze dryer.

8.3.5 Bulkware Innovation Potential: Supply Chain Flexibility

As previously outlined in Section 8.2, the supply chain in conventional freeze drying is comparably long and rigid and shows specific limitations.

The availability of free-flowing, dust-free, homogenous lyophilized bulk forms a buffer in the supply chain that gets held at a point where the product is already stabilized. The filling step and the lyophilization process are beneficially decoupled. Still a high degree of flexibility is maintained, as in this manner it is possible to fill the bulk product when required, independent from the liquid prep process, with the dosing and the unit quantities as required, and allows the filling into any primary packaging that may be chosen freely rather than constricted by the lyophilization process or equipment.

In sum, time to market is significantly reduced. Furthermore, bulkware with the properties described opens new options for formulation. By compounding of various components on the filling line, combinatory products with flexible dosing of single components can be formulated. Finally, applications in the solid dosage area, like for orally disintegrating tablet (ODTs) or for multi-particulate dosage form, including coating, are also available.

8.4 Conclusion

Due to geometrical considerations of droplets/particles vs. solution/cake, more efficient heat transfer, mass transfer, and product handling are possible with spray freeze drying compared with traditional shelf drying. Using QbD to describe the desired attributes of a lyophilized process and product, more attributes are met by this novel processing route compared with traditional methods.

Spray freeze drying is a new approach to lyophilization, with innovation potential for both the product as well as for the manufacturing logistics, introducing flexibility in the supply chain in various aspects of value to producers and patients.

References

1 Meryman, H.T. (1976). Historical recollections of freeze-drying. *Developments in Biological Standards* 36: 29–32.

2 Wallen, A.J., Van Ocker, S.H., Sinacola, J.R., and Phillips, B.R. (2009). The effect of loading process on product collapse during large-scale lyophilization. *Journal of Pharmaceutical Sciences* 98: 997–1004.

3 Pikal, M.J., Cardon, S., Bhugra, C. et al. (2005). The nonsteady state modeling of freeze drying: in-process product temperature and moisture content mapping and pharmaceutical product quality applications. *Pharmaceutical Development and Technology* 10 (1): 17–32.

4 Trappler, E.H. (2005). Assure batch uniformity for freeze-dried products. Pharmaceutical Manufacturing. https://www.pharmamanufacturing.com/articles/2005/191/ (accessed 27 July 2018).

5 Ganguly, A., Varma, N., Sane, P. et al. (2017). Spatial variation of pressure in the lyophilization product chamber part 1: computational modeling. *AAPS PharmSciTech* 18 (3): 577–585.

6 Khan, M. and Jameel, F. (2009). Quality-by-design as applied to the development and manufacturing of a lyophilized protein product. *American Pharmaceutical Review* www.americanpharmaceuticalreview.com/Featured-Articles/117782-Quality-by-Design-as-Applied-to-the-Development-and-Manufacturing-of-a-Lyophilized-Protein-Product/ (accessed 28 July 2018).

7 Wanning, S., Süverkrüp, R., and Lamprecht, A. (2015). Pharmaceutical spray freeze drying. *International Journal of Pharmaceutics* 488 (1–2): 136–153.

8 Okuda, T., Suzuki, Y., Kobayashi, Y. et al. (2015). Development of biodegradable polycation-based inhalable dry gene powders by spray freeze drying. *Pharmaceutics* 7 (3): 233–254.

9 Schiffter, H. (2007). Spray freeze-drying in the manufacture of pharmaceuticals. *European Pharmaceutical Review* www.europeanpharmaceuticalreview.com/article/2325/spray-freeze-drying-in-the-manufacture-of-pharmaceuticals/ (accessed 28 July 2018).

10 Schiffter, H., Conliffe, J., and Vonhoff, S. (2010). Spray-freeze-drying of nanosuspensions: the manufacture of insulin particles for needle-free ballistic powder delivery. *Journal of the Royal Society Interface* 7 (supplement 4): S483–S500.

11 Alqurshi, A., Chan, K.L., and Royall, P.G. (2017). In-situ freeze-drying: forming amorphous solids directly within capsules: an investigation of dissolution enhancement for a poorly soluble drug. *Scientific Reports* https://www.nature.com/articles/s41598-017-02676-2 (accessed 28 July 2018).

12 Wagh, M.A., Kothawade, P.D., Salunkhe, K.S. et al. (2010). Techniques used in orally disintegrating drug delivery system. *International Journal of Drug Delivery* 2: 98–107.

13 Lammens, J., Mortier, S.T.F.C., DeMeyer, L. et al. (2018). The relevance of shear, sedimentation and diffusion during spin freezing, as a potential first step of a continuous freeze-drying process for unit doses. *International Journal of Pharmaceutics* 25 (1–2): 1–10.

14 Kahn, A. H. (1987). Kaltlufttrocknung von pharmazeutischen Präparaten und von gefrorenen Lösungen in der Wirbelschicht. PhD thesis. Basel University (CH).

15 Mumenthaler, M. and Leuenberger, H. (1991). Atmospheric spray-freeze drying: a suitable alternative in freeze-drying technology. *International Journal of Pharmaceutics* 72 (2): 97–110.

16 Plitzko, M. (2006). Gefriertrocknung in der Wirbelschicht. PhD thesis. Basle University (CH).

17 Leuenberger, H., Plitzko, M., and Puchkov, M. (2006). Spray freeze drying in a fluidized bed at normal and low pressure. *Drying Technology* 24 (6): 711–719.

18 Luy, B., Plitzko, M., and Struschka, M. (2011). Process line for the production of freeze-dried particles. European Patent EP2764309B1, filed 2012 and granted 2016.

19 Struschka, M., Plitzko, M., Gebhard, T., and Luy, B. (2011). Rotary drum for use in a vacuum freeze-dryer. European Patent EP2764310B1, filed 2012 and granted 2016.

20 Plitzko, M., Struschka, M., Gebhard, T., and Luy, B. (2011). A process line for the production of freeze-dried particles. European Patent EP2764311B1, filed 2012 and granted 2015.

21 Y.Z., Garcia, A.S., Johnston, K.P., and Williams, R.O. (2004). Spray freezing into liquid nitrogen for highly stable protein nanostructured microparticles. *European Journal of Pharmaceutics and Biopharmaceutics* 58 (3): 529–537.

22 Mishra, M. (ed.) (2015). *Handbook of Encapsulation and Controlled Release*, 185. Boca Raton, FL: CRC Press.

9

Microwave Drying of Pharmaceuticals

Tim Durance[1], *Reihaneh Noorbakhsh*[2], *Gary Sandberg*[3], *and Natalia Sáenz-Garza*[1]

[1] *Food Nutrition and Health, University of British Columbia, 2205 East Mall, Vancouver, BC V6T 1Z4, Canada*
[2] *BC Hops, 1905 Cole Rd, Abbotsford, BC V3G 1T3, Canada*
[3] *BC Institute of Technology, 3700 Willingdon Ave., Burnaby, BC V5G 3H2, Canada*

9.1 Fundamentals of Microwave Heating and Drying

9.1.1 Theory of Microwave Heating and Drying

Microwave heating is a subcategory of dielectric heating. The use of microwaves for processing is not new as the technology has been in use since the 1940s. Microwaves are electromagnetic radiation with wavelengths from 1 mm to 1 m in length and with frequencies from about 300 MHz to 300 GHz. The principal frequencies of microwaves used for industrial and domestic heating in North America are 915 and 2450 MHz.

Microwaves interact with a material by being transmitted (which is the dominant interaction for glass, paper, and nonpolar plastics), reflected (dominant interaction with metals), or absorbed. For a material to absorb the microwave energy, the molecules or atoms must be able to accept the energy by increasing their energy state – e.g. water in foods (dipolar rotation/vibration). An additional form of energy transfer in many biological materials occurs through ionic conduction.

The interpretation of microwave effects being considered as a form of heat transfer is incorrect as microwaves do not possess intrinsic heat. Rather the heating is a result of the absorption of the electromagnetic waves by the material. As with all electromagnetic radiation, microwaves have electric and magnetic components that oscillate at right angles to each other while propagating through space at the speed of light (Figure 9.1) [1].

The electric and magnetic fields are perpendicular to each other and to the direction of travel. This is called a plane wave. Note that the wave changes its energy content as it travels through a medium and photons are absorbed. It is the periodic oscillation of the wave's polarity and its decay through zero that causes the stress upon ions, atoms, and molecules and results in heating. The energy of the radiation (E) is directly related to the frequency (ν), by Planck's constant

Drying Technologies for Biotechnology and Pharmaceutical Applications, First Edition.
Edited by Satoshi Ohtake, Ken-ichi Izutsu, and David Lechuga-Ballesteros.

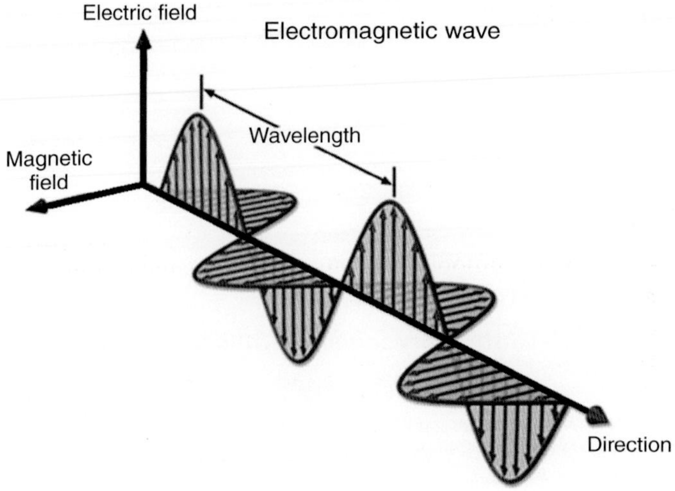

Figure 9.1 Electromagnetic wave components [1]. Source: Adapted from Coyne and Murphy [1].

$(h) = 6.63 \times 10^{-34}$ J/s:

$$E = h\nu \tag{9.1}$$

The frequency (ν) is inversely related to the wavelength (λ) by

$$\nu = c/\lambda \tag{9.2}$$

where c is the velocity of the radiation. The stress induced is manifested in two forms: (i) ionic conduction, a minor effect in most biological materials, and (ii) dipole rotation/vibration, a major effect. Due to the great molar abundance of dipolar molecules, especially water, in most biological materials, the dipole rotation effect is predominant. The greater the field strength, the greater the entire effect observed.

9.1.2 Ionic Conduction

Ions in materials exposed to microwaves are accelerated electrophoretically by the oscillating electric field of the microwaves and collide with other neighboring molecules, imparting agitation, which we define as heat. In a solution of salt in water, sodium, chloride, hydrogen, and hydroxyl ions will all move in the direction opposite to their charge. As the electric field oscillates 2.45×10^9 times per second in a typical microwave oven, ions attempt to change direction at the same rate. Depending upon the viscosity of the material, such motion may be more or less impeded. The motion of ions and the resulting collisions constitute a transfer of electric field energy to molecular kinetic energy, i.e. heat.

9.1.3 Dipolar Rotation/Vibration

Many molecules such as water and most biological molecules are dipolar in nature, i.e. they possess an asymmetric charge center, resulting in permanent partial charges at different positions on the molecules. Stresses due to an electric field also may cause otherwise nonpolar molecules to become induced dipoles. Similar to the effects of an electric field on ions, dipoles also react to the changing polarity of an electric field. Rather than electrophoretic motion however, dipoles are induced to reorientate so as to align partial charges with the electric field. Dipole movement is subject to relaxation events. The time needed for effective molecular motion is a reciprocal function of frequency, defined as the relaxation time $\tau = 1/2\pi f_c$ where f_c is the maximum absorption frequency or relaxation frequency. If τ is substantially greater than the oscillation period, then the dipole will be essentially immobilized; thus absorption and heating will not occur. In organic solids and liquids irradiated at 2450 MHz, τ is too long to allow true molecular rotation. Instead, dipolar molecules are induced to vibrate in various modes. The resulting energy conversion is a temperature-dependent, molecular-size-dependent process that defines a relaxation frequency. Small molecules (water and monomers) exhibit a relaxation frequency higher than the microwave frequency, which may rise higher as the temperature rises and thus may slow energy conversion. Large molecules, such as polymers, exhibit the opposite and as a result can exhibit runaway heating with increasing temperature. Both processes occur concurrently. Since liquids, such as water and monomers, absorb heat better than polymers, the problems with polymers can be dealt with [2]. In other words, in most processes it is the small molecules that require heating, and therefore the process can be done at a lower temperature to avoid the problems of runaway heating exhibited by large molecules. In fact, drying materials, such as food and therapeutics, can be performed at cold or subfreezing temperatures with vacuum applied to reduce the boiling point of water.

9.1.4 Microwave Application at Low Pressures

Microwave freeze drying is being developed in pharmaceutical manufacturing to recover the active pharmaceutical ingredients (and the accompanying excipients) from an aqueous solution in a relatively shorter time compared with lyophilization or conventional freeze drying. It is known that lyophilizing has many advantages over other drying techniques. These include minimal loss in product quality due to the absence of oxygen during drying, low drying temperatures, reduction of moisture content to a very low value, and easy rehydration due to the spongelike structure of the dried product. However, major disadvantages of the freeze-drying process are high energy consumption and long drying times. This is due to poor heat supply from the exterior to the interior of the frozen material being dried as well as the poor heat transfer rate associated with the conventional electric heating method that transfers heat for drying by conduction. The rate of heat transfer is a bottleneck of lyophilization because the rate of heat transfer is rate limiting. Furthermore, thermal conductivity decreases as the mass fraction of water decreases in the material being dried [3]. Microwave heating could be an ideal approach to improving internal heat transfer during drying, due to its unique volumetric heating capability. Microwave energy penetrates into the interior of biological materials, whether frozen or not, at the speed of light. If absorption and conversion to heat is adequate, then energy transfer limitations are removed, and mass transfer of water vapor becomes the bottleneck of dehydration. If a porous structure can be created and maintained, rapid drying and low final moistures can be achieved. Studies on microwave freeze drying have demonstrated advantages such as reliability and high quality, fast drying rate, and low cost [4].

9.2 Equipment Used for Microwave Freeze Drying

9.2.1 Microwave Generators

Two main types of microwave generators are possible: klystrons and magnetrons. Both consist of a tube and a DC power supply. In the case of the klystron, an electron flow is generated and flows into two cavities. The first cavity functions to regulate the speed of the electrons into "bunches," which then pass into the output cavity and produce microwaves that are then directed though a waveguide. Klystrons are characterized by high power, large size, high stability, high gain, and high operating voltages and to our knowledge have not been used for microwave-freeze-drying studies.

Magnetrons consist of a vacuum diode surrounded by a permanent magnet. Inside is a central cathode surrounded by a coaxial anode with vanes extending toward the cathode. The anode structure consists of an even number of vanes and thereby creates a number of resonance cavities (microwave resonators), for which the alternating segments have opposite polarity and are connected with conducting straps. When a DC is applied to the cathode, electrons are generated. The permanent magnets around the vacuum tube create a magnetic field that causes the electrons to be deflected into a circular pattern between the cathode and anode. The electron "cloud" exhibits spokes that touch every other vane of the anode, inducing an alternating current in the resonance cavities at microwave frequencies.

An antenna in the resonant cavity transmits the microwaves to a waveguide. The resulting characterization of microwaves generated by the magnetron is high peak power, small size, efficient operation, and relatively low operating voltage. The other significant difference between the two generators is that the magnetron produces a noncoherent transmission, whereas the klystron produces a coherent transmission. This means that for the magnetron the starting phase of each pulse is not the same for the different successive pulses but is rather a random function related to the start-up process of the oscillator.

9.2.2 Chambers

Transportation of the microwaves generated to the application is facilitated by a waveguide. Waveguides are typically constructed of aluminum although any highly conductive metal can be used. The waveguide itself may serve as the method of application of microwaves to the material. Such is the case of a traveling-wave applicator for which the application is basically a "lossy" extension of the inputting waveguide (Figure 9.2) (although usually positioned transversely to the input waveguide).

The waveguide can also be used as an applicator of microwave energy. The material to be heated is introduced by wall slots, and the waveguide is terminated

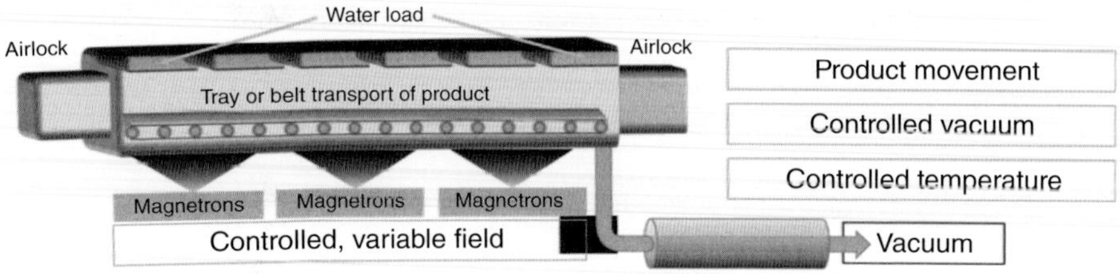

Figure 9.2 Continuous "traveling-wave" vacuum microwave dehydration system.

by a matched load (such as water) to absorb the excess energy. This configuration is called a traveling-wave design as the field maxima change with time. In the traveling wave the load can be positioned in the center of the microwave field, where the energy is at a maximum. Very efficient energy transfer and thus resultant heating can occur at this location although there may be some side-to-side nonuniformity.

Alternatively the microwaves may be directed to a cavity, often referred to as a resonant cavity, of which the home microwave is an example. For this type, the application load is usually quite small in comparison with the size of the chamber, resulting in a 3D exposure of the sample to the microwave field.

The major problem with this type of application is the lack of uniformity of heating due to the high and low values of electric field intrinsic to the cavity structure. This lack of uniformity is due to the microwaves entering the cavity being reflected from the walls. At the walls, the energy becomes "short-circuited" and the value is forced to zero. Internal to the cavity the value is other than zero. Amplitudes of the microwaves in the cavity add and subtract from each other, thus producing regions of high and low electric fields (hot and cold spots). The distribution of these stationary patterns of electric fields within the three-dimensional space of the cavity is called standing waves as contrast to traveling waves. To create a more even exposure of the load to these hot and cold spots necessitates a number of steps, usually in combination, such as moving or turning the load in some fashion, providing mode stirrers, using multiple inputs for the microwave energy, using multiple inputs with slight differences in frequency that cause different mode patterns, and choosing the cavity dimensions to support the maximum number of modes (resonant multimode cavity) [2].

9.2.3 Vacuum Systems

As mentioned earlier in this chapter, the microwave drying of food and therapeutics with vacuum can be effectively done at low temperatures and thus avoid the problems of heating polymers.

Polymers represent a "structural memory" to a material. Above the glass transition temperature, amorphous polymers become pliable or "relaxed." The relaxation behavior of polymer chains at long times (low frequencies) depends on the orientation of the dipoles of bonds, or groups of bonds, relative to the chain contour. Stockmayer [5] classified polymer dipoles into three types: A, B, and C. Polymer dipoles of types A and B are rigidly fixed to the polymer

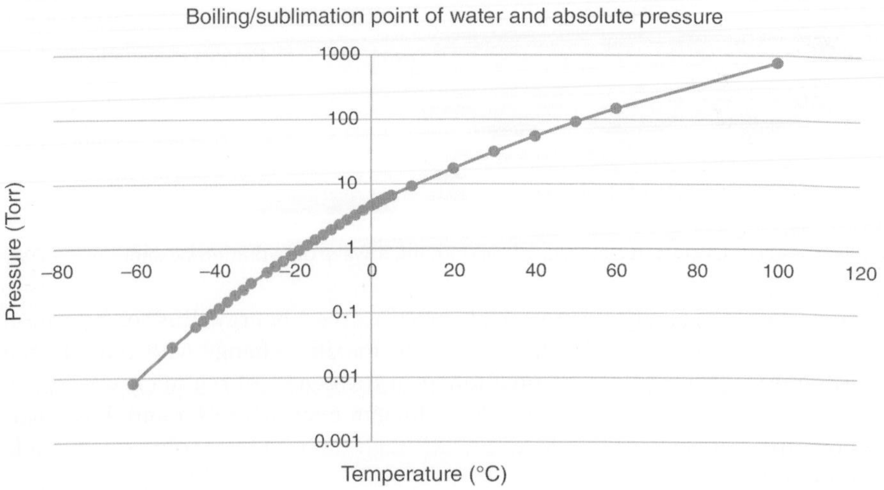

Figure 9.3 Relationship of boiling point and sublimation points of water vs. absolute pressure.

chain backbone such that their mobility in the force field requires motion of that backbone. Type C dipoles are located in flexible side chains and move independently of the backbone.

Since water is the primary molecule targeted for removal during drying, a decrease in pressure also results in a decrease in its boiling/sublimation point. This further serves to reduce the potentially damaging effects of heat on desirable components of pharmaceutical formulations. The relationship between pressure and boiling point of water can be seen in Figure 9.3. For example, at a pressure of 30 Torr, the boiling point of water is approximately 29 °C.

Depending on the system chosen for creating the vacuum in the microwave chamber, low pressures within the freeze-drying range can be created. This allows for accelerated freeze drying of materials using microwaves as the source of the sublimation energy relative to traditional freeze drying. The challenge with this application is that plasma discharges are much more likely to occur at this pressure range (0.003–0.2 kPa) [6, 7] with the result of thermal damage to the product surface due to the large energy discharges.

Generally plasma discharge will occur if the electric field intensity in the vacuum chamber exceeds the breakdown voltage, which is the minimum voltage that causes an insulator to become electrically conductive. The occurrence of this phenomenon is responsible for considerable energy losses and excessive heating of the material's dry zone, seriously damaging the final product [6, 8]. The threshold value of the breakdown voltage is dependent on the vacuum. The minimum is within the vacuum pressure range used by conventional freeze drying (see Figure 9.4).

The avoidance of plasma discharges is necessary, which requires optimization of process parameters such as chamber pressure and microwave power. On the equipment side, the design of the vacuum chamber itself and good coupling between the microwave generator and the vacuum chamber containing the

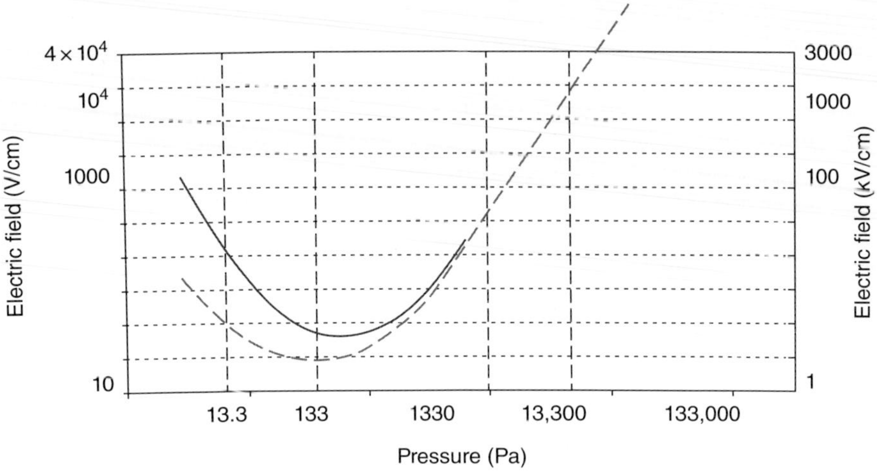

Figure 9.4 Typical breakdown electric field responses in air as a function of pressure for two frequencies, 915 MHz (solid line) and 2450 MHz (dashed line).

product are also important [9]. Generally, traveling-wave applicators are less likely to create plasma than resonant cavity applicators.

9.2.4 Safety and Microwave Leakage Control

Leakage from the microwave system must be controlled in order to contain radio-frequency (RF) interference within acceptable levels and also for personnel safety. In North America frequencies allowed for microwave cooking and processing were originally allocated in 1946 in the United States by the Federal Communications Commission (FCC). Safety issues can be summarized in four categories [10]: interference to communication and electronic systems, exposure of users to microwave radiation, safety of the cooking or preparation processing, and the safety of the prepared or processed material.

There are many methods of microwave containment that can be used at conveyor openings, doors, windows, seams, etc. and, coupled with good engineering design, make it possible to keep leakage within the limits and guidelines set by various regulatory organizations. This is required to be verified during equipment manufacture as well.

With well-designed and well-maintained equipment, the exposure of users to microwave energy should not cause concern. It is important to note that microwaves cause human body tissues to heat in the same way they heat "other biological materials." However, the legal limit of microwave energy allowed to leak from a domestic microwave oven is 5 mW/cm^2 measured at a distance of 5 cm under very specific conditions [11]. Humans cannot sense any heating at this exposure level, and any heat that might be generated is rapidly dissipated by the homeothermic mechanisms of the human body; hence there is no marked temperature rise much less burning of the flesh. Experiments to determine the point at which a human can sense warming by microwaves indicated that satisfactory warmth is experienced at exposure level of 35–50 mW/cm^2 [12]. Accidental exposure to high levels of microwave energy has been shown to alter or kill sperm, producing temporary sterility. But these types of injuries – burns, cataracts, temporary sterility – can only be caused by exposure to large amounts of microwave radiation, much more than the 5 mW limit for microwave leakage [11].

Additional controls are typically installed to prevent damage to magnetrons through increased reflected power as the materials become drier or if a plasma discharge is created. As described earlier, ionic conduction is a response of charged molecules to the electric field generated. This also carries over to those charged molecules in the cavity air (since the process is never under absolute vacuum). As a result, these accelerated molecules collide with their neighbors and with sufficient energy will cause further ionization. As the process repeats the resulting flow of ions creates a "lightning bolt"-like arc. Magnetron power on its own cannot create arcing. To produce arcing there must be some means of concentrating the electric field. In metals, electrons or electric charges move freely and arcing may result. Electrons also concentrate at sharp points or edges. Other inducements to arcing may occur due to very low pressures and small product loads or from products with high salt contents or exhibiting sharp edges.

Since microwaves are of low photon energy and entirely nonionizing, there is no residual radiation in the materials being dried as the microwaves are not retained in the material. Due to the low boiling points for water under low pressure, the retention of nutritional components and bioactivity of therapeutics are minimally affected. Interlocks can be installed such that magnetrons cannot be energized when the door is open; there is insufficient vacuum, insufficient cooling water flow, etc. as effective safety measures.

9.3 Formulation Characterization

Defining the composition profile of a pharmaceutical product to be microwave-freeze-dried is a crucial step. This composition should be determined taking into consideration factors such as dielectric properties, glass transition temperature, and various excipients that may be included to increase stability of bioactive compounds during subsequent storage.

9.3.1 Dielectric Properties, Microwave Absorption, and Depth of Penetration

As was mentioned earlier in this chapter, energy is transferred by the interaction of electromagnetic fields with the sample at a molecular level. The permittivity dielectric constant (ε') and loss factor (ε'') quantify the capacitive and conductive components of the dielectric response to microwave exposure [13]. They are usually expressed as a complex permittivity (ε^*) number of the form

$$\varepsilon * = \varepsilon' - i\varepsilon'' \tag{9.3}$$

where "i" is the imaginary component. Or they can also be expressed as the loss tangent equation

$$\tan\delta = \frac{\varepsilon''}{\varepsilon'} \tag{9.4}$$

The loss tangent equation is useful since it shows how "lossy" a material is. In other words, the higher the loss tangent, the higher the material's capacity to convert microwave energy into heat.

Knowing the dielectric properties of a material is also useful for calculating the depth of microwave penetration. Depth of penetration (d_p) is defined as the depth below a large flat surface of a compound at which the power density of a propagating electromagnetic wave that has impacted perpendicularly has decayed to $1/e$ or 36.8% of the surface value [14, 15].

The depth of penetration can be calculated by the following equation:

$$d_p = \frac{\lambda_o \sqrt{\varepsilon'}}{2\pi\varepsilon''} \tag{9.5}$$

where λ_o is the free space microwave wavelength (for 2.45 GHz, λ_o is 12.2 cm).

Depth of penetration is an important parameter to consider when processing thick samples. If the depth of penetration of microwaves is much lower than the thickness of the material, then only a fraction of the sample (surface mainly) will be directly heated/dried [13].

Dielectric properties depend on sample composition. Moisture and salt concentration can heavily influence these properties. Salt can depress the freezing point of a solution, leaving more unfrozen water at a given temperature. Salt provides ions that can interact with microwave fields. Adding salt usually decreases the dielectric constant while increasing the loss factor [9, 14] when compared with the behavior of pure water. The loss factor increase is a result of the addition of conductive charge carriers.

Physical structure of the samples may also affect dielectric properties but to a lesser degree than chemical composition. Laminated and fibrous structures seem to have higher dielectric constants than granular structures, for example [14].

The efficiency of microwave drying is material dependent and relies heavily on moisture content. Above the freezing point, the higher the moisture, the higher the loss factor and the capacity of the sample to convert microwaves into heat. This is an advantage over conventional drying since heat transfer is higher when the sample is more moist and lower when the sample is dry [16]. Depth of penetration increases significantly as moisture is removed from the matrix [9]. Changes in the dielectric properties of the sample throughout the drying process modulate the capacity of microwaves to generate heat. This can increase the complexity of modeling and controlling the process [13].

In complex pharmaceutical formulations, the sample may consist of several ingredients (active compounds, buffers, excipients). Dielectric properties of a mixture are not additive [4]. Rather the loss factor is more likely affected by the fraction of the volume that the components occupy [17]. The mixture's dielectric properties will change as the process proceeds, due to decreasing moisture content and changes in temperature [18].

As in freeze drying, microwave freeze drying is usually divided into three stages: freezing, primary drying (ice sublimation), and secondary drying (removal of unfreezable bound water) [19]. Microwave freeze drying may encounter issues in the secondary stage of drying if the loss factor of the excipient is smaller than that of the active compound. When this is the case, the

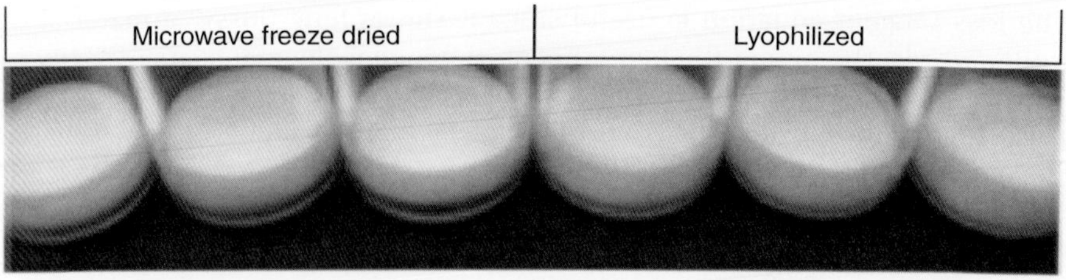

Figure 9.5 Solid, porous, non-shrunken "cakes" left after microwave freeze drying and traditional lyophilization.

temperature of the active compound will rise faster (microwave selectivity) than the excipient to potentially undesirable levels where it may decompose [20].

Therefore, formulations (for the drying) should be adjusted by an expert who has particular knowledge about excipients and their dielectric properties.

9.3.2 Glass Transition Temperature and Collapse

In microwave freeze drying, frozen samples have a solid structure, imparted by ice crystals. Water is removed via sublimation. The rigidity of the sample prevents collapse, and a solid, porous, non-shrunken matrix is left behind, usually referred to as a "cake" (see Figure 9.5). This porous structure allows for rapid and almost complete rehydration when water is added [9].

During the primary stage of drying, the temperature of the sample should not go above the glass transition temperature (T_g'); otherwise viscous flow of the amorphous phase takes place, with the frozen matrix losing its structure and collapsing. Usually collapse will occur by the time the sample is at the collapse temperature (T_c), which is usually about two degrees higher than T_g' [21].

The ice crystals formed in the freezing stage will determine the size of the pores in the cake. The bigger the ice crystals, the more efficient the drying process during the primary stage. Ice crystal size can be established by controlling the ice nucleation temperature and through the process of "annealing." Annealing, or the process of holding a sample at a predetermined temperature for a period of time after freezing, can also increase the T_g' of the amorphous phase of a sample [21].

9.3.3 Excipients for Microwave Freeze Drying of Pharmaceutical Products

The formulation and choice of the right excipients in optimal quantities can affect the glass transition temperature of the materials and characteristics of each step such as freezing and length of primary and secondary steps. Processing parameters that should be considered are microwave intensity, pressure, and temperature of the material dried. Post-processing considerations include storage conditions and degree of reconstitution of pharmaceutical products.

Pharmaceutical formulations may utilize excipients for different purposes. They can be added as bulking agents, stabilizers, antioxidants, emulsifiers, cryoprotectants, structure modifiers, collapse inhibitors, chemical/biological stabilizers, etc. [21]. Common excipients include mannitol, glycine, tris-HCl, sodium phosphate, sodium metabisulfite, lactose, glucose, dextran, etc. Phosphate buffers, particularly sodium phosphate, should be avoided as they tend to change pH significantly during freezing [21, 22]. When the active ingredient is a protein, nonreducing excipients such as trehalose, mannitol, and sucrose are ideal since they avoid potential Maillard reactions [23].

Proteins can suffer damage in both the freezing step and the drying step. In the process of freezing, solutes concentrate in the non-ice fraction. Without cryoprotectants, this concentration can lead to protein denaturation.

Hydrogen bonding between the sugar (excipient) and the protein (active agent) is essential for stabilization, since it helps retain native conformation even in the dry state. Carbohydrates will bond with the dried protein and serve as a water substitute, retaining its native state when water is removed [22].

The effects of the excipients depend on their concentration in the formulation, but in some cases high concentration of excipients may cause adverse effects due to their high loss factor as was mentioned earlier. Knowledge of dielectric properties of the excipients is a very useful parameter for quick identification and selection of different formulations with dielectric responses suitable for the intended application of microwave technology. From the practical point of view, application of scientific and engineering knowledge to the industry requires extensive research and development effort.

9.4 Dehydration Process Using Microwave Freeze Drying

Controlled microwave power can be used as a source of energy to reduce the primary and secondary drying time of conventional freeze drying.

9.4.1 Primary Drying

During the primary drying stage, sublimation occurs mainly as a result of the heat supplied by controlled microwave power to the sublimation interface through the dried and frozen layers. It is worth noting that frozen water has a low dielectric loss factor; therefore energy will mainly be absorbed by the organic molecules of the product, while the solution is still frozen. The dielectric loss factor of water can be ignored during the primary phase of microwave freeze drying when the temperature is under the glass transition temperature (T_g') of the solution and penetration depth is significant. Under these conditions, more energy can be transferred due to the dielectric losses of the organic product. Knowledge of the dielectric properties of pharmaceutical materials is thus essential during the primary phase of drying. It is crucial to control the microwave absorbance and temperature of the sample during the primary drying stage. Increasing the temperature of the frozen sample above T_g' will cause viscous flow of the amorphous phase, and the frozen matrix will lose its pore structure, leading to the collapse of the material. The water vapor formed by sublimation is transported by convection and diffusion through the porous dried layer until it enters the vacuum chamber and finally is collected on the condensers. Drying chamber pressure is an important parameter that affects microwave freeze drying; a high chamber pressure increases the heat transfer rate but significantly reduces the mass transfer rate inside the porous dried layer. The primary drying stage in freeze microwave drying is a mass transfer limited process. The chamber pressure must be maintained well below the ice vapor pressure of the sample to increase water vapor mass flux through the pores of the dried material.

9.4.2 Secondary Drying

The last stage in the microwave-freeze-drying process is known as the secondary drying stage and involves the removal of bound water inside the sample by physical desorption and chemical desorption. The heat of desorption required by the bound water molecules during the secondary drying stage is supplied by the controlled microwave power. Secondary stage critical factors that determine product quality include distributions of bound water within the sample, product temperature (which depends on dielectric and thermal properties of the sample), microwave density, chamber pressure, the thickness and geometrical shape of the sample, and the temperature of the condenser. During the secondary stage, the rate of increase in microwave power is crucial in order not to have significant losses in chemical stability and bioactivity of the material, especially at the end of the process when the active materials are dry and the dielectric properties of the formulation could lead to temperature increase due to higher microwave absorption. The final distribution of bound water in the microwave-freeze-dried product is important to determine its quality. Large variations in bound water distribution at the end of the secondary drying are not desirable since they may lead to serious problems in heat distribution and chemical stability of the product after drying. In recent years, several successful lab-scale microwave-freeze-drying attempts have been reported by EnWave Corporation. There, researchers have successfully dried various probiotic bacteria (see Figure 9.6), enzymes, and proteins with bioactivity comparable with

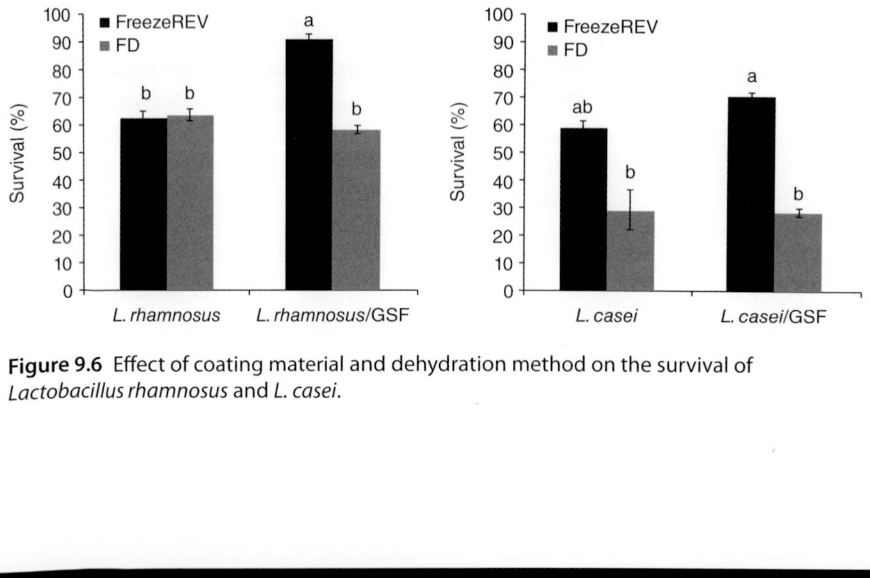

Figure 9.6 Effect of coating material and dehydration method on the survival of *Lactobacillus rhamnosus* and *L. casei*.

traditional freeze drying. Industrial-scale equipment for microwave-assisted freeze drying is reportedly under development by this company [24].

9.4.3 Control of Drying

Microwave freeze drying in particular requires a combined understanding of process science, formulation, and drying container choices. During the primary and secondary stages, the sample's microwave absorption ability changes as drying proceeds. Optimal process control of the primary and secondary stages leads to more uniform temperature and bound water distributions at the end of the drying. The use of scientific and engineering knowledge in the design and operation of industrial microwave freeze dryers contributes to this state-of-the-art technology at optimum conditions that will lower the cost and operation time of the process.

9.5 Advantages and Challenges of Pharmaceutical Microwave Freeze Drying

9.5.1 Advantages

Microwave freeze drying offers several advantages over conventional thermal methods of drying such as air drying, vacuum drying, and freeze drying. Air drying exposes samples to relatively high temperatures and oxygen that may lead to degradation of sensitive compounds. Freeze drying and vacuum drying are lengthy processes due to low drying rates [9].

The advantages of microwave freeze drying include (i) the capacity to adjust microwave power at different drying stages and moisture contents, (ii) the possibility for selective heating of materials [13] such as "dielectric cores" that can function as heat sources [25], (iii) rapid energy dissipation, and (iv) higher efficiency in secondary drying due to the use of microwaves [9]. Higher throughputs and shorter processes translate into higher energy and monetary savings.

Due to the low T_g' of a lot of therapeutic formulations, having a low loss factor (and thus a low microwave absorption) in the frozen portion of the sample is ideal since it allows for better control during the primary drying stage. Microwave freeze drying has the capacity of heating up samples volumetrically [15, 25], rather than by thermal gradient through conduction as would occur in conventional freeze drying.

9.5.2 Challenges

Drawbacks of microwave freeze drying include potential for plasma discharge and potential for nonuniformity of the electromagnetic field [13, 18] that can lead to uneven heating and potential for degradation during processing.

Since dielectric properties of liquid water are much more favorable to microwave absorption than in frozen water, localized melting in the sample can lead to thermal runaway (hot spots), thus resulting in a heterogeneous temperature profile [9], if not carefully controlled.

As was explained in past sections of this chapter, the appearance of arcing may cause burns on the product surface, energy losses, and excessive heating, which can translate into losing the final product. To avoid the occurrence of this phenomenon, strict control of process parameters (chamber pressure and power intensity) is required. Designing a chamber that minimizes the localized concentration of the electromagnetic field is also essential [9].

Since dielectric properties are temperature dependent, having even samples that are uniform in concentration and temperature is essential for even drying.

Field concentration of standing waves or the sample being in close proximity to the power feed point can cause an uneven distribution of the microwave field [20]. These can be avoided with appropriate cavity shape design and adequate location of the microwave inlet point. It should be noted that a sample's loss factor, depth of penetration, size/shape, and thickness may affect the microwave field as well and vary from product to product [13].

9.6 Some of the Published Patents for Application of Microwave Freeze Drying

Title	Inventors	Patent no.	Priority date
Process for Drying Medicinal Plants	Timothy Douglas Durance, Alex N. Yousif, Hyun-Ock Kim, Christine H. Scaman	US 6128831	10 October 2000
Method for Producing Hydrocolloid Sponges and Foams	Timothy D. Durance, Jaya Sundaram, Mareike Ressing	AU 2005266812 CA 2571232 CN ZL200580025500.X EP 1771503 DE 602005044655.9 HK1115503 IN 268059 US 8722749	30 July 2004
Method of Drying Biological Material (Vaccines)	Timothy D. Durance, Parastoo Yaghmaee, Shafique Ahmad, Guopeng Zhang	CA 2673589 CN ZL200780052152.4 CN ZL201210024322.0 HK1135715B US 8877469	1 February 2007
Apparatus and Method for Dehydrating Biological Materials (bioREV)	Timothy D. Durance, Jun Fu, Parastoo Yaghmaee, Robert L. Pike, Vu Truong, Binh Pham	CA 2699120 US 8718113	13 September 2007

Title	Inventors	Patent no.	Priority date
Apparatus and Method for Dehydrating Biological Materials with Freezing and Microwaving (freezeREV)	Timothy D Durance, Jun Fu, Parastoo Yaghmaee, Robert L. Pike	CA 2736317 CN ZL200980136008.8 HK1156655	12 September 2008
Apparatus and Method for Dehydrating Biological Material (powderREV I)	Timothy D. Durance, Jun Fu	CA 2755039	28 April 2009
Apparatus and Method for Dehydrating Biological Material (powderREV II)	Jun Fu, Timothy D. Durance, Parastoo Yaghmaee	AU2010342753 CA 2781644 CN ZL201080061581.X EP 2525675 EP 2526776 DE 60 210 027 821.2 HK 1172214 JP 5778175 MX 332017 NZ 600723	18 January 2010
Apparatus and Method for Microwave Drying of Organic Materials (powderREV III)	Jun Fu, Timothy D. Durance, Parastoo Yaghmaee	CA 2833280	19 July 2011
Continuous Microwave Freeze-Drying Device	Chaohui Liu, Chuan Zhou, Yi Liu, Qi Kang, Jun You, Kun Zhou	US 20130333237 A1	9 June 2011
Accelerated Freeze-Drying of Produce Using Microwaves	Sebastian MONCKEBERG	WO2015008153A3 CN 105611838A EP 3021676A2 US 20160157501 WO2015008153A2	19 July 2013
Microwave Freeze Drying Method and Apparatus	Toai Le Viet	US 4204336A DE 2818646A1 DE 2818646C2	27 April 1977
Process for Microwave-Freeze-Drying Dendrobium Stem Decoction Medicine Pieces	罗春丽, 廖晓康, 廖方华, 杨继勇, 邓贤芬, 亢俊峰	CN 103920018 A	13 May 2014
Production Process of Vacuum Microwave Freeze-Dry Orally Disintegrating Tablet	王小树	CN 101324397 A CN 200710112381	13 June 2007
Microwave Vacuum Freezing Dryer	陈金传	CN 201476476 U	7 August 2009

References

1 Coyne K, and Murphy T. (2016) Faraday cage: MagLab [Internet]. https://nationalmaglab.org/about/around-the-lab/what-the/faraday-cage (accessed 15 July 2018)

2 Schiffman, R.F. (2015). Microwave and dielectric drying. In: *Handbook of Industrial Drying*, 4e (ed. A.S. Mujumdar), 283–302. New York: CRC Press.

3 Rahman, M.S. (1995). *Food Properties Handbook*, 292. New York: CRC Press.

4 Yaghmaee, P. and Durance, T. (2002). Predictive equations for dielectric properties of NaCl, D-sorbitol and sucrose solutions and surimi at 2450 MHz. *Journal of Food Science* 67 (6): 2207–2211.

5 Stockmayer, W.H. (1967). Dielectric dispersion in solutions of flexible polymers. *Pure and Applied Chemistry* 15 (3–4): 539–554.

6 Gould, J.W. and Kenyon, E.M. (1971). Gas discharge and electric field strength in microwave freeze-drying. *The Journal of Microwave Power* 6: 151–167.

7 Karel, M. (1974). Fundamentals of dehydration processes. In: *Advances in Preconcentration and Dehydration of Foods* (ed. A. Spicer), 45–94. New York: Wiley.

8 Arsem, H.B. and Ma, Y.H. (1985). Aerosol formation during the microwave freeze dehydration of beef. *Biotechnology Progress* 1 (2): 104–110.

9 Duan, X., Zhang, M., Mujumdar, A.S., and Wang, R. (2010). Trends in microwave-assisted freeze drying of foods. *Drying Technology* 28 (4): 444–453.

10 Buffler, C.R. (1993). *Microwave Cooking and Processing: Engineering Fundamentals for the Food Scientist*. New York: Van Nostrand Reinhold.

11 FDA. (2014) Radiation-emitting products [Internet]. http://www.fda.gov/Radiation-EmittingProducts/ (accessed 15 July 2018)

12 Buffler, C.R. (1998). Whole body microwave heating of humans and livestock. *Harvard Graduate Society Newsletter*: 11–13.

13 Thostenson, E.T. and Chou, T.-W. (1999). Microwave processing: fundamentals and applications. *Composites Part A: Applied Science and Manufacturing* 30 (9): 1055–1071.

14 Ryynänen, S. (1995). The electromagnetic properties of food materials: a review of the basic principles. *Journal of Food Engineering* 26 (4): 409–429.

15 Venkatesh, M.S. and Raghavan, G.S.V. (2004). An overview of microwave processing and dielectric properties of agri-food materials. *Biosystems Engineering* 88 (1): 1–18.

16 Loh, Z.H., Liew, C.V., Lee, C.C., and Heng, P.W.S. (2008). Microwave-assisted drying of pharmaceutical granules and its impact on drug stability. *International Journal of Pharmaceutics* 359 (1–2): 53–62.

17 McLoughlin, C.M., McMinn, W.A.M., and Magee, T.R.A. (2003). Microwave-vacuum drying of pharmaceutical powders. *Drying Technology* 21 (9): 1719–1733.

18 Kelen, A., Ress, S., Nagy, T. et al. (2006). Mapping of temperature distribution in pharmaceutical microwave vacuum drying. *Powder Technology* 162 (2): 133–137.

19 Nastaj, J.F. and Witkiewicz, K. (2009). Mathematical modeling of the primary and secondary vacuum freeze drying of random solids at microwave heating. *International Journal of Heat and Mass Transfer* 52 (21–22): 4796–4806.

20 Kelen, A., Pallaivarsanyi, E., Ress, S. et al. (2006). Practical method for choosing diluent that ensures the best temperature uniformity in the case of pharmaceutical microwave vacuum drying of a heat sensitive product. *European Journal of Pharmaceutics and Biopharmaceutics* 62 (1): 101–109.

21 Sadikoglu, H., Ozdemir, M., and Seker, M. (2006). Freeze-drying of pharmaceutical products: research and development needs. *Drying Technology* 24 (7): 849–861.

22 Arakawa, T., Prestrelski, S.J., Kenney, W.C., and Carpenter, J.F. (2001). Factors affecting short-term and long-term stabilities of proteins. *Advanced Drug Delivery Reviews* 46 (1–3): 307–326.

23 Anhorn, M.G., Mahler, H.-C., and Langer, K. (2008). Freeze drying of human serum albumin (HSA) nanoparticles with different excipients. *International Journal of Pharmaceutics* 363 (1–2): 162–169.

24 Durance, T. and Yaghmaee, P. (2011). 4.51—Microwave dehydration of food and food ingredients. In: *Comprehensive Biotechnology* [Internet], 2e (ed. M. Moo-Young), 617–628. Burlington: Academic Press http://www.sciencedirect.com/science/article/pii/B9780080885049003068. (accessed 15 July 2018)

25 Tao, Z., Wu, H., Chen, G., and Deng, H. (2005). Numerical simulation of conjugate heat and mass transfer process within cylindrical porous media with cylindrical dielectric cores in microwave freeze-drying. *International Journal of Heat and Mass Transfer* 48 (3–4): 561–572.

10

Foam Drying

Phillip M. Lovalenti and Vu Truong-Le

Aridis Pharmaceuticals, Inc., 5941 Optical Ct., San Jose, CA 95138, USA

10.1 Introduction

Pharmaceutical drying technologies are often employed to enhance the storage stability of thermally labile biopharmaceutical products, as well as the handling efficiency or delivery convenience of the finished product. However, it is becoming more understood that the thermal history provided by a particular drying method can have a major impact on both the solid-state properties and storage stability of a biopharmaceutical product [1]. While a multitude of drying technologies with varying level of maturity have been developed (many are discussed elsewhere in this book), each with its advantages and disadvantages, only a select few that have demonstrated the ability to preserve the bioactivity of biologic drugs have been implemented commercially. Such technologies are, namely, lyophilization and, to a much more limited extent, spray drying. Among the lesser known and less developed drying technology is vacuum foam drying. While it has some disadvantages, it also has some very compelling benefits primarily stemming from the substantial improvement in storage stability at elevated temperatures that it has provided to some biologics. This summary will reference several studies demonstrating substantial biopharmaceutical stabilization and a discussion on the process science behind this drying method. The merits of this drying technology and its possible future role in commercial implementation for biopharmaceutical products will also be discussed.

Vacuum drying is a vitrification process where moisture removal is enabled by the application of vacuum. A foamed solid is not necessarily the final product and could include, for example, the processes of film drying or even freeze drying. Foam drying can refer to any process that involves a foamed state, either as an intermediate or the final product, and can also produce the foamed liquid by incorporating air through agitation. In order to define the scope of this chapter, it is important to distinguish between three similar, if not overlapping, drying methods for producing a glassy matrix: vacuum drying, foam drying, and vacuum foam drying. Vacuum foam drying is the focus of this chapter, especially as it applies to biopharmaceuticals. Vacuum foam drying is a subset of general

Drying Technologies for Biotechnology and Pharmaceutical Applications, First Edition.
Edited by Satoshi Ohtake, Ken-ichi Izutsu, and David Lechuga-Ballesteros.

foam drying whereby the liquid is "foamed" by the application of vacuum to lower the pressure below the vapor pressure of the liquid to cause boiling. It lends itself to more rapid drying than general vacuum drying because of the increased surface area for moisture removal via evaporation and even sublimation when significant evaporative cooling is present. Vacuum foam drying also provides a lower temperature for boiling to produce the foams and can enable aseptic processing in commercially available freeze driers, both of which are not necessarily amenable to general foam drying processes.

10.1.1 Challenges in Developing Stable Dosage Forms for Biopharmaceuticals

The demand exists for biologic drug products and vaccines to exhibit a commercially useful stability profile, particularly for live vaccines being implemented for the developing world markets. Improved product stability not only removes the need for the cold chain requirements but can also lower costs for shipping, handling, and long-term storage. Producing a room-temperature stable vaccine, for example, would facilitate mass immunization program to areas unreachable without refrigeration. Also, the need to store these drugs for long-term stockpiling can pose a significant challenge.

10.1.2 Chapter Overview

This chapter will provide a basic introduction to the science and practice of vacuum foam drying. A case will be presented to suggest that this technology can be a viable drying option for difficult to stabilize biologics. The historical background of this drying process will be discussed that traces its early origins in the food industry and its first application for pharmaceutical preparations. This will be followed by a brief discussion of other drying technologies to illustrate where foam drying fits in and where it has shown advantages. Section 10.4 will give more details on the foam-drying process and its several iterations, as well as a presentation of the challenges that will need to be overcome for the process to be successful at commercial scale. Sections 10.5 and 10.6 will provide some strategies for formulating a stable foam-dried drug product and techniques for its characterization. The chapter ends with case studies and concluding remarks.

10.2 Comparison of Drying Methods

10.2.1 Brief Description of Established Pharmaceutical Drying Methods

Here we provide a brief overview of the essential elements of the leading drying methods used in the pharmaceutical industry with research or commercial application, i.e. freeze drying and spray drying, and how they compare with foam drying. In general, the reader can find more details on a particular drying method in other chapters of this book.

10.2.1.1 Freeze Drying

Lyophilization or freeze drying is carried out by first freezing the liquid formulation to very low temperatures, followed by lowering the pressure to near vacuum until the water is removed by sublimation (primary drying). Additional residual moisture is removed by raising the temperature in a controlled fashion (secondary drying). This method can achieve very low moisture content and results in a fine microporous structured solid or "cake" as the final product (see Figure 10.2).

10.2.1.2 Spray Drying

Spray drying is performed by emitting the liquid formulation from a nozzle to produce a fine aerosol of liquid droplets. Heated, dry air is used to carry the aerosol through a chamber where the water is removed from the droplets by rapid evaporation. The small droplet size and associated high surface area facilitate the rapid drying and the formation of solid particles. The carrier gas then drives the gas–solid suspension through a centrifugal separator to allow collection of the resulting powder product (see Figure 10.2).

10.2.1.3 Vacuum Foam Drying

This approach is similar to freeze drying (and some have referred to it as "freeze drying done under a cake collapsed conditions"), but with the primary drying step not carried out entirely by sublimation. Here the water is removed at least partially by boiling through the application of vacuum before the solid structures are locked in. This approach is made possible by the higher shelf temperatures used, which are generally near ambient conditions. Although the product is not initially frozen, as in freeze drying, freezing can take place transiently owing to evaporative cooling. As the moisture content drops, the formulation becomes more viscous and begins to form a static foam. Further application of vacuum and mildly elevated temperatures provide additional moisture removal (secondary drying). In contrast to the microstructured product from freeze drying, the resulting dried product is typically a closed-cell foam with macroscopic structures (see Figure 10.2).

Figure 10.1 shows a comparison of the drying pathways for the above three methods. In freeze drying the liquid product is first cooled to its melt temperature T_m (A–B′). With continued cooling below T_m (B′–C′), there is separation into two phases, one a growing accumulation of essentially pure ice crystals and the other a progressively more concentrated product solution containing the excipients. After the liquid product phase cools below its glass transition temperature T_g (C′–D′), primary drying proceeds by application of high vacuum to remove the ice by sublimation. This is followed by a ramp in temperature to allow for secondary drying (D′–E′), i.e. removal of water from the solid concentrated product by evaporation. When the final product returns to room temperature (E′–F), the resulting high T_g protects against collapse of its porous microstructure.

With spray drying the water evaporates rapidly from the liquid product droplets such that the temperature is maintained near ambient conditions by a balance between evaporative cooling and the heat supplied by the warm, dry carrier gas (Figure 10.1, A–B″). At some point when enough water is removed, the dissolved solids reach their solubility limit and begin to precipitate out (B″–C″),

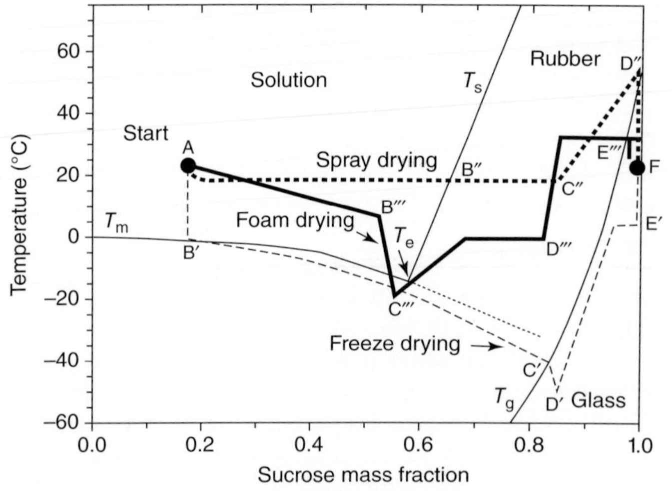

Figure 10.1 Sucrose–water state diagram comparing illustrative pharmaceutical drying pathways for a sucrose-based formulation undergoing freeze, spray, and foam drying. T_m is the melt temperature, T_s represents the solubility limit, T_g is the glass transition temperature, and T_e is the eutectic temperature of the solution.

until finally the rate of evaporation slows and the temperature of the now solid particle begins to rise and approach the carrier gas temperature (C″–D″). When the powder is collected, it cools back to room temperature (D″–F).

For the foam drying depicted in Figure 10.1, the process starts with a lower solids content than is typical, i.e. less than 20%, and requires a concentration step by the application of a low vacuum and near ambient temperatures. During this period the sample temperature may drop due to lowering shelf temperature and/or evaporative cooling as moisture is removed (A–B‴). Once the product solution is sufficiently concentrated and more viscous, a high vacuum can be applied without risk of excessive boiling/splattering. The resulting rapid water removal produces a sharp drop in product temperature due to the latent heat of vaporization and leads to the transient product freezing and locking in the foam structure (B‴–C‴). During freezing, moisture removal could also involve sublimation that is progressing under a high surface area. With the rapid vaporization now halted, the product begins to warm, and additional moisture is removed by a combination of sublimation and evaporation, eventually approaching the shelf temperature when moisture is removed primarily by evaporation (C‴–D‴). A rise in shelf temperature above ambient conditions brings about additional moisture removal until the T_g of the product approaches the shelf temperature (D‴–E‴). The product then cools to room temperature (E‴–F).

Examples of the finished product from these drying methods are provided in Figure 10.2a.

10.2.1.4 Other Drying Methods

While there are a host of other hybrid drying methods that have been studied, some of the more common include microwave vacuum drying, spray freeze

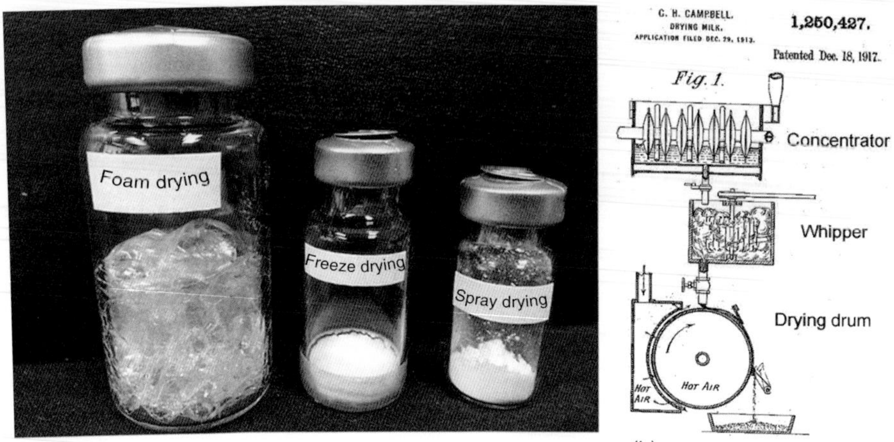

(a) (b)

Figure 10.2 (a) Representative samples of dried product from foam, freeze, and spray drying. Source: Lovalenti et al. 2016 [11]. Reproduced with permission of Springer Nature. (b) Foam drying of milk in 1917.

drying, and supercritical freeze drying, with several of these processes covered in other chapters of this book. Closely related to vacuum foam drying, vacuum film drying utilizes vacuum less aggressively to prevent foaming and has been applied with some success to biologic formulations [2–4].

10.2.2 Advantages of Foam Drying over Other Methods

Foam drying offers a number of advantages over both freeze drying and spray drying for the preservation of biologic activity of a biopharmaceutical product, particularly for thermal labile products and those with susceptibility to damage at phase interfaces. Compared with freeze drying, foam drying's primary advantage is that the product is not frozen during primary drying, so the instabilities associated with the formation of ice crystal can be avoided. This also prevents freeze concentration of solutes, which can lead to, for example, large shifts in pH and damage to the biologic product [5]. In addition, during freeze drying there is larger surface area at phase interfaces between frozen ice crystals and the concentrated liquid, which offers sites for denaturation of the biologic material. Further, because moisture is removed by boiling rather than sublimation, in many cases foam drying can offer shorter drying cycles than lyophilization.

When compared with spray drying, the advantage of foam drying is the significant reduction in the amount of air–water interface during drying. This interface can attract surface active regions of the biologic and lead to degradation of the product, both from the drying process and during storage. Studies have shown a correlation between the specific surface area (SSA) of the dried product and the stability of the incorporated bioactive agent [6, 7]. In addition, foam drying avoids the thermal and high shear stresses that can be generated during spray drying by product preheating and by the aerosolizing nozzle during the liquid formulation's discharge under high pressure.

Because foam drying operates at near ambient conditions, the energy consumption costs associated with processing are expected to be lower than other drying processes [8]. In addition, foam drying can be performed with formulations with high concentration of dissolved solids, e.g. sugars, which allows for better protection of the biologic during processing. Freeze drying is limited in initial solids concentration by the requirements of sublimation for effective drying and good cake structure, while spray drying can be similarly limited because of constraints on nozzle pressure and particle size.

In addition, although not the focus of this chapter, the application of foam drying to poorly soluble active pharmaceutical ingredients (APIs) has been used to enhance tablet dissolution and oral bioavailability [9, 10].

Many of the above advantages associated with foam drying (ambient processing temperatures, lower SSA, minimized ice crystal formation) result in the superior preservation of biologic activity, both following processing and during storage, relative to freeze or spray drying. A number of studies have demonstrated this for bacterial and viral vaccines as well as monoclonal antibodies [6, 7, 11–13]. More detailed discussion of biostabilization is provided in Section 10.5, and Section 10.6 identifies other possible mechanisms for foam drying's stabilization effectiveness.

10.3 Foam Drying: Historical Perspective

10.3.1 Foam Drying in the Food Industry

The food industry has a rich history of understanding the amorphous glassy state and how it is useful to preserve food products. Perhaps the earliest record of the application of foam drying in an industrial setting is associated with the production of foam-dried milk in the early part of the twentieth century. In this early process the foam was generated by agitation of a pre-concentrated stock of increased viscosity. The moisture was then removed at elevated temperatures, by, for example, heated drum drying [14] (Figure 10.2b). This type of drying technology, where foam is produced by agitation, has continued in other forms and included the addition of edible additives, such as egg whites and methyl cellulose, to serve as foaming agents and stabilizers, which allows for a lower concentrated liquid. Most notably is the process of foam mat drying [15], which has been applied to a wide variety of food products, from papaya pulp [16] to carrageenan [17], because of its improvement in drying time and retention of product quality. In this process the foam is generated by mixing and then cast onto a sheet (or "mat") where it is dried by heat and/or convection.

In as early as the 1940s, with the goal of improved manufacturing of a shelf stable product that not only reconstituted quickly but also retained its original flavor profile, processes to produce foam-dried food products began to be developed with the use of vacuum [18]. This approach was essentially defined by boiling off the water at lower temperatures until the moisture content was reduced sufficiently to increase in viscosity and produce a stable foam, with further drying yielding a glassy state. The approached was refined beginning in the

1950s toward continuous processes to lower manufacturing costs, driven largely from the goal of producing a quality foam-dried milk product by a research and development division of the US Department of Agriculture [19, 20]. The use of vacuum foam drying in the food industry continues to be studied today with its advantage of faster drying; the retention of color, flavor, and nutritional content; and enhanced shelf life [21, 22].

Other vacuum-drying technology is applied to fruits and vegetables with similar advantages using approaches that utilized alternative forms of energy, such as microwave vacuum drying [23] or far-infrared vacuum drying [24]; although the products may have considerable porosity they may not necessarily be "foam-dried."

10.3.2 Foam Drying in the Pharmaceutical Industry

Perhaps the earliest records of foam-dried biologics were for the preservation of bacteria. In the 1930s the Russian biologist Olga Lepeshinskaya published her finding that bacteria recovered their activity following reconstitution with water after days suspended in a foamy solid [25, 26]. Later, in the 1940s, the microbiologist Lord Stamp described a foam-drying process that involved applying a mild vacuum combined with a desiccant for a few days, which provided a major enhancement in preserving bacterial activity relative to lyophilization [27]. In a more extended effort, the microbiologist Douglas Annear published a series of articles starting in the mid-1950s through 1970s [28–31]. This pioneering work on the preservation of cells demonstrated that a significant improvement in the retention of biologic activity could be provided by foam-drying bacteria into a glassy matrix. Upon rehydrating the dried foam even after days of storage at 100 °C, a significant portion of several bacteria's activity was found to be retained.

Renewed interest in this technology did not resurface until the 1990s with the use of this approach on both bacterial and viral vaccines. Both Roser and Gribbon and Victor Bronstein patented a vacuum process for producing foam-dried biologics such as viruses and bacteria that retained their potency [32–34]. Truong et al. followed in the 2000s with the development of a vacuum-foam-drying process for the potency preservation of viral vaccines such as live attenuated flu virus and parainfluenza virus [7, 35] that demonstrated a substantial improvement in storage stability relative to other conventional methods such lyophilization. Such process was applied to monoclonal antibodies as well, which showed it had similar advantages over spray drying or lyophilization [6]. Workers at Aridis refined the Truong et al. foam-drying process further for the stabilization of both live viral and bacterial vaccines [36].

A more detailed comparison for these processes is provided in Section 10.4.

10.4 The Foam-Drying Process

10.4.1 Detailed Thermal Cycle and Equipment Parameters

Although there are a variety of methods to perform foam drying, we provide here details on the parameters used successfully for biologics preservation. By analogy

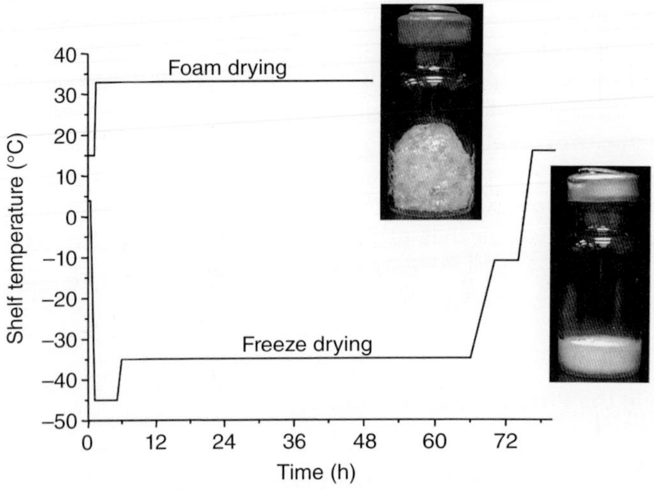

Figure 10.3 Comparison of representative foam- and freeze-drying shelf temperature profiles in a conventional lyophilizer.

to freeze drying, there is typically a primary drying step and a secondary drying step. However, in foam drying the primary drying step is performed near ambient temperatures such that the liquid formulation is either supercooled or not (completely) frozen before the application of vacuum. This allows the bulk of the moisture to be removed by boiling, leading to the formation of a static foam. Then, similar to freeze drying, the temperature is generally raised to perform secondary drying also under vacuum. Foam drying can be carried out in stoppered vials so that the equipment and facilities will be the same as those for freeze drying. Examples of temperature profiles comparing foam drying to freeze drying are provided in Figure 10.3.

Drying equipment for foam drying needs to be able to tightly control temperature and pressure to be successful [8]. If the pressure is lowered too rapidly for a given shelf temperature, evaporative cooling can dominate heat transfer from the shelf, leading to freezing and foaming suppression. If pressure is lowered too slowly, moisture removal will occur more by evaporation than boiling, which will simply thicken the liquid and hinder the foaming action.

Figure 10.4a illustrates a foam-drying process in a standard lyophilizer used successfully for the preservation of a live attenuated flu vaccine. In this method, prior to lowering the pressure and initiating the foaming/drying process, the product is first equilibrated at the approximate phase transition temperature of the lipid membrane surrounding the virus or bacteria (~15 °C) to facilitate penetration of excipient stabilizers in the formulation [35]. This method also illustrates the multiple water loss phenomena that can occur during a foam-drying cycle depending on the process parameters, which can include evaporation, boiling, and sublimation, sometimes occurring simultaneously.

Compared with freeze drying, typically a foam-drying cycle will have a very short primary drying step when the bulk of the moisture is removed. Therefore, in order to carry out foam drying effectively, the freeze dryer used must have

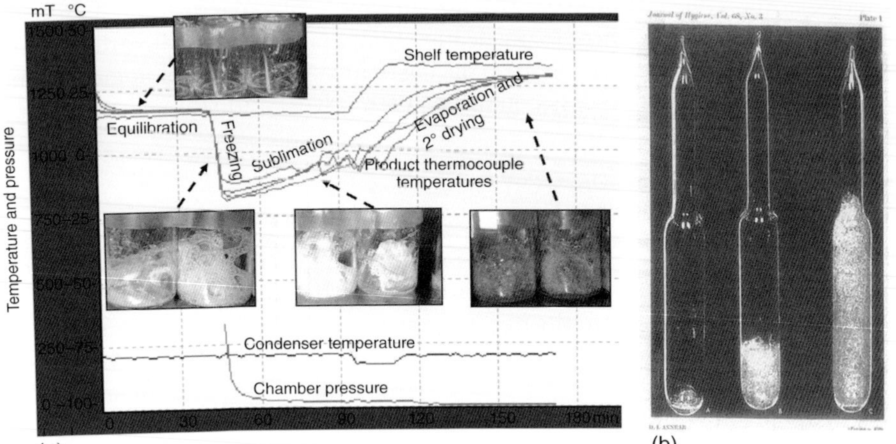

Figure 10.4 (a) Foam-drying process conditions for the preservation of live attenuated flu vaccine, including product temperature profiles. Source: Truong-Le and Abdul-Fattah (2010) [1]. Reproduced with permission of John Wiley & Sons. (b). Stages of the foam-drying process of Annear. Source: Annear 1970 [31]. Reproduced with permission of Cambridge University Press..

adequate capacity to handle the high moisture load during the rapid primary drying phase. Secondary drying in a foam drying cycle may be similar to or longer than that of a typical freeze-drying cycle, because the removal of residual moisture from foam-dried solids is more limited by the lower SSA.

10.4.2 Wet Blend Requirements

The liquid properties of the formulation to be dried into the solid state are critical to producing an effective foam-dried solid. The concentration of dissolved solids in a liquid wet blend to be foam-dried is typically much higher than that associated with the wet blend to be freeze-dried or spray-dried. A wet blend for foam drying will typically contain 20–50% dissolved solids, while a wet blend for freeze drying or spray drying may contain less than 10%. For freeze drying, the lower solids content is needed to generate a sufficiently porous cake that can be rapidly reconstituted; for spray drying the concentration can be limited by constraints on nozzle pressure and/or particle size. Since these constraints do not apply to foam drying, the formulator can take advantage of a wet blend with higher solids loading to reduce the moisture load and energy input and possibly improve throughput for the drying equipment, increasing viscosity to facilitate generating a stable foam structure, in addition to providing a greater stabilizing environment for the biologic to reduce activity loss during processing. The mechanism for this reduced process loss with high stabilizer concentration can be explained by its impact on (i) suppressing the damaging ice crystal formation through freezing point depression and the promotion of super cooling, (ii) reducing ice crystallization rate and ice crystal size, (iii) stabilization of viral or bacterial membrane structure, and (iv) osmotic pressure-induced mass transfer to increase the concentration of protein and low molecular weight stabilizers inside membranes while lower ice nucleation temperature there. More discussion on the specific excipients used in foam drying to further stabilize biologics during processing (beyond the process conditions themselves) and storage is provided in Section 10.5.

10.4.3 Variants of the Foam-Drying Process

There is a variety of process condition pathways that can achieve a foam-dried solid state, and a number of researchers have developed their own methods for foam drying, often tailored to the needs of their specific biologic. Advancements in the process were brought about with the use of the modern freeze dryer, which provided tighter controls on the process conditions and allowed for more efficient drying while maintaining temperature closer to ambient. A few of the better known or patented methods are described further below. A summary is provided in Table 10.1.

10.4.3.1 Annear

As mentioned previously, this was one of the earliest documented foam-drying methods for preserving a biologic agent. It can be seen that Annear's process evolved somewhat over the several papers he published. The more refined method described in his 1970 paper [31] included a concentration step where bacteria suspended in a 40% solution of sodium glutamate was loaded into a glass ampoule and placed in a 25 °C bath for about one hour while under pump vacuum, which concentrated the liquid and brought about some boiling. This was followed by placing the ampoule in a 100 °C bath for about one hour while still under pump vacuum, which brought about significant foaming and the final foamed glassy product (see Figure 10.4b). Given the somewhat uncontrolled environment, in terms of a specified and measured level of vacuum, it is unclear whether the formulation remained liquid or went through a freezing transition as a result of evaporative cooling.

10.4.3.2 Roser and Gribbon

The method described in a patent application by Roser and Gribbon [32] for producing foamed glass matrices followed the same process of Annear but with the more sophisticated controlled drying using a commercially available freeze dryer. Here effort was made to develop a process that did not go through a freezing transition, which was prevented by maintaining a lower vacuum initially and/or a shelf temperature sufficiently high to offset evaporative cooling. In some cases a first step concentrated the formulation at low vacuum (e.g. 10–30 Torr) for less than hour. This was then followed by a second step of foaming and drying at a high vacuum for several hours and optionally at elevated temperatures.

10.4.3.3 Bronshtein (PFF)

Bronshtein detailed a very similar process to Annear for vacuum foam drying in his 1998 patent [33] and referred to it as preservation by foam formation (PFF). This method of drying a bioactive agent from an aqueous solution (e.g.

Table 10.1 Examples of process parameters associated with various foam-drying methods.[a)]

Method	Annear [31]	Roser/Gribbon [32]	Bronshtein (PFF) [33]	Truong et al. (FFD) [35]	Truong et al. – Aridis (CFD) [36]	Bronshtein (PBV) [37]
Concentration/ evaporation/ equilibration step	"Boil" Vacuum = pump max; $T = 25\,°C$ (bath); $t = 1$ h	"Evaporate" Vacuum = 10–30 Torr; $T = 10–30\,°C$ (shelf); $t = 10–40$ min	"Evaporate/boil" Vacuum = 7.6–152 Torr; T = ambient; $t = 4$ h	"Equilibrate" Vacuum = none; $T = 15\,°C$ (shelf); $t = 10–60$ min	"Boil" Vacuum = reduced stepwise to 100 mTorr; $T = 15\,°C$ (shelf); $t = 10–180$ min	"Partial freeze" Vacuum = none; $T = -20–0\,°C$; $t = x$ min
Primary drying/ foaming step	"Foam" Vacuum = pump max; $T = 100\,°C$ (bath); $t = 1$ h	"Foam" Vacuum = 10–30 mTorr; $T = 25–60\,°C$ (shelf); $t = 16–20$ h	"Foam" Vacuum < 7.6 Torr; $T = 5–25\,°C$; $t = 0.5–4$ h	"Foam/freeze/sublime" Vacuum = 50 mTorr; $T = 12–30\,°C$ (shelf); $t = 0.5–2$ h	"Foam" Vacuum ≤ 100 mTorr; $T = 15\,°C$ (shelf); $t = 24$ h	"Foam/sublimate" Vacuum < 3 Torr; $T = -20–0\,°C$; $t = x$ h
Secondary drying	None	None	Vacuum = x mTorr; T ≥ ambient; t = up to 8 d with DRIERITE	Vacuum ≤ 50 mTorr; $T \geq 30\,°C$ (shelf); $t = 1–4$ d	Vacuum = 50 mTorr; $T = 33\,°C$ (shelf); $t = 24$ h	Vacuum = x mTorr ("high vacuum"); $T \geq$ ambient; $t = x$ h
Highlights	Stabilized bacteria 1 y at 4 °C, ≥1 d at 100 °C	Foam-dried HepB surf antg; polio, measles, blood, bacteria [32]	Stabilized enzyme >100 d at 37 °C; bacteria 16 d at 50 °C, >150 d at 37 °C; processed >10 l in one vessel	Stabilized live viral vaccines >16 mo at 25 °C, >3 mo at 37 °C, >1 mo at 50 °C	Foam-dried live bacterial and viral vaccines	Foam-dried rabies vaccine

a) "x" represents values unspecified by this patent. T=temperature, t=time, y=years, mo=months, d=days, h=hours, min=minutes.

containing 25% sucrose), also known as VitriLife™ technology, comprised four steps: (i) dehydration/concentration at low vacuum >7.6 Torr (e.g. four hours at 152 Torr) at room temperature, (ii) boiling/foaming at high vacuum <7.6 Torr until a stable foam forms (e.g. four hours at room temperature), (iii) secondary drying of stable foam (e.g. eight days over DRIERITE under vacuum at room temperature), and (iv) cooling final product below the glass transition temperature. Similar to Roser and Gribbon, the process was designed to prevent the formulation from going through a freezing transition as a result of evaporative cooling.

10.4.3.4 Truong (FFD)

The process developed by Truong et al. a few years later [35] was referred to as freeze foam drying (FFD) and differs from the above methods in two ways. First, the liquid is initially formulated with high solids content, and no low vacuum concentration step is employed. Instead the liquid is equilibrated at a lowered temperature (e.g. 15 °C) near the glass transition temperature of the lipid membrane of the biologic present (i.e. bacteria or virus lipid bilayers). Second, the primary drying is performed under high vacuum (e.g. 50 mTorr) for up to two hours with the shelf temperature maintained at the same lowered temperature. This leads to rapid evaporation, boiling, and foaming. The cooling brought about by the rapid evaporation quickly freezes the foam, and further moisture is removed by sublimation. Secondary drying then follows with a ramp in temperature to as high as 45 °C and a hold for up to 96 hours. The moisture content of the resulting glassy solid can be 2% or less. To perform this process a high capacity condenser is required to handle the moisture load.

10.4.3.5 Truong (CFD)

Truong et al. later modified the FFD process by performing the drying at higher shelf temperatures to arrest the freeze transition resulting from rapid evaporative cooling, similar to the earlier approaches [36]. Their process, termed "cavitation" foam drying (CFD), also maintained a liquid state and continued evaporative boiling by lowering pressure in a slower stepwise fashion with brief equilibration between each step. The process is designed to generate an open cell foam for improved drying kinetics. Preventing the formulation from freezing also reduces the process loss likely associated with damage from ice crystal formation and denaturation at phase interfaces. It was successfully applied to a number of biologics, including bacterial and viral vaccines [11–13], and shown to minimize process losses.

10.4.3.6 Bronshtein (PBV)

More recently Bronshtein proposed a new process for foam drying called preservation by vaporization (PBV) [37], which more fully embraced the idea of the FFD process of allowing the liquid to freeze. In the PBV process the progression of lower shelf temperatures was continued; by prescribing levels below −5 °C, the liquid was to be partially frozen into a slushy state prior to initiating high vacuum to bring about simultaneous foaming of the liquid and sublimation of the ice.

10.4.4 Challenges to Commercialization

There a number of challenges that will need to be overcome before a foam-dried pharmaceutical product can reach the marketplace.

10.4.4.1 Process Stresses

The surface tension or shear stresses associated with liquid bubbling or boiling could potentially damage a biopharmaceutical agent, particularly resulting from denaturation of proteins at interfaces. In addition, the overall impact of dehydration stresses can lead to protein aggregation. However, the use of appropriate glass formers, surfactants, and other stabilizers can minimize these issues.

10.4.4.2 Scalability and Process Robustness

In contrast to lyophilization the foam structure following foam drying can be nonuniform and highly variable in appearance and cake height and within a batch can vary from vial to vial; some vials may not foam at all with a dried viscous film resulting instead. Therefore, it would be difficult to enforce the same Quality Control (QC) acceptance criteria of "cake elegance" applied to lyophilization without imposing a high reject rate on the product; this potential for higher reject rate would negatively impact throughput and yield. In some cases, the inhomogeneity in foam density and moisture between and within vials can cause some vials to experience foam collapse either during or after processing. This inhomogeneity can lead to variability in biologic stability as well. Further, without sufficient headspace the splattering of product during the foaming phase of drying can deposit product near the vial opening, risking issues with container-closure integrity.

Scalability can be improved by controlling the foaming action. This can be achieved to some degree by a more gradual, controlled vacuum ramp down rate while tuning the shelf temperature profile. Carefully navigating the path through the parameter space of time/temperature/pressure is necessary in order to avoid sacrificing too much of the low cycle time benefit of foam drying over lyophilization. Also the introduction of foaming agents and foam stabilizers can address some of these variability challenges. Attempts to address some of these scalability issues, including bubble nucleation and equipment limitations, have been proposed by Bronshtein with variable successes as described in a series of patents [38–40], although there is likely still more research and development necessary in this area. In addition, continuous vacuum-drying equipment exists for food and pharmaceuticals to increase throughput and improve economics [41, 42], which potentially could be applied to vacuum foam drying of biologics.

With the bulk of mass and heat transfer occurring in the first minutes of primary drying, it should be recognized that a foam-drying process can put a significant moisture load on a freeze dryer's condenser, and as a result it is critical that the equipment is scaled appropriately to handle the proposed batch size. Also, owing to the larger closed-cell foam structures and lower surface to volume ratio, the secondary drying cycle time associated with a foam-drying process can sometimes exceed that of freeze drying to achieve the same moisture level. However, the formulation's moisture target will ultimately depend on the demands of the particular product, because foam-dried formulations can be more stable even with higher moisture content than their freeze-dried counterparts [11]. That is, the moisture content of the dried cake and its glass transition temperature (T_g) alone are not always good predictors of storage stability.

10.4.4.3 Drug Delivery Requirements

Because a foam-dried product has lower surface to volume ratio, it can have longer reconstitution times compared with either a lyophilized or spray-dried counterpart. However, the reconstitution time for most foam-dried products is still generally less than a minute.

One challenge for foam drying is converting the final product into a powder; the vial format is not conducive to this. Alternative methods such as foam mat drying could facilitate a milling step to produce powders; however, making this an aseptic process (generally required for a biologic) can be challenging. Although spray drying produces powders directly, this issue holds true for lyophilized products as well. Methods for converting foam-dried glasses to powders and for formulating convenient delivery systems from the resulting powders have been proposed [40, 43]

10.4.4.4 Barriers to Change in the Pharmaceutical Industry

As with any new process to be introduced to an established industry, the resistance to change is often the result of the lack of infrastructure, equipment, and overall process knowledge and experience, in addition to the fact that discomfort with potential risks (known or unknown) often outweigh even a substantial demonstrated benefit, financial or otherwise. However, it is expected that aseptic processing of biologics via foam drying is feasible given the fact that commercial production could be conducted with existing freeze-drying equipment and infrastructure.

10.5 Application of Foam Drying to Biostabilization

As discussed above, the primary advantage offered by foam drying is the enhanced thermal stabilization of bioactive agents that is frequently unrivaled with other pharmaceutical drying processes. Since the successful preservation of a number of bacteria was demonstrated with foam drying by Annear a half century ago, several researchers have used this approach for stabilization of a number of biologics in the dried state. For example, live attenuated vaccines for rinderpest and peste des petits ruminants viruses [44], Newcastle disease virus [45], parainfluenza virus [7], *Francisella tularensis* bacteria [12], *Salmonella* Typhi bacteria [13], rabies virus [46], porcine reproductive and respiratory syndrome virus [47], and influenza virus [11] have all been successfully foam-dried showing superior stabilization relative to lyophilization and/or spray drying. Similar results were found with foam drying an IgG monoclonal antibody [6]. More detailed results for a few of these biologics are presented in case studies in Section 10.5.2.

10.5.1 Formulation Considerations

As important as the drying method is to produce a stable product, optimum stability can only be achieved with the appropriate combination of pharmaceutical excipients. Indeed, the advancement in the use of better stabilizers for drying processes has been as important as the improvements in freeze-drying equipment for the preservation of biologic activity. The excipients that are often included in a foam-dried formulation are not uncommon to other pharmaceutical drying processes and include buffers, glass formers, polymers, plasticizers, proteins, surfactants, amino acids, etc. However, the concentration of the base stabilizer, i.e. the glass former or polyol, is used at significantly higher concentration. Some of the important considerations for each of these are discussed further below.

10.5.1.1 Moisture Content

Water acts as a very effective plasticizer lowering the T_g of an amorphous glass and increasing its molecular mobility [48]. Thus, moisture may be the most important component determining the storage stability of a dried solid formulation, although, as mentioned above, it is not always a reliable predictor of storage stability on its own. Perhaps no other drying process methods have emphasized this exception more than foam drying, because minimizing moisture content (with the goal of maximizing T_g) does not necessarily monotonically improve stability [11].

10.5.1.2 Buffers and pH

As with any formulation development process, finding a suitable buffering system and pH is generally the first step. In addition to controlling pH, buffers can serve as a stabilizer or solubilizer and may participate in the foaming process itself. The pH of the formulation is generally in a physiological range, e.g. pH 6–8. Because foam drying is at near ambient conditions, the tendency to form ice crystals, to freeze-concentrate excipients, and to create large pH shifts is minimized. Thus, the constraints on buffer selection for freeze drying are often not present for foam drying. In a study of foam-dried bovine serum albumin (BSA), sodium phosphate was found more stabilizing than potassium phosphate [49], a result that would not be expected for a freeze-dried product because of the pH shift observed with sodium phosphate-buffered formulations during processing [5].

10.5.1.3 Glass Formers

Glass formers inhibit protein unfolding and slow degradation reactions by surrounding the biologic with an amorphous solid environment and reducing molecular mobility. The more commonly employed amorphous excipients are disaccharides such as sucrose or trehalose, which stabilizes the biologic both during drying and in the final product when encased in the resulting glassy matrix. Sucrose and other polyols can also protect the biologic against drying-induced denaturation by replacing the lost water of hydration through hydrogen bonding to charged regions of the protein. Sugar alcohols such as mannitol generally do not stabilize biologics as effectively as sucrose in foam-dried powders because of their tendency to crystalize instead of forming an amorphous glass

[50]. However, in combination with other sugar alcohols, mannitol has been shown to remain amorphous and provide enzyme and protein storage stability superior to trehalose in vacuum-dried foams [51]. Glass formers also thicken the formulation to enhance bubble formation and stabilization, ultimately providing the structural integrity to the thin films that form the bubble interfaces.

10.5.1.4 Foaming Agents

Some researchers have included foaming agents, such as surfactants or foam stabilizers, to enhance the generation of the foams for a more controlled and reproducible process. In addition to facilitating foaming action, surfactants provide large cake volume and larger foam bubbles. Surfactants can also improve potency retention and stability by (i) reducing surface adsorption of the protein/biologic, driving them to the interior by displacement, (ii) altering the glass phase dynamics (see Section 10.6), and (iii) lowering SSA. In addition, surfactants can enhance the solubility of certain constituents. Tween® and Pluronic® surfactants are common in biologic formulations in low concentration of less than 1%. However, in some cases the addition of surfactants can reduce the stability of certain biologics by, for example, destabilizing the lipid membrane of bacteria [12]. Foam stabilizers such as carboxymethyl cellulose (CMC) [15] and polyvinylpyrrolidone (PVP) [49] provide foam stability by inhibiting foam collapse and reducing the final foam brittleness while also facilitating the drying process. Viscosity modifiers such as guar gum serve a similar purpose [32]. Other foaming agents such as dissolved gasses, suspended bubbles, or gas forming chemicals can serve to initiate the foaming process. Researchers in the food industry have used egg white (albumin) as a foaming agent for a foam-mat-drying application [17].

10.5.1.5 Polymers

Polymers generally enhance the formulation viscosity and therefore improve "foamability." Gelatin (a peptide or protein polymer) is often included in biologic formulations to improve storage stability [11–13]. Polymers such as PVP can interact with glass formers to enhance recoveries of the biologic from processing [49]. Some lower molecular weight polymers, such as Pluronics, serve the dual role as both a surfactant-based foaming agent and stabilizer by displacing the biologic from the phase interfaces of the foam where surface tension-induced denaturation can take place.

10.5.1.6 Plasticizers

The addition of a plasticizers will not only lower the glass transition temperature of the dried solid but can also serve to dampen the fast dynamics associated with the molecular mobility of the glass matrix. Lower molecular weight additives such as sorbitol, glycerol, or dimethyl sulfoxide (DMSO) when included in the right amount relative to glass formers have been used successfully for these purposes to improve the storage stability of solid dosage form biologics [13, 52, 53].

10.5.1.7 Proteins and Amino Acids

While gelatin also fits in this category, other proteins such as human albumin or fetal bovine serum have also been included in several dry vaccine formulations [42].

Although amino acids such as glutamate have been used historically in foam drying as the glass former [31], amino acids such as arginine have also been demonstrated to provide stabilization of flu virus [11] and a bacterial vaccine [12]. Potentially acting as mild antioxidant, methionine has shown benefit in stabilizing foam-dried bacterial vaccines as well [12, 13]. Mattern et al. studied the use of amino acids for improved vacuum-drying kinetics and high-temperature stabilization of proteins both as an additive to sugar glass formulations [54] and as mixtures of certain pure amino acid combinations to produce high T_g solids [55].

In some cases, excipients can interact synergistically to enhance the stabilization of the biologic. Combinations such as sucrose and phosphate [56] or surfactant in the presence of gelatin [12] have shown this effect.

10.5.2 Examples of Foam-Dried Biopharmaceuticals: Case Studies

10.5.2.1 *Protein*: IgG_1 Monoclonal Antibody

In a study to explore the differences in physicochemical properties and the resulting stability of an IgG_1 monoclonal antibody from alternative drying methods, Abdul-Fattah et al. employed several analyses to characterize dried formulations produced by spray, freeze, and foam drying [6]. The excipients used in the formulations, other than the 1 mM potassium phosphate buffer in all of the wet blends prior to drying, were sucrose and the surfactant Pluronic F68 at varying concentrations. Moisture content of all formulations was maintained in the same range of about 1–2% by mass; the authors claimed stability of the formulations varied little over this range. Specifically, they assessed surface composition for protein accumulation, SSA, and the molecular mobility of the dried product. These results were then correlated with storage stability of the protein in the formulations. The findings from this study demonstrated the significant impact thermal history has on both the properties and the storage stability of biologics embedded in glassy matrices of similar composition.

With regard to surface properties, the foam-dried formulations with higher sucrose content had the lowest SSA, while spray-dried formulations had the highest SSA, although their SSA tended to decrease with increasing sucrose content. The presence of surfactant did not have a strong impact on SSA. On the other hand, the presence of surfactant significantly reduced the protein surface coverage of all formulation (independent of drying method) as determined by electron spectroscopy for chemical analysis (ESCA). Therefore, the total protein surface exposure was lowest for the foam-dried formulations with higher sucrose content. Regarding molecular mobility, data indicated that the foam-dried formulations with higher sucrose content had the lowest molecular mobility, which included both long-range global motions and shorter-range fast dynamics. Storage stability data at elevated temperatures showed good (inverse) correlation with total surface coverage of antibody and the molecular mobility from fast dynamics such that the higher sucrose foam-dried formulation was most stable. Conversely, preservation of protein secondary structure (as measured by Fourier transform infrared (FTIR) spectroscopy) in sucrose-rich formulations did not correlate well with stability; the foam-dried formulations were least effective in preserving protein secondary structure.

10.5.2.2 *Viral Vaccine*: Influenza

Lovalenti et al. compared the effectiveness of different drying methods to produce a stable solid dosage form of live attenuated influenza vaccine (LAIV) [11]. Prior to the comparison, some effort was made to produce individually optimized foam-dried, spray-dried, and freeze-dried formulations of an H1N1 strain of flu virus through excipient screening. While the addition of arginine and gelatin had a stabilizing effect in the foam-dried formulation, it had negligible impact on the spray-dried formulation, which exhibited some stabilization benefit from the nonionic surfactant Pluronic F68. Each of the formulations was then evaluated for their storage stability at 4, 25, and 37 °C (Figure 10.5). A commercial freeze-dried formulation (NASOVAC™) was also included in the comparison. Although the NASOVAC formulation performed similarly to the foam-dried formulation at 4 °C (potency loss rate of 0.007 vs. 0.006 log $TCID_{50}$/ml/wk, respectively), the foam-dried formulation exhibited as much as an order of magnitude lower potency loss rate than all formulations at 25 and 37 °C (Table 10.2). In fact, while the spray- and freeze-dried formulations lost more than 1 log_{10} in potency after one week at 37 °C, the foam-dried formulation

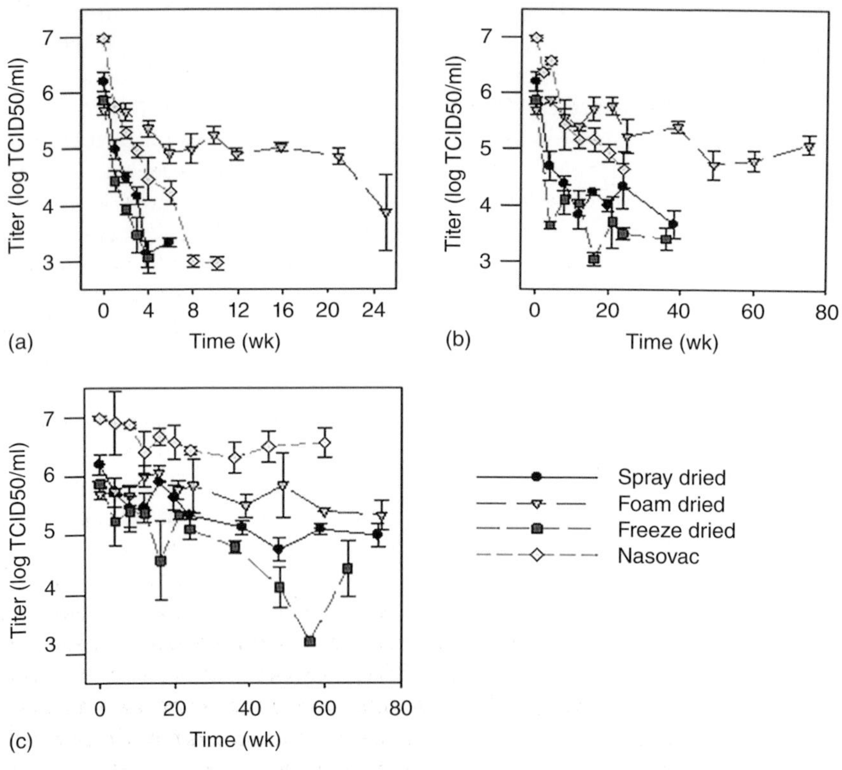

Figure 10.5 Storage stability at 37 °C (a), 25 °C (b), and 4 °C (c) for H1N1 LAIV formulations manufactured using spray-drying (•), foam-drying (▾), and freeze-drying processes (□), along with a commercial freeze-dried product, NASOVAC™ (◇). Data represents average of three measurements and the error bars the standard deviation. Source: Lovalenti et al. (2016) [11]. Reproduced with permission of Springer Nature.

Table 10.2 Physical properties and H1N1 LAIV stability in foam-dried, freeze-dried, and spray-dried formulations.

Formulation	Moisture (%)	T_g (°C)	Process loss (log $TCID_{50}$/ml)	Rate of titer loss (log $TCID_{50}$/ml/wk)		
				4 °C	25 °C	37 °C
Spray dried	2.0 ± 0.3	51.5 ± 0.5	0.3 ± 0.2	0.014 ± 0.003	0.23 ± 0.09	0.72 ± 0.09
Foam dried	2.9 ± 0.4	40.1 ± 0.5	0.4 ± 0.4	0.006 ± 0.002	0.013 ± 0.003	0.055 ± 0.011
Freeze dried	0.3 ± 0.2	48.5 ± 0.2	0.5 ± 0.2	0.028 ± 0.006	0.22 ± 0.19	0.66 ± 0.12
NASOVAC™	0.1 ± 0.0	N/A	N/A	0.007 ± 0.003	0.18 ± 0.05	0.58 ± 0.09

Results are the average of three measurements, except T_g measured in duplicate, and include the standard deviation.
Source: Lovalenti et al. (2016) [11]. Reproduced with permission of Springer Nature.

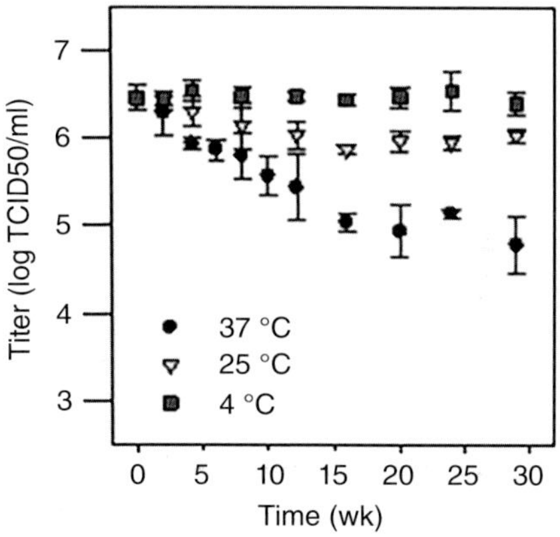

Figure 10.6 Stability profile of foam-dried formulation for type-B LAIV strain. Data represents average of three measurements and the error bars the standard deviation. Source: Lovalenti et al. (2016) [11]. Reproduced with permission of Springer Nature.

took more than 20 weeks to lose the same amount. It may be surprising that even though the foam-dried formulation had the lowest glass transition temperature (T_g) and highest moisture content of the formulations, it was able to excel in stabilizing the vaccine at elevated temperatures (see Table 10.2). As will be discussed in the Section 10.6, there may be other physical properties such as molecular mobility that may be more significant in dictating stability, and the foam-dried formulation is more effective in imparting those desired properties. These formulations were further evaluated for their immunogenicity in a ferret model. All formulations were found to elicit an equivalent immune response to the frozen LAIV control, indicating the potency of the vaccine was retained in the drying process. The foam-dried formulation was also used with a type-B LAIV and showed similar storage stability (Figure 10.6).

10.5.2.3 *Bacterial Vaccine*: Ty21a

The effectiveness of foam drying to preserve the potency and immunogenicity of a *Salmonella* Typhi live bacterial vaccine (Ty21a) was demonstrated in a study by Ohtake et al. [13] who investigated the impact of not only formulation and detailed drying cycle on process and storage stability but also the culturing of the

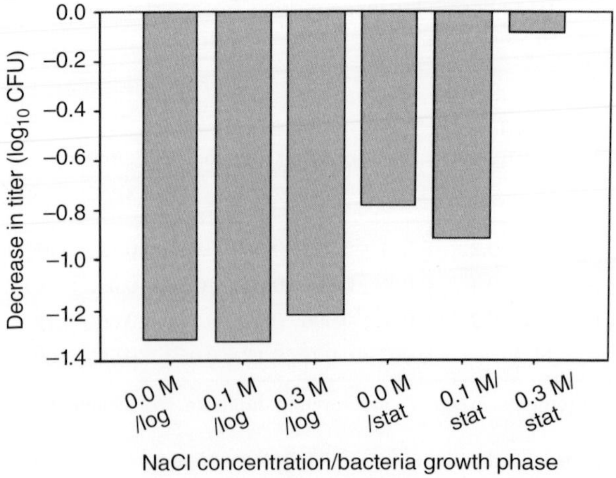

Figure 10.7 The process recovery of Ty21a upon foam drying. Bacteria were grown in brain heart infusion (BHI) growth media containing varying amounts of NaCl, ranging from 0 to 0.3 M NaCl, and were harvested either in the log phase (log) or the early stationary phase (stat), as indicated. Source: Ohtake et al. (2011) [13]. Reproduced with permission of Elsevier.

bacteria itself. They found that by exposing the bacteria to osmotic stress by the addition of sodium chloride to the growth media and by harvesting during the stationary phase of growth (as opposed to the lag or log phase) enhanced the bacteria's resistance to stresses during foam drying (see Figure 10.7) and subsequent storage.

One of the important factors in minimizing the process loss associated with foam drying the bacteria was found to be the careful control of the rate of foaming and drying by reducing the pressure from atmospheric to less than 100 mTorr in a stepwise fashion while controlling shelf temperature to minimize freezing caused by evaporative cooling. Initial studies found most of the process loss to occur in the early part of the cycle when most of the moisture removal takes place. Thus, through cycle optimization by making stepwise reductions in the system pressure with short equilibration holds, the process loss was reduced from 0.8 to 0.3 log_{10} CFU. Stabilization of the bacteria in the foam-dried state was further improved by the addition of the stabilizers: the amino acid methionine, the plasticizer DMSO, and gelatin all contributed to reduce process and storage losses in potency. Gelatin had the added benefit of enhancing the foaming action during drying. The optimized formulation stabilized the vaccine for over four weeks at 37 °C with less than 0.5 log_{10} CFU loss in potency and for 12 weeks at 25 °C with no loss in titer. The significantly improved stabilization provided by foam drying relative to either freeze drying (note: the commercial Ty21a product Vivotif™ is freeze-dried) or spray drying is further illustrated in Table 10.3.

In order to evaluate the retention of immunogenicity of the foam-dried vaccine, the formulation was tested in mice for its ability to elicit an immune response and protect the mice against a lethal dose challenge. Interestingly the foam-dried vaccine not only demonstrated an enhanced immune response (as measured by antibody titers) but also provided better protection against infection relative to the either the unformulated vaccine or the commercial freeze-dried product Vivotif.

10.5.2.4 *Human Cells*: T Cells

Recent studies conducted at Pfizer have shown superior stabilization of human T cells by foam drying [57]. The process loss in cell viability associated with

Table 10.3 Process-associated loss and storage stability at 25 °C for freeze-dried, spray-dried, and foam-dried Ty21a.

Process	Process loss ($\log_{10}$ CFU)	Stability loss after 1 wk at 25 °C ($\log_{10}$ CFU)
Freeze drying[a)]	0.8 ± 0.1	0.5 ± 0.0
Spray drying[b)]	0.7 ± 0.1	1.7 ± 0.1
Foam drying[c)]	0.3 ± 0.2	No loss[d)]

All data represent the average (±scanning electron microscopy [SEM]) of duplicate experiments.

a) Formulation contained 28% (w/v) sucrose, 1% (w/v) gelatin in 25 mM KPO_4, pH 7.
b) Formulation contained 7% (w/v) sucrose.
c) Formulation contained 25% (w/v) sucrose, 0.5% (w/v) methionine, 2.4 wt% DMSO, 25 mM KPO_4, pH 8.
d) Storage stability following 4 wk at 25 °C.

Source: Ohtake et al. (2011) [13]. Reproduced with permission of Elsevier.

foam drying was significantly less than that of the freeze-dried formulation of the same composition, 42.4% vs. 61.2%, respectively. Also, the foam-dried formulation showed less than 1% loss in cell viability after one week of storage at 5 °C, compared with the corresponding liquid formulation losing ~9% over the same period. The same formulation composition that was freeze-dried lost 22% per week. Remarkably, after more than 160 days at 5 °C, the cell viability of the foam-dried formulation was similar to that of the frozen liquid held at −70 °C for the same period of time.

10.6 Physiochemical Characterization of the Foam-Dried Product

Analytical techniques have been used to characterize the solid-state properties of the foam-dried product and the nature of the stabilization of the encased biologic. A few of the more relevant approaches are discussed further below.

10.6.1 Thermal Analysis and Protein Secondary Structure

The most common physiochemical characterization is the measurement of the glass transition temperature (T_g) of the dried solid formulation using differential scanning calorimetry (DSC). The general expectation is that a formulation with higher T_g will have better storage stability. However, it has been found that despite the T_g of a foam-dried formulation often being lower than an equivalent freeze-dried or spray-dried formulation with the same moisture content, the foam-dried formulation can provide significantly better storage stability [11]. Findings such as this emphasize the point that other physicochemical characterization beyond T_g of solid dosage forms are as, if not more, important for correlating with the stabilization of bioactive agents. Bronshtein contends that the T_g of a foam-dried glass formulation cannot be above its highest drying temperature and recommends using a "Thermally Stimulated Depolarization Current (TSDC) technique designed for measurements of T_g in polymeric materials, which permits reliable monitoring of vitrification processes in biological materials stabilized using sugar polymers" [38]. Abdul-Fattah et al. used modulated differential scanning calorimetry (MDSC) to not only evaluate the T_g of similar sucrose-based formulations of a viral vaccine produced by spray, freeze, and foam drying but also their enthalpy recovery during the thermal scan [7]. They found excellent correlation between high enthalpy recovery (which was linked to low molecular mobility) and storage stability at elevated temperatures, with the foam-dried formulation having highest enthalpy recovery and best storage stability despite having lower T_g.

FTIR spectroscopy can be used to probe protein secondary structure while embedded in a glassy matrix. Dried formulations that preserve proteins with secondary structures more closely resembling their native state are expected to have greater stability. However, in studies of foam-dried formulations of IgG_1 antibody, the greater apparent preservation of native structure (as determined by FTIR) did not correlate with improved storage stability [6]. In contrast, Pisal et al. has used IR spectra to probe secondary structure of foam-dried human serum albumin in the presence of different excipients [50] and found correlation with protein stability [49].

10.6.2 Specific Surface Area and Surface Composition Analysis

Here, Brunauer–Emmett–Teller (BET) analysis and ESCA can provide SSA and surface nitrogen content, respectively. These measurements can combine to give a measure of the surface exposure of the biologic for a given drying method [1]. The low values for foam drying, relative to either spray or freeze drying, have been pointed to as being at least partly responsible for the associated improved storage stability of foam-dried formulations [6, 7].

10.6.3 Molecular Mobility and Amorphous Structure Analysis

The techniques used to evaluate molecular mobility provide an indication of both the global (slow) dynamics and local (fast) dynamics and include the use of a thermal activity monitor (TAM) for tracking rates of enthalpy relaxation and a high-flux backscattering spectrometer (HFBS) for measuring incoherent elastic neutron scattering, respectively [1]. It is the significantly reduced molecular mobility associated with local fast dynamics that has been most significantly correlated with foam-dried formulations and the superior storage stability they provide for biologic actives [6, 7].

X-ray powder diffraction (XRPD) analysis has also been used to measure and monitor the amorphous character of the glassy matrix. Pisal et al. used XRPD on foam-dried formulations of LaSota virus to screen excipients for inhibiting crystallization of the disaccharides they contained [45]. For example, the inclusion of polymers such as polyvinylpyrrolidone or polyethylene glycol aided in maintaining the amorphous character of the glass-forming sucrose, which correlated with improved storage stability relative to formulations showing some crystallization of the sucrose.

10.7 Conclusions and Future Prospects

Foam drying represents an attractive drying technology that can produce solid dosage forms for biologics with enhanced storage stability, especially for very unstable biopharmaceuticals such as live viral or bacterial vaccines. The "science" behind often extraordinary stability properties of the foam formulation is related to its "mild" thermal history and the solid-state property that seems to suggest longer glass relaxation time and lower local molecular motions as compared with the same formulation that has been dried using more common pharmaceutical drying processes such as freeze drying and spray drying. Of course, the specific formulation excipients are also critical to the final stability profile, but it is useful to note that many of the basic formulation parameters used with foam drying are those that are commonly used in typical pharmaceutical formulations. Scaled-up processing at pilot plant or commercial scale remains a challenge with foam drying. But the clear demonstration of a strong stability profile seems consistent across many researchers who have used foam drying, such that additional process research is warranted to advance this technology to a manufacturing reality.

References

1 Truong-Le, V. and Abdul-Fattah, A.M. (2010). The impact of formulation and drying processes on the characteristics and performance of biopharmaceutical powders. In: *Formulation and Process Development Strategies for Manufacturing Biopharmaceuticals* (eds. F. Jameel and S. Hershenson), 565–586. Hoboken, NJ: Wiley.

2 Schroeder, A.L. and Schwarz, H.W. (1949). Low temperature vacuum dehydration. *Chemical Engineering Progress* 45: 370–376.

3 Franks, F., Hatley, R., and Mathias, S. (1991). Material science and the production of shelf-stable biologics. *Biopharm* 4: 38–55.

4 Abdul-Fattah, A.M., Lechuga-Ballesteros, D., Kalonia, D.S. et al. (2008). The impact of drying method and formulation on the physical properties and stability of methionyl human growth hormone in the amorphous solid state. *Journal of Pharmaceutical Sciences* 97 (1): 163–184.

5 Pikal-Cleland, K.A., Rodríguez-Hornedo, N., Amidon, G.L. et al. (2000). Protein denaturation during freezing and thawing in phosphate buffer systems: monomeric and tetrameric beta-galactosidase. *Archives of Biochemistry and Biophysics* 384 (2): 398–406.

6 Abdul-Fattah, A.M., Truong-Le, V., Yee, L. et al. (2007). Drying-induced variations in physico-chemical properties of amorphous pharmaceuticals and their impact on stability I: stability of a monoclonal antibody. *Journal of Pharmaceutical Sciences* 96: 1983–2008.

7 Abdul-Fattah, A.M., Truong-Le, V., Yee, L. et al. (2007). Drying-induced variations in physico-chemical properties of amorphous pharmaceuticals and their impact on stability II: stability of a vaccine. *Pharmaceutical Research* 24: 715–727.

8 Walters, R.H., Bhatnagar, B., Tchessalov, S. et al. (2014). Next generation drying technologies for pharmaceutical applications. *Journal of Pharmaceutical Sciences* 103: 2673–2695.

9 Sprunk, A., Page, S., and Kleinebudde, P. (2013). Influence of process parameters and equipment on dry foam formulation properties using indomethacin as model drug. *International Journal of Pharmaceutics* 465: 189–196.

10 Sawatdee, S., Atipairin, A., Sae Yoon, A. et al. (2019). Enhanced dissolution of sildenafil citrate as dry foam tablets. *Pharmaceutical Development and Technology* 24 (1): 1–11.

11 Lovalenti, P.M., Anderl, J., Luisa, Y. et al. (2016). Stabilization of live attenuated influenza vaccines by freeze drying, spray drying, and foam drying. *Pharmaceutical Research* 33: 1144–1160.

12 Ohtake, S., Martin, R.A., Saxena, A. et al. (2011). Formulation and stabilization of *Francisella tularensis* live vaccine strain. *Journal of Pharmaceutical Sciences* 100: 3076–3087.

13 Ohtake, S., Martin, R.A., Saxena, A. et al. (2011). Room temperature stabilization of oral, live attenuated *Salmonella enterica* serovar typhi-vectored vaccines. *Vaccine* 29: 2761–2771.

14 Campbell, C.H. (1917) Drying milk. US Patent 1250427, filed 1917 and issued 1913.

15 Hardy, Z. and Jideani, V.A. (2017). Foam-mat drying technology: a review. *Critical Reviews in Food Science and Nutrition* 57: 2560–2572.

16 Kandasamy, P., Varadyaraju, N., Kalemullah, S. et al. (2014). Optimization of process parameters for foam-mat drying of papaya pulp. *Journal of Food Science and Technology* 51: 2526–2534.

17 Djaeni, M., Prasetyaningrum, A., Sasongko, S.B. et al. (2015). Application of foam-mat drying with egg white for carrageenan: drying rate and product quality aspects. *Journal of Food Science and Technology* 52: 1170–1175.

18 Heyman, W.A. (1941) Porous expanded citrus fruit products. US Patent 2328554, filed 1943 and issued 1941.

19 Aceto, N.C., Sinnamon, H.I., Schoppet, E.F. et al. (1962). Continuous vacuum drying of whole milk foam. *Journal of Dairy Science* 45: 501–507.

20 Turkot, V.A., Aceto, N.C., Schoppet, E.F. et al. (1969). Continuous vacuum drying of whole milk foam. *Food Engineering* 59–64 (97): 41.

21 Sramek, M., Schweiggert, R.M., van Kampen, A. et al. (2015). Preparation of high-grade powders from tomato paste using a vacuum foam drying method. *Journal of Food Science* 80: 1755–1762.

22 Hertzendorf, M.S., Moshy, R.J., and Seltzer, E. (2009). Foam drying in the food industry. *C R C Critical Reviews in Food Technology* 1: 25–70.

23 Cui, Z., Xu, S., and Sun, D. (2004). Microwave–vacuum drying kinetics of carrot slices. *Journal of Food Engineering* 65: 157–164.

24 Mongpraneet, S., Abe, T., and Tsurusaki, T. (2002). Accelerated drying of welsh onion by far infrared radiation under vacuum conditions. *Journal of Food Engineering* 55: 147–156.
25 Lepeshinskaya, O. (1939). The origin of the cell. *Pod znamenem marksizma (USSR)* 5: 130–145.
26 Katkov, I.I., Isachenko, V., Isachenko, E. et al. (2006). Low- and high-temperature vitrification as a new approach to biostabilization of reproductive and progenitor cells. *International Journal of Refrigeration* 29: 346–357.
27 Stamp, L. (1947). The preservation of bacteria by drying. *Journal of General Microbiology* 1: 251–265.
28 Annear, D.I. (1954). Preservation of bacteria. *Nature* 174: 359–360.
29 Annear, D.I. (1956). The preservation of bacteria by drying in peptone plugs. *Journal of Hygiene* 54: 487–508.
30 Annear, D.I. (1962). The preservation of leptospires by drying from the liquid state. *Journal of General Microbiology* 27: 341–343.
31 Annear, D.I. (1970). Recoveries of bacteria after drying and heating in glutamate foams. *Journal of Hygiene* 68: 457–459.
32 Roser, B.J. and Gribbon, E.M. (1996) Methods for stably incorporating substances within dry, foamed glass matrices and compositions obtained thereby. Patent WO 1996040077, filed 1996 and issued 1996.
33 Bronshtein, V. (1998) Preservation by foam formation. US Patent 5766520, filed 1998 and issued 1997 .
34 Bronshtein, V. (2004). Preservation by foam formulation, an alternative to freeze-drying. *Pharmaceutical Technology* 28 (5): 86–92.
35 Truong-Le, V. (2006) Preservation of bioactive materials by freeze dried foam. US Patent 7135180, filed 2006 and issued 2003.
36 Truong-Le, V., Ohtake, S., Chiueh, G. et al. (2011) Formulation for room temperature stabilization of a live attenuated bacterial vaccine. US 2011/0064723, issued 2010.
37 Bronshtein, V. (2016) Preservation by vaporization. US Patent 9469835, filed 2016 and issued 2005.
38 Bronshtein, V. (2003) Scalable long-term shelf preservation of sensitive biological solutions and suspensions. US Patent 6509146, filed 2003 and issued 1997.
39 Bronshtein, V., Bracken, K.R., and Cambell, J.G. (2005) Bulk drying and the effects of inducing bubble nucleation. US Patent 6884866, filed 2005 and issued 2002.
40 Bronshtein, V., Bracken, K.R., Livers, R.K. et al. (2001) Industrial scale barrier technology for preservation of sensitive biological materials at ambient temperatures. US Patent 6306345, filed 2001 and issued 1999.
41 Santivarangkna, C., Kulozik, U., and Foerst, P. (2007). Alternative drying process for the industrial preservation of lactic acid starter cultures. *Biotechnology Progress* 23: 302–315.
42 Otake, S., Lechuga-Ballestero, D., Truong-Le, V. et al. (2015). Strategies for heat-stable vaccines. In: *Vaccine Development and Manufacturing* (eds. E.P. Wen, R. Ellis and N.S. Pujar), 287–318. Hoboken, NJ: Wiley.

43 Bronshtein, V. (2006) Preservation and formulation of bioactive materials for storage and delivery in hydrophobic carriers. US Patent 7153472, filed 2006 and issued 2000.
44 Worrall, E.E. (2003) Method for the preservation of viruses and mycoplasma. US Patent 6664099, filed 2003 and issued 2000.
45 Pisal, S.S., Wawde, G.M., Salvankar, S. et al. (2006). Vacuum foam drying for preservation of LaSota virus: effect of additives. *AAPS PharmSciTech* 7 (3): E30–E37.
46 Smith, T.G., Siirin, M., Wu, X. et al. (2015). Rabies vaccine preserved by vaporization is thermostable and immunogenic. *Vaccine* 33: 2203–2206.
47 Fang, L., Yu, L., Zheng-lin, H. et al. (2016). Preparation and heat resistance study of porcine reproductive and respiratory syndrome virus sugar glass vaccine. *Vaccine* 34: 3746–3750.
48 Ohtake, S. and Shalaev, E. (2013). Effect of water on the chemical stability of amorphous pharmaceuticals: I. Small molecules. *Journal of Pharmaceutical Sciences* 102: 1139–1154.
49 Jangle, R.D. and Pisal, S.S. (2012). Vacuum foam drying: an alternative to lyophilization for biomolecule preservation. *Indian Journal of Pharmaceutical Sciences* 74: 91–100.
50 Hajare, A.A., More, H.N., and Pisal, S.S. (2011). Effect of sugar additives on stability of human serum albumin during vacuum foam drying and storage. *Current Drug Delivery* 8: 678–690.
51 Roser, B.J. and De Castro, A.G. (1999) Amorphous glasses for stabilizing sensitive products. Patent WO 99/047174, filed 1999 and issued 1999.
52 Cicerone, M.T., Tellington, A., Trost, L. et al. (2003). Substantially improved stability of biological agents in dried form: the role of glassy dynamics in preservation of biopharmaceuticals. *Bioprocess International* 1: 36–47.
53 Cicerone, M.T., Soles, C.L., Chowdhuri, Z. et al. (2005). Fast dynamics as a diagnostic for excipients in preservation of dried proteins. *American Pharmaceutical Review* 8: 22–27.
54 Mattern, M., Winter, G., Rudolph, R. et al. (1997). Formulation of proteins in vacuum-dried glasses. Part 1. improved vacuum-drying of sugars using crystallizing amino acids. *European Journal of Pharmaceutics and Biopharmaceutics* 44: 177–185.
55 Mattern, M., Winter, G., Kohnert, U. et al. (1999). Formulation of proteins in vacuum-dried glasses. Part II. Process and storage stability in sugar-free amino acid systems. *Pharmaceutical Development and Technology* 4: 199–208.
56 Ohtake, S., Schebor, C., Palecek, S.P. et al. (2004). Effect of pH, counter ion, and phosphate concentration on the glass transition temperature of freeze-dried sugar-phosphate mixtures. *Pharmaceutical Research* 21: 1615–1621.
57 Balthazor, B. (2018) Development of foam drying and application to novel biotherapeutic modalities. *SP LyoLearn Webinar*, May 16th, 2018. https://www.spscientific.com/WebinarDetail.aspx?id=4198 (accessed 16 May 2018).

11

Effects of Electric and Magnetic Field on Freezing

Arun S. Mujumdar[1] *and Meng W. Woo*[2]

[1] *McGill University, MacDonald College, Bioresource Engineering Department, 2111 Lakeshore Road, Sainte-Anne-De-Bellevue, QC H9X 3V9, Canada*
[2] *University of Auckland, Department of Chemical and Materials Engineering, Auckland CBD, Auckland 1010, New Zealand*

11.1 Introduction

The freeze-drying process is commonly used in the preservation of food, biologicals, and pharmaceutical materials. This is particularly important for heat-sensitive materials to prevent degradation or structural changes typically encountered in thermal dehydration and preservation of materials [1–3]. A key step in freeze drying, the first process actually, is the freezing of the material that determines the size and structure of the water crystals formed within the material of interest. The size of water crystals will affect the quality of the material in different ways. For food or biological material preservation applications, very often, the requirement is to have smaller ice crystals so that the structure of the food or biological material is preserved [4–7]. This is because the water crystals from the unbound water (intercellular) and the water within the cells (intracellular) may grow and rupture the adjacent cell wall of the materials. This will also be particularly important for the freezing and preservation of biological materials. Conversely, for pharmaceutical applications, the freezing of protein-based formulation may benefit from having larger crystals [8–11]. This is because the water crystals in the formulation will create an interface from which surface-active proteins may bind and denature. In such a scenario, larger crystals will translate to smaller surface area, leading to less denaturation of the proteins. Therefore, there is a strong need to be able to control the size of the water crystals formed during the initial freezing process.

There are many different alternatives to control the size of the water crystals during freezing. These include the pressure shift method, ultrasonic method, mechanical agitation, manipulation of the cooling rate, etc. [12–15]. A comprehensive review specific for applications in the pharmaceutical industry is given by Geidobler and Winter [16]. Manipulation of the cooling rate of the material is the most direct and common approach to control the size of the crystals. In general, faster cooling rate will result in smaller crystals, while slower

Drying Technologies for Biotechnology and Pharmaceutical Applications, First Edition.
Edited by Satoshi Ohtake, Ken-ichi Izutsu, and David Lechuga-Ballesteros.

cooling rate will result in larger crystals. The pressure shift method, ultrasonic method, and mechanical agitation are mainly mechanical approaches at the relatively larger scale to manipulate the ice crystals or nuclei formed to generate small crystal particulates. This review aims to discuss another approach to "mechanically" manipulate the formation of the crystals at the molecular scale by the use of electric and magnetic wave.

The premise of the effect of magnetic and electric field on the freezing process is that water consists of dipole molecules. The oxygen end of the molecule is more negative, while the hydrogen end is more positive. When an electric or magnetic field is applied to water, this dipole behavior will cause the molecules to rotate with the negative end of the molecule toward the positive end of the magnetic or electric field [17]. Depending on how the field is applied, this can then be used to manipulate the structure of the water in the liquid state as well as during the formation or solidification of water. This phenomenon will be the focus of the first half of this chapter (Sections 11.3 and 11.4).

Most reported work in the literature focuses on how the electric and magnetic field affects the freezing process. However, the freezing-drying process also consists of the lyophilization process in which the ice crystals are sublimed under vacuum. In most commercial freezing-drying process, the sublimation process is typically the rate limiting step and has the most significant effect on the economics of the process due to the relatively long sublimation time. The size of the ice crystals will have direct influence on the diffusivity of water vapor during the sublimation stage [18–20]. Section 11.5 will focus on how the electric and magnetic field can affect this latter stage in the freeze-drying process.

While there is no doubt that the magnetic and electric fields do affect the properties of water, there are contrasting views on the significance of this approach in translating to beneficial gains in actual preservation or freezing of materials [21]. This is because a real sample is not just water and the range of the magnetic field used in actual commercial units is relatively low. Section 11.4.2 provides a brief review in this and identifies areas to look into.

11.2 The Different Stages and Parameters of Freezing

The freezing process can be divided into three distinct stages [22]. Figure 11.1 illustrates a typical freezing curve of water at ambient pressure. Firstly, water is cooled down from the ambient temperature at a certain cooling rate. The freezing point of pure water at ambient pressure is typically at 0 °C. However, the formation of the water crystal is a stochastic and time-dependent process. Therefore, at high cooling rate, the water may not start crystallization at 0 °C and can be cooled further below the freezing point. The difference in temperature below the freezing point is called the degree of supercooling. At certain degree of supercooling, the crystallization process will spontaneously occur. When the water crystallizes at a large degree of supercooling, the driving force for crystallization is more "intense" because the water molecules would be closer to each other. Hence, more nucleates will be formed, leading to the formation of a larger number of smaller crystals. Conversely, when crystallization occurs at a smaller degree of supercooling, less nucleates will be formed. This will then lead to the propagation and formation

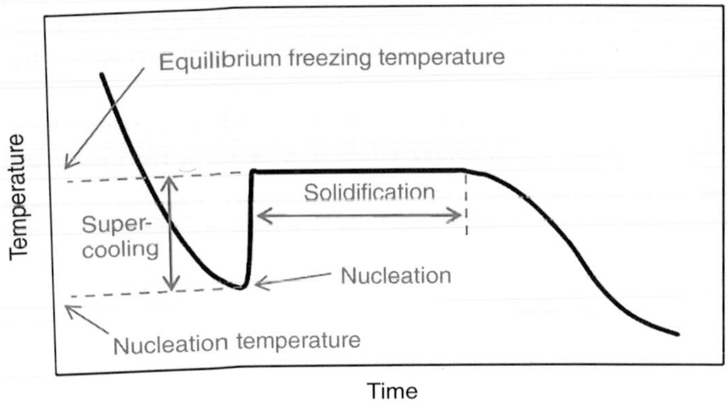

Figure 11.1 The different stages of freezing.

of smaller number of crystals albeit with a larger size. Due to the liberation of the energy of formation, there will be a sudden spike in the temperature of the water. Beyond this point, the water crystals will then progressively grow controlled by the rate in which heat is removed from the water. Hence, a plateau in the temperature profile will be observed as the energy liberated from the formation of the crystals balances with the energy removed via cooling. Once all the dendrites are formed, progressive cooling to the sample will then effectively reduce the temperature of the sample. There are various views on how all the different process parameters affect the morphology of the ice crystals formed [23]. The electric and magnetic field, in general, have direct effect mainly on extending or reducing the degree of supercooling of water. Changes in the degree of supercooling, from which nucleation occurs, will also affect the subsequent processes of freezing, which will be discussed in detail in subsequent sections of this chapter.

11.3 Effect of Electric Field on Freezing

11.3.1 Application to Water and Systems with Dissolved Solute

Earlier scientific reports on the application of the DC field to freezing were undertaken on pure water systems. The application of pulsed or continuous DC electric field was reported as a possible approach to reduce the supercooling of the water sample [24–27]. With the reduced supercooling, in general, larger water crystals are then formed. Such phenomenon of the electric field on the freezing process was also extensively investigated from research groups in the area of meteorology trying to understand the formation of hailstorm and ice. Therefore, the effect of the electric field on water freezing is widely established.

The mechanism behind this reduction in the supercooling was attributed to the realignment of the water molecules following the polarity of the DC electric field giving stronger hydrogen bonds in the direction of the electric field. This closer alignment between the molecules then induces spontaneous nucleation of ice at a certain degree of supercooling alleviating the need for a closer packing of the water molecules at high degree of supercooling. Brief mathematical description based on the thermodynamics of nucleation under the influence of an electric field was given by describing the critical size of the ice crystal for effective use of the DC [27]. Sun et al. [22] provided a base case theory showing that the orientation of the water molecules under the effect of an electric field will provide the most conducive condition for nucleation. A more detailed review of the possible mechanisms involved is provided by Dalvi-Isfahan et al. [28]. Jha et al. [29] provided a detailed thermodynamic description on the mechanism of freezing assisted by a static electric field.

It can argued that the increment of the nucleation temperature can also be achieved by using a slower cooling rate, without the need for more complicated equipment in using the DC electric field. This approach has been the conventional approach used in freezing control [16]. In this respect, the DC electric field may be used as an additional avenue, on top of cooling rate control, to provide a wider range of manipulation to nucleation temperature control. The homogeneous nucleation process is widely known to be stochastic, and repeated operations may lead to significant fluctuations in the nucleation temperature [24]. Application of the DC electric field was reported to reduce the stochastic nature of homogenous nucleation [30]. This will be a significant advantage particularly in product quality control.

In a real system, there are bound to be dissolved solutes within the aqueous sample to be frozen. Generally, it is widely established that the presence of dissolved solutes, organic and nonorganic materials, will decrease the homogeneous nucleation temperature and the equilibrium freezing temperature of water [31]. Similar phenomenon will also be encountered when the DC electric field is applied to the freezing process. The application of the DC field will then be advantageous in overcoming the depression of the homogeneous nucleation temperature particularly when there is a need to have a higher nucleation temperature. This has been demonstrated by Petersen et al. [30, 32] examining the applicability of this technique for the freezing of common cryoprotectants such as hydroxyethyl starch, glucose, and glycerol. There could be a limit, however, on the effect of the DC electric field in controlling or increasing the nucleation temperature of water with dissolved ionic solutes. In the experiments by Petersen et al. [30], the DC electric field was capable of inducing nucleation at relatively low salt concentration. Such electric field-induced nucleation was however not achievable (when cooled down to the temperature of −14 °C) when the salt concentration was extended to mimic physiological conditions. As a result, an alternative pure water nucleation control system was required to induce crystallization in the high salt content samples. The new system allows the ice crystals from the pure water sample to propagate into the high salt content samples. More details on this method can be found in the references cited. Although this observation may be specific within the boundary of their experimental conditions, electric pulsed strength, and cooling rates, it does illustrate the possible constrains that may be encountered in using this technique for real systems.

There are certain benefits, depending on the industrial applications, to making relatively large water crystals. In general larger crystals will allow higher diffusivity of water vapor in the subsequent sublimation stage of freeze drying. This will be particularly important to reduce the operation cost of the overall freeze-drying process [12]. Similarly, larger ice crystals may also help in ensuring fast rehydration of the freeze-dried materials, as the movement of moisture will work in both directions. However, on the flip side, large water crystals may cause structural changes due to the breakage of the cell structures by the penetrating crystals. For pharmaceutical applications, particularly drug formulations with proteins, which are surface active, might tend to attach on to the interface between the crystals and the solute, leading to the loss of its tertiary structure causing denaturation [8–11]. Production of smaller crystals will minimize such denaturation of the protein. Nevertheless, in the evaluation on the need to minimize ice crystal size, it should be noted that these denaturation may be reversible upon thawing of the sample. Another possible damage to pharmaceutical materials, necessitating the formation of smaller crystals, is due to the freeze-concentration effect [33]. When ice crystals are formed, the process tends to expel the protein and solutes from the crystals matrix. This will concentrate the materials that may lead to undesired reactions. Formation of smaller crystals will minimize the concentration buildup as the solutes are expelled to "smaller pocket" within the matrix of relatively smaller ice crystals.

11.3.2 Application to Solid Materials

There are limited reports pertaining to the application of the DC electric field in the freezing of these materials. Xanthakis et al. [34] reported on the use of DC electric field assisted freezing in producing smaller ice crystals in frozen pork. In their report, stronger static DC field (between 6 and 12 kV, electrodes at ~8 mm apart) resulted in smaller degree of supercooling, which led to the formation of smaller crystals. Similarly, Dalvi-Isfahan et al. [35] also found that higher static DC electric field also led to smaller ice crystals. In their experiments, the dripping of the meat samples decreased at higher electrostatic field, while the hardness becomes progressively increasing. There was no significant color change within the range of DC electric field evaluated ($1.9–5.8 \times 10^4$ V/m).

These findings by Xanthakis et al. [34] and Dalvi-Isfahan et al. [35] that smaller degree of supercooling led to smaller ice crystals and vice versa are consistent with the other nonconventional methods in assisting the nucleation process in freezing of solid food and biological materials such as meat and other substrates. For example, Xanthakis et al. [36] reported a similar finding in their experiments, microwave assisted freezing in reducing the degree of supercooling. Within their range of microwave power used, the freezing rate in the solidification phase reduced when compared with the conventional freezing without microwave. However, at higher microwave power, there was no significant decrease in the freezing rate. Similar trend was also observed when ice-nucleating bacteria were incorporated into the freezing of Tylose gel, which is commonly used as a model material for meat [37]. The smaller degree of super cooling led to small crystals.

It is noteworthy that this effect of DC electric field on the freezing of solid materials is in contrast when applied to aqueous or water systems discussed in Section 11.3.1. Theoretically, from studies of freezing pure water and aqueous matrix, smaller degree of supercooling should lead to the formation of less nuclei allowing the growth of these nuclei into relatively larger crystals. In solid samples, for example, meat, the growth of these crystals may have been limited by the structure of the meat and therefore is affected even more so by the heat distribution and transport within the meat samples. This also highlights some possible limitations in the report pertaining to the use of the DC electric field for the freezing of solid samples. In the report by Xanthakis et al. [34] and Dalvi-Isfahan et al. [35], samples in the length-scale order of millimeters were used. More work will need to be undertaken to evaluate the use of the DC electric field on larger samples in which the transport gradient will be more significant. In view that the DC electric field "directionally" orientates the water molecule (even when a pulsed field is used), it is unclear how this affects the propagation of the crystals within the structure.

For future work in this area, particularly when applying this technique to meat, it will also be important to evaluate the advantage of this technique to pre-rigor and post-rigor meat samples. Wu et al. [38] noted that the effect of freezing rate of the formation of ice crystals in salmon is different when compared with fish pre-rigor or post-rigor. For pre-rigor, the formation of the ice crystals is smaller when faster cooling rates were applied. However, for post-rigor samples, the reverse was observed. This is because in pre-rigor fish, the binding of the water to the intracellular protein is higher, leading to lower diffusion of water during freezing. Similar finding was observed by Kaale et al. [39]. When pre-rigor fish salmon fillet was frozen in a fast manner, smaller ice crystals were observed, when compared with the sample frozen slowly. As discussed, it will be important to evaluate how the DC electric field, with its "directional" orientation of water molecules, affects the diffusion of water and the propagation of ice crystals in such different matrix.

11.3.3 Application of AC Field to Freezing

The application of the AC electric field is in contrast to that of the DC electric field. Due to the oscillating behavior of the AC electric field, the water molecules will tend to rotate continuously, and this will then disturb the structure of the water molecule cluster, leading to lower nucleation temperature. There are numerous patents utilizing this phenomenon to control the quality of the frozen product [40, 41] or to maintain products in the supercooled state [42]. On top of that, there are also numerous patents that apply both (or either) the magnetic and AC electric field in assisting the freezing process (to be discussed later).

In view of these commercial patents, it may seem that the technology has already reached maturity. Recent fundamental studies assessing the technology, however, revealed that there may be an alternate mechanism in which the AC electric field assists the control of the freezing process, differing from the well-accepted mechanisms claimed in these patents. Jha et al. [29] also noted and provided a review on the different mechanisms proposed in the literature.

One possible alternate mechanism is the possible effect of the AC electric field on the hydrated ions found in water, which indirectly affects the crystallization of the water molecules. Sun et al. [43] undertook freezing experiments of diluted salt solution with an AC field with different magnitudes of frequencies, ranging from 50 kHz to 5 MHz. It was found that higher frequency reduced the degree of supercooling. Within the range evaluated, there is a critical level at 500 kHz, in which the lowest degree of supercooling was achieved. Interestingly, at subsequent higher frequency, there is a reversed effect in which a larger supercooling was then observed. Most reports in the use of AC electric field to freezing did not comment on such a reversed effect at higher frequency of the AC electric field. One can then question on the existing understanding on how the AC electric field assists the freezing process. If the AC field does cause the water molecules to wiggle, why then, at the higher frequency evaluated, a reversed effect was observed?

Additionally, Sun et al. [43] repeated the experiments with deionized water and found that the application of the AC electric field did not significantly affect the nucleation temperature. On this basis, it was proposed that the AC electric field assisted the freezing process by inducing flow behavior of the Na^+ and Cl^- ions. These may have generated nonuniform electric field within the water system with hot spots of higher field intensity that may have assisted the nucleation process. These results suggest that alternate mechanisms may be involved for the AC electric field to affect the freezing process.

Ma et al. [44] similarly found that there is a critical threshold in the AC electric field frequency in which the maximum cryopreservation of rat liver samples can be achieved. Analogous to the explanation by Sun et al. [43], it was suggested that the optimal frequency of 2.45 MHz observed in their work was because it approximated the dielectric relaxation frequencies of the NaCl ions in the solutions. As a result, there will be a slight lag in the oscillation of the ions, relative to the change in the AC electric field, leading to disturbances in the samples. Such disturbances may have mitigated the formation of the ice crystals. This explanation was derived and supported by an earlier report on how the crystallization of dilute salt solutions can be controlled by the AC electric field. In that earlier paper, the frequency and the strength of the AC electric field were varied. At the extremes of the frequency tested, in regions where the dielectric relaxation frequency of the saline solution is significantly different from the AC field frequency, larger crystal grains were formed. Only between the regions in which the dielectric relaxation frequency was in the same order with the field frequency that smaller ice grains are achieved. It is unclear if these alternative mechanisms are the reasons why the AC electric field does display positive effect on ice crystal manipulation, despite a report estimating that for the AC electric field to affect the homogenous nucleation of water droplet, a relatively high strength electric field in the range of 10^7–10^8 V/m may be required [45]. The maximum AC electric field strengths typically encountered in commercial patents are in the order of 10^6 V/m [46]. Coincidentally, the optimal 2.45 MHz AC electrical field frequency also falls within the preferred range of AC electric field of 250 kHz and 3 MHz in the patent by Owada [47].

11.3.4 Important Additional Considerations

As discussed above, there are existing commercial freezing units utilizing the AC electric field for food application. Therefore, the reliability of the commercial units, from a safety perspective, was demonstrated. At the moment in preparing this chapter, to the best of the authors' knowledge, the application of the DC field is yet to be commercialized to the extent of the AC electric field. From the reports available in the literature, only small-scale experimental rigs were reported, utilizing samples in the order of millimeter or centimeter in length scale. In scaling up this process, care has to be taken in the control of the DC electric field strength. Currently, relatively high field strength was reported and is certainly achievable with small gaps or length scales investigated in the reports. In most of the experiments evaluated, very high voltage field (in the order of kilovolts) is used, and this has to be limited to avoid corona discharge which may burn or may cause electrical hazards to the system [48]. On top of that, in the report by Sun et al. [22], it was highlighted the importance of keeping the DC voltage to a limit to prevent breakdown of the electrodes.

In applying this technique to pharmaceutical materials, more work needs to be undertaken to evaluate if this technique changes the material of interest. Much of the focus of this technique is mainly focusing on cryogenic and refrigeration applications. There are minimal results reported on how the strong electric field will affect pharmaceutical materials, for example, such as those observed in the polymorph of ultrasonic nucleated mannitol solutions [12]. There is also no report on how the electric field will affect the freezing of emulsions that is also affected by the freeze-concentration squeezing effect during freezing [49].

11.4 Effect of Magnetic Field on Freezing

11.4.1 Patent Claims and Studies on Magnetic Field Assisted Freezing

There are many patents available in introducing the magnetic field, static and dynamic field, into the freezing chamber to assist the freezing process. The rationale provided by most patents is that the imbalance spin of the water molecules, when placed under the magnetic field, will tend to break up the water cluster allowing smaller crystals to be formed [46]. As a result, this will minimize drip loss and preserve the quality of the frozen sample. Similar to the discussion on the application of the AC electric field, this will then provide an avenue to produce small ice crystals without the need for excessive rapid cooling. At the moment, fast freezing is still prescribed for certain cryopreservation applications [50]. This aspect will be particularly advantageous in freezing relatively large samples or when slow cooling is required.

Over the years, several modifications and improvements to the technology were patented. Owada [47] and Fujisaki and Amano [51] stressed on the importance of achieving uniform magnetic field within the freezing chamber and proposed revised designs to achieve this. Owada and Saito [52] proposed the incorporation of inert gas into the electromagnetic field freezer. It was claimed that this is essential in preventing any subtle reactions between the material that is to be frozen and the surrounding air; for example, to allow the preservation of live tissues, inert gas was introduced to minimize reactions. Sato and Fujita [53] proposed a method of magnetic field assisted freezer in which the samples to be frozen is preferred to be rotated and moved relative to the static magnetic field. This is akin to a dynamic magnetic field. Nevertheless, common between these patents is that the magnetic field is commonly applied in conjunction with an AC electric field or other forms of energy such as ultrasound waves or microwaves.

This aspect will be further discussed later on in this section. A detailed list and discussion of existing patents for this technology can be found in the report by Otero et al. [21].

Subsequent to the commercialization of this technology, there is now a growing interest in the research community in evaluating this technology, particularly for cryopreservation by freezing. Most of the recent scientific evaluation focused on the Cells Alive System (CAS) technology patented by ABI Co. Ltd. In cryopreservation applications, the advantage claimed is that slow crystallization is sometimes required to allow sufficient transport of water in a low cryoprotectant environment. The low concentration of cryoprotectant is typically used to prevent toxicity effect to biological cells. The use of the magnetic field was claimed to prevent or mitigate the nucleation at low supercooling, which is typical at such slow cooling rates.

Iwasaka et al. [54], in partnership with ABI Co. Ltd., also undertook some fundamental studies on the effect of the magnetic field on the formation of the ice crystals. With the application the magnetic field, rotation and mechanical agitation of the ice crystals were observed *in situ* during cooling, giving smaller ice crystal grain size. Abedini et al. [55] tested the CAS magnetic freezer for teeth samples and found that there was no significant difference between the controlled group (noncryopreserved) and the CAS frozen teeth samples. This follows a very similar finding from the same group reporting the effectiveness of the approach for preserving periodontal ligament cells [56]. It was claimed that the magnetic field can be used to manipulate the formation of ice during the relatively slow freezing required for the preservation of the periodontal ligament cells. Similar positive effect of the CAS freezer was reported by the group [57] on the preservation of rat bone marrow-derived mesenchymal stem cells. In an earlier publication as claimed in the later paper, it was found that the magnetic freezing, however, did not produce positive results in the proliferation of the cells; it only helped in the survival rate [58]. The thawing process with magnetic field also helped in the proliferation rate.

It is noteworthy that in the use of the CAS freezer, also discussed earlier, there is also a presence of AC electric field within the chamber. Iwasaka et al. [54] also mentioned in their paper that in using the Helmholtz coil to generate the magnetic field, inevitably, electric field was also generated during their freezing experiments. Therefore common between all these experimental reports, it may not be so conclusive that the effect of magnetic field is the sole factor that helped in manipulating the ice crystal formation and subsequently contributed to the preservation of the biological samples. Along this line, it will be important to be aware of the arguments on whether or not the magnetic field is significant in controlling the water crystallization process, which will be discussed in Section 11.4.2.

11.4.2 Debate on the Possible Nonsignificant Effect of Magnetic Field to Freezing

Based on existing reports in the literature, this debate can be examined from two different arguments. The first angle questions the significance of the magnetic field in controlling the orientation of water molecules. The second angle, partially following from the first angle, hypothesizes that perhaps the magnetic field affects the solutes in the freezing process rather than the water molecules.

Let us start with the first angle. There has been considerable interest from the academic field on the effect of magnetic field on the properties or water. A significantly thorough review on this area can be found in the report by Jha et al. [29]. Because of its diamagnetic property, water can be magnetized by a magnetic field [59–61]. In general, diamagnetic fluids (including water) display an increase in stability and an increase in the level of hydrogen bonding when placed under a magnetic field. One may expect this to lead to a similar effect observed in the application of an electric field on water, in which it leads to lower degree of supercooling. Indeed, this was demonstrated in an experiment by Aleksandrov et al. [62]. When water droplets were frozen with magnetic fields of 0–0.5 T, lower degree of water supercooling of water was observed. Therefore, the scientific claims by the patents described earlier, particularly on how the magnetic field manipulates the orientation and movement of the water molecules during freezing, seemed to contradict the well-established fundamental understanding in this area. On this basis, there are opinions that perhaps the AC electric field is the main factor contributing to the positive effect on ice crystal manipulation in commercial patents.

Wowk [63] questioned the effect of the low strength magnetic field on the water molecules (as claimed by patents) while acknowledging the effect of the electric field. One of the bases of this argument is that the effect of the magnetic moment of water is proportional to the square of the magnetic field, while the effect of the electromagnetic moment of water is directly proportional to the electric field, proposing that the electric field is more significant in affecting the orientation and movement of water molecule. Further amplifying this difference, as noted by Wowk [63], is that the magnetic field used in the CAS machines are relatively low, even lower that the Earth's magnetic field. It was further postulated that the moving magnetic field used in the machine could also have, inevitably, induced a moving electric field, which may have contributed to the manipulation of ice crystals. Extending the discussion by Wowk [63] and Kobayashi and Kirschvink [64] further postulated that both the electric and magnetic field may not significantly affect the "wiggle" of the water molecules. In contrast, the electric field may have caused a corona wind at the boundary of the system, leading to higher rate of heat transfer away from the system that subsequently led to larger supercooling. Zhao et al. [65] also presented a set of statistical analysis that showed that the magnetic field does not have any significant effect on the nucleation temperature, delineating no significant effect on the supercooling process. Comprehensive details on this angle of the debate can be found in the review by Otero et al. [21].

There is very little attention in systematically investigating the combined magnetic and electric on the freezing process. Mok et al. [66] incorporated a static magnetic field and a pulsed electric field in their report. When only the pulsed electric field was used, as expected, higher frequency led to shorter phase transition time and also resulted in smaller and rounder ice crystals with a more uniform distribution. Higher supercooling was also shown to produce smaller ice crystals. Interestingly, when only the static magnetic field was used, irregular crystal shapes were produced. Surprisingly, the attractive static magnetic field prolonged the phase transition time, while only the repulsive field decreased the phase transition time by about 30% when compared to the control experiments. These results certainly provided more evidence on the effect of the magnetic field on the freezing process. The more important aspect from this report is that there is a need to control the attractive state or the repulsive state of the magnetic field. It is unclear if this aspect was considered in the past reports in this area. Mok et al. [66] further showed that the combined repulsive magnetic field with the pulsed electric field produced a synergistic effect in reducing the phase transition time.

In the second angle of the debate, assuming that the magnetic field does not directly affect the orientation of the water molecules, what are then the possible mechanisms in which it may affect the freezing mechanism? Kobayashi and Kirschvink [64] suggested that the mechanical vibration of the ferromagnetic materials in the fluid, induced by the magnetic field, may be the main cause, resulting in the breakup of the water cluster. In similar veins, Zhao et al. [65] reported that while the magnetic field did not significantly affect the supercooling of their freezing process, the magnetic field did reduce the phase transition time for NaCl solution by about >50%. They attributed this to the effect of the magnetic field on the movement and diffusion of the ionic solutes that will subsequently affect the overall freezing process, particularly in the solidification phase.

Higashi et al. [67] noted that biological cells may be affected by magnetic field. The red blood cells evaluated in that report was found to orientate under the influence of a magnetic field of up to 8 T. This effect however is expected to not be as strong as the effect of electric field due to the diamagnetic property of human tissues [68]. Lin et al. [69] investigated the effect of magnetic field in the slow freezing of red blood cells. They found that the magnetic field produced particles with the same morphology, volume, and cell activity when compared to the control group without magnetic field. However, in addition, they found that the membrane fluidity reduced significantly, indicating that magnetic field produced a more rigid and less permeable cell wall. This may have contributed to two factors in improving the survival of the cell wall. Firstly, the more rigid cells may have improved the resistance toward stresses imposed by the crystallizing water. Secondly, the more rigid membrane may reduce dehydration by the reduction in the transport of water in the cryoprotectant solutions. They suggested that this may be one mechanism in which magnetic field provides positive effect on freezing preservation and not due to the manipulation of ice. Direct investigation on the ice formation was however not performed or reported in that study.

Kobayashi and Kirschvink [70] claimed in their patent that the stabilization and oscillation of magnetite particles in biological samples, when exposed to a magnetic field, will be able to enhance the preservation of the samples during freezing. It was claimed that the oscillation of the magnetite particles will minimize the formation and growth of the ice clusters on the surface of these particles and subsequently minimize the formation of large ice crystals. Magnetite particle are prevalent in many living organisms including human.

Therefore, these are evidences that the magnetic field may produce contributing effect to the freezing preservation process that may not be linked directly to the manipulation or orientation of the ice molecules. In the opinion of the authors, this area may be important for further investigation.

11.5 Possible Effect of Electric and Magnetic Field on the Sublimation Process

Most of the reports on the application of the electric field and magnetic field on the freezing process focused on the preservation of material that is to be subsequently thawed. To the best of the author's knowledge, there are minimal direct studies on how the electric and magnetic field affect the sublimation process, the second part of the freeze-drying process. In contrast, the effect of various other forms of "assisted freezing," such as the use of ultrasonic wave, microwave, and bacterial ice nucleating, on the sublimation process has been thoroughly investigated [71, 72]. Regardless of the method in which the freezing process is assisted, one may expect the same main physical constrains controlling the sublimation process, which is the structure of the ice formed in the freezing process. It is hoped that the subsequent discussion will provide a guide for future worker intending to undertake further investigation to provide direct evidence on the applicability of the electric and magnetic field in this area.

The lyophilization process involves the sublimation of ice under vacuum condition and the simultaneous transport of the sublimed water vapor across the porous structure of the frozen sample. This can be divided into two distinct steps: (i) the initial sublimation and transport of free water that is called primary drying stage and (ii) the latter sublimation and transport of bound water called the secondary drying stage. The total sublimation process is a very time-consuming process when compared with the freezing process and will significantly affect the economics of a product manufacturing.

In the primary drying process, the bulk of the frozen water unbound to the surface of the solute in the matrix of the sample is sublimed and transported away. The size of the ice crystals is the predominant factor controlling the rate of transport of the sublimed vapor; larger crystal will allow higher rate of sublimation as it offers less resistance and vice versa. Cheng et al. [71] noted that ultrasonic field used in controlling the nucleation process to produce larger crystals led to high sublimation rates. This was also demonstrated in the freezing of pharmaceutical vials in which larger mean ice crystals resulted in less mass transfer resistance (Hottot et al. 2007). Passot et al. [72] also undertook a systematic study on freeze-drying sucrose and catalase mixtures by using various cooling rate and also including different methods to control earlier nucleation. Similar findings of ice crystal size on the primary drying stage were obtained.

Apart from the primary size of the ice crystals, the connectivity of the ice crystals will also affect the transport of the sublimed water vapor. For the drying of aqueous system (nonsolid systems), this can be controlled by inducing directional solidification to the ice crystals during the freezing process. A very detailed investigation on the effect of nucleation temperature on the crystal morphology and growth behavior is given by Searles et al. [73]. They found that the cooling rate between 0.05 and 1 °C did not exhibit any significant difference in the primary drying rate delineating that the cooling did not significantly affect the size of the crystals. This is because the crystal size and the crystal connectivity closely affect the mass transfer of water vapor during the lyophilization stage. Smaller degree of supercooling led to higher primary drying rate. It was found that the lower supercooling resulted in a structured lamellar crystal structures with spacing around 10 μm; this is directional ice formation. This could have contributed to the significantly higher primary drying rate. It was suggested that the solidification rate was partly controlled by the initial supercooling. This is because, relative to the shelf temperature, a larger supercooling will give a larger temperature driving force for solidification post nucleation, and vice versa. It will be interesting to see how the magnetic and electric field can be used to control this aspect of crystallization. Searles et al. [73] further suggested that there is a critical nucleation temperature in which ice crystal is generated by global supercooling and crystallization vs. directional solidification. This is because relatively large thermal gradient is required for directional freezing. More complex modeling technique may be able to assist in such control of the freezing process [74].

On top of the ice crystal size and connectivity affecting the sublimation rate in the drying process, it also indirectly affects the behavior of the product temperature rise during the primary drying stage and the operation temperature [72]. A slower sublimation stage may results in faster temperature rise and vice versa. The temperature of the product will have to be controlled such that it does not result in the collapse of the freeze-dried matrix.

In the secondary drying stage, the ice bound to the solute is sublimed and transported away from the porous frozen matrix. The surface area available for the bound water to be sublimed then becomes the physical limitation controlling the process. Smaller ice crystals that will give a larger surface area for sublimation will then provide a higher rate of moisture removal. This requirement is in contrast to the requirements of the primary stage of drying, and there is a need to find a balance between the two stages of the process that may be material specific as well. Awotwe-Otoo et al. [75] investigated both the primary and secondary sublimation stage of freezing drying using sucrose and antibody solutions. In samples with controlled nucleation (earlier nucleation), the size of the pores was larger, which resulted in faster primary stage of drying, measured by the change in the pressure of the chamber and the temperature of the product in approaching the shelve temperature. Conversely, the samples with non-controlled nucleation (larger supercooling) resulted in smaller pores, and this led to slower primary drying stage. Smaller pores however led to slightly lower final moisture after secondary drying treatment by putting in an oven at 25 °C at eight hours, by about 0.5 wt% moisture, when compared with that of the larger pores. This is because the samples containing smaller pores have higher surface area for desorption of the bound moisture. Although such small moisture content difference may seem trivial, such small changes may cause significant change in the glass transition temperature of the sample, which determines its stability. In contrast, Passot et al. [72] did a systematic study but found that the in their runs, the difference in crystal size did not affect the final moisture content. Secondary stage drying of 10 hours at 30 °C was undertaken.

11.6 Future Outlook for Pharmaceutical Application

A comprehensive list of the patents and reported work in this area can be found in the review cited here [21]. The bulk of the technological development and fundamental studies in the application of magnetic and electric field to freezing has been undertaken for non-pharmaceutical products, mainly for food-related products or for the cryopreservation of medical-related samples. Nevertheless, it is envisaged that this technology can be translated to pharmaceutical product applications, and a few important guidelines and suggestions are provided here, summarized from the discussion in this chapter:

1. The production of smaller ice crystals during freezing will in general be advantageous for pharmaceutical product formulations. This recommendation is suggested on the basis that smaller ice crystals will potentially lead to lower solute freeze concentration and will need to be balanced with the need for feasible subsequent sublimation rates.
2. Application of the AC electric field will provide the potential to produce smaller ice crystals during freezing, while, in contrast, the DC electric will potentially lead to larger ice crystals.
3. There are evidences to suggest that the effect of the AC electric field on the ice crystals size may be indirectly caused by its effect on the movement of the dissolved solutes, rather than having a direct effect on the water molecules. This suggests that the application or potential effectiveness of the AC field to the freezing of pharmaceuticals may be significantly product specific.
4. There are evidences to suggest that the reported effect of the magnetic field on the ice crystal size may actually be due to the AC electric field generated from the moving magnets or due to the AC electric field concurrently applied in most of the commercially available magnetic field freezers. This aspect will need to be considered when designing future pharmaceutical product freezing trials with the magnetic field freezer.
5. To the best of the authors' knowledge, during the preparation of this chapter, there is yet to be any reported commercial pharmaceutical freezing trials using the DC electric field. In the authors' opinion, innovative design in the position of the electrodes (and its operation) to cater for the different vial sizes and at the same time avoiding the potential problems highlighted in Section 3.4 will allow more inroads to be made in this area to provide an avenue for a better control of the stochastic nature of nucleation.

References

1 Alves-Filho, O., Eikevik, T.M., and Goncharova-Alves, S.V. (2008). Single- and multistage heat pump drying of protein. *Drying Technology* 26: 470–475.

2 Rahman, S.M.A. and Mujumdar, A.S. (2008). A novel atmospheric freeze-drying system using a vibro-fluidized bed with adsorbent. *Drying Technology* 26: 393–403.

3 Tambunan, A.H., Yudistira, Kisdiyani, and Hernani (2001). Freeze drying characteristics of medicinal herbs. *Drying Technology* 19: 325–331.
4 Han, Y., Quan, G.B., Liu, X.Z. et al. (2005). Improved preservation of human red blood cells by lyophilisation. *Cryobiology* 51: 152–164.
5 Jackel, T., Dautel, K., and Ternes, W. (2008). Preserving functional properties of hen's egg yolk during freeze-drying. *Journal of Food Engineering* 87: 522–526.
6 Li, J., Zhang, L.L., Liu, Q.H. et al. (2009). Extra- and intra-cellular ice formation of red seabream (*Pagrus major*) embryos at different cooling rates. *Cryobiology* 59: 48–53.
7 Stephenson, J.L. (1956). Ice crystal growth during the rapid freezing of tissues. *Journal of Biophysical and Biochemical Cytology* 2: 45–52.
8 Bhatnagar, B.S., Bogner, R.H., and Pikal, M.J. (2007). Protein stability during freezing: separation of stresses and mechanisms of protein stabilization. *Pharmaceutical Development and Technology* 12: 505–523.
9 Cao, E., Chen, Y., Cui, Z., and Foster, P.R. (2003). Effect of freezing and thawing rates on denaturation of proteins in aqueous solutions. *Biotechnology and Bioengineering* 82: 684–690.
10 Maa, Y.F. and Prestrelski, S.J. (2000). Biopharmaceutical powders: particle formation and formulation considerations. *Current Pharmaceutical Biotechnology* 1: 283–302.
11 Roy, I. and Gupta, M.N. (2004, 2004). Freeze-drying of proteins: some emerging concerns. *Biotechnology and Applied Biochemistry* 39: 165–177.
12 Hottot, A., Nakagawa, K., and Andrieu, J. (2008). Effect of ultrasound-controlled nucleation on structural and morphological properties of freeze-dried mannitol solutions. *Chemical Engineering Research and Design* 86: 193–200.
13 Hozumi, T., Saito, A., Okawa, S., and Kumano, H. (2002). Freezing device for supercooled water. US6354102 B1, filed 26 July 2000 and issued 3 December 2002.
14 Lebail, A., Chevalier, D., Mussa, D.M., and Ghoul, M. (2002). High pressure freezing and thawing of foods: a review. *International Journal of Refrigeration* 25: 504–513.
15 Takahashi, K. (2004). Method of preserving food and method of producing non-frozen water. EP1454541A1, filed 26 November 2002 and issued 17 May 2007.
16 Geidobler, R. and Winter, G. (2013). Controlled ice nucleation in the field of freeze-drying: fundamentals and technology review. *European Journal of Pharmaceutics and Biopharmaceutics* 85: 214–222.
17 Shevkunov, S.V. and Vegiri, A. (2002). Electric field induced transitions in water clusters. *Journal of Molecular Structure* 593: 19–32.
18 Araki, T., Sagara, Y., Abdullah, K., and Tambunan, A.H. (2001). Transport properties of cellular food materials undergoing freeze-drying. *Drying Technology* 19: 297–312.
19 Hottot, A., Vessot, S., and Andrieu, J. (2004). A direct characterization method of the ice morphology. Relationship between mean crystal size

and primary drying times of freeze-drying processes. *Drying Technology* 22: 2009–2021.

20 Pikal, M.J. (2007). Freeze drying. In: *Encyclopedia of Pharmaceutical Technology* (ed. J. Swarbick), 1807–1832. Bosa Roca, US: Taylor & Francis Inc.

21 Otero, L., Rodriguez, A.C., Perez-Mateos, M., and Sanz, P.D. (2016). Effects of magnetic fields on freezing: application to biological products. *Comprehensive Reviews in Food Science and Food Safety* 15: 646–667.

22 Sun, W., Xu, X.B., Zhang, H., and Xu, C.X. (2008). Effects of dipole polarization of water molecules on ice formation under an electrostatic field. *Cryobiology* 56: 93–99.

23 Sadikoglu, H., Ozdemir, M., and Seker, M. (2006). Freeze-drying of pharmaceutical products: research and development needs. *Drying Technology* 24: 849–861.

24 Hottot, A., Andrieu, J., Vessot, S. et al. (2009). Experimental study and modelling of freeze-drying in syringe configuration. Part 1: Freezing step. *Drying Technology* 27: 40–48.

25 Hozumi, T., Okawa, S., Saito, A., and Eshita, Y. (2005). Effects of shape of electrodes on freezing of supercooled water in electric freeze control. *International Journal of Refrigeration* 28: 389–395.

26 Hozumi, T., Saito, A., Okawa, S., and Watanabe, K. (2003). Effects of electrode materials on freezing of supercooled water in electric freeze control. *International Journal of Refrigeration* 26: 537–542.

27 Orlowska, M., Havetm, M., and Le-Bail, A. (2009). Controlled ice nucleation under high voltage DC electrostatic field conditions. *Food Research International* 42: 879–884.

28 Dalvi-Isfahan, M., Hamdami, N., Xanthakis, E., and Le-Bail, A. (2017). Review on the control of ice nucleation by ultrasound waves, electric and magnetic fields. *Journal of Food Engineering* 195: 222–234.

29 Jha, P.K., Xanthakis, E., Jury, V., and Le-Bail, A. (2017). An overview on magnetic and electric field interactions with ice crystallization; application in the case of frozen food. *Crystals* 7: 299.

30 Petersen, A., Schneider, H., Rau, G., and Glasmacher, B. (2006). A new approach for freezing of aqueous solutions under active control of the nucleation temperature. *Cryobiology* 53: 248–257.

31 Mackenzie, A.P. (1977). Non-equilibrium freezing behaviour of aqueous systems. *Philosophical Transactions of the Royal Society of London, Series B: Biological Sciences* 278: 167–189.

32 Petersen, A., Rau, G., and Glasmacher, B. (2006). Reduction of primary freeze-drying time by electric field induced ice nucleus formation. *Heat and Mass Transfer* 42: 929–938.

33 Wang, W. (2000). Lyophilization and development of solid protein pharmaceutics. *International Journal of Pharmaceutics* 203: 1–60.

34 Xanthakis, E., Havet, M., Chevallier, S. et al. (2013). Effect of static electric field on ice crystal size reduction during freezing of pork meat. *Innovative Food Science and Emerging Technologies* 20: 115–120.

35 Dalvi-Isfahan, M., Hamdami, N., and Le-Bail, A. (2016). Effect of freezing under electrostatic field on the quality of lamb meat. *Innovative Food Science and Emerging Technologies* 37: 68–73.

36 Xanthakis, E., Le-Bail, A., and Ramaswamy, H. (2014). Development of an innovative microwave assisted food freezing process. *Innovative Food Science and Emerging Technologies* 26: 176–181.

37 Zhang, S.Z., Wang, H.Y., and Chen, G.M. (2010). Addition of ice-nucleation active bacteria: *Pseudomonas syringae* pv. *panici* on freezing of solid model food. *LWT Food Science and Technology* 43: 1414–1418.

38 Wu, C.H., Yuan, C.H., Ye, X.Q. et al. (2014). A critical review on superchilling preservation technology in aquatic product. *Journal of Integrative Agriculture* 13: 2788–2806.

39 Kaale, L.D., Eikevik, T.M., Rustad, T. et al. (2013). Ice crystal development in pre-rigor Atlantic salmon fillets during superchilling process and following storage. *Food Control* 31: 491–498.

40 Kim, S.C., Shin, J.M., Lee, S.W., et al. (2007). Non-freezing refrigerator. WO2007/094556A2, filed 20 December 2006 and issued 23 August 2007.

41 Kim, S.C., Shin, J.M., Youn, D.H., et al. (2008). Supercooling apparatus. WO2008/004763A1, filed 01 June 2007 and issued 10 January 2008.

42 Kim, S.C., Shin, J.M., Lee, S.W., et al. (2009). Ice maker and method of making ice. US20090165467A1, filed 27 September 2006 and issued 2 July 2009.

43 Sun, W., Xu, X.B., Zhang, H., et al. eds. (2006). The mechanism analysis of NaCl solution ice formation suppressed by electric field. *Proceedings of the 8th International Conference on Properties and Applications of Dielectric Materials*, Denpasar, Indonesia (26–30 June 2006).

44 Ma, Y.H., Qin, G.F., Li, J. et al. (2016). AC electric field enhances cryopreservation efficiency of Sprague-Dawley rat liver during a slow freezing procedure. *Biopreservation and Biobanking* 14: 23–28.

45 Stan, C.A., Tang, S.K.Y., Bishop, K.J.M., and Whitesides, G.M. (2011). Externally applied electric fields up to 1.6×10^5 V/m do not affect the homogenous nucleation of ice in supercooled water. *Journal of Physical Chemistry B* 115: 1089–1097.

46 Owada, N. and Kurita, S. (2001). Super-quick freezing method and apparatus therefore. US 6250087 B1.

47 Owada, N. (2005). Highly-efficient freezing apparatus and highly-efficient freezing method. US 20050005611A1, filed 1 November 2002 and issued 13 January 2005.

48 Mandal, G. and Kumar, P.P. (2002). A laboratory study of ice nucleation due to electrical discharge. *Atmospheric Research* 61: 115–123.

49 Degner, B.M., Olson, K.M., Rose, D. et al. (2013). Influence of freezing rate variation on the microstructure and physicochemical properties of food emulsions. *Journal of Food Engineering* 119: 244–253.

50 Al-Hasani, S. (2007). Three years of routine vitrification of human zygotes: is it still fair to advocate slow-rate freezing? *Reproductive BioMedicine Online* 14: 288–293.

51 Fujisaki, Y. and Amano, M. (2012). Core unit for refrigeration unit and refrigeration unit including the core unit. US8127559B2, filed 7 August 2007 and issued 13 August 2009.

52 Owada, N. and Saito, S. (2010). Quick freezing apparatus and quick freezing method. US7810340B2, filed 31 March 2005 and issued 12 October 2010.

53 Sato, M. and Fujita, K. (2006). Refrigeration device, refrigeration method and refrigerated object. US2006/0112699A1, filed 8 May 2003 and issued 2 September 2008.

54 Iwasaka, M., Onishi, M., Kurita, S., and Owada, N. (2011). Effects of pulsed magnetic fields on the light scattering property of the freezing process of aqueous solutions. *Journal of Applied Physics* 109: 07E320.

55 Abedini, S., Kaku, M., Kawata, T. et al. (2011). Effects of cryopreservation with a newly-developed magnetic field programmed freezer on periodontal ligament cells and pulp tissues. *Cryobiology* 62: 181–187.

56 Kaku, M., Kamada, H., Kawata, T. et al. (2010). Cryopreservation of periodontal ligament cells with magnetic field for tooth banking. *Cryobiology* 61: 73–78.

57 Shitaka, H., Kaku, M., Kojima, S.I. et al. (2016). The effect of magnetic field during freezing and thawing of rat bone marrow-derived mesenchymal stem cells. *Cryobiology* 73: 15–19.

58 Kojima, S., Kaku, M., Kawata, T. et al. (2013). Cryopreservation of rat MSCs by use of a programmed freezer with magnetic field. *Cryobiology* 67: 259–263.

59 Iwasaka, M. and Ueno, S. (1998). Structure of water molecules under 14T magnetic field. *Journal of Applied Physics* 83: 6459–6461.

60 Tagami, M., Hamai, M., Mogi, I. et al. (1999). Solidification of levitating water in a gradient strong magnetic field. *Journal of Crystal Growth* 203: 594–598.

61 Ueno, S. and Iwasaki, M. (1994). Parting of water by magnetic fields. *IEEE Transactions on Magnetics* 30: 4698–4700.

62 Aleksandrov, V.D., Barannikov, A.A., and Dobritsa, N.V. (2000). Effect of magnetic field on the supercooling of water drops. *Inorganic Materials* 36: 2000.

63 Wowk, B. (2012). Electric and magnetic fields in cryopreservation. *Cryobiology* 64: 301–303.

64 Kobayashi, A. and Kirschvink, J.L. (2014). A ferromagnetic model for the action of electric and magnetic fields in cryopreservation. *Cryobiology* 68: 163–165.

65 Zhao, H.Z., Hu, G.Q., Liu, S., and Han, J.T. (2017). Experimental study on freezing of liquids under static magnetic field. *Chinese Journal of Chemical Engineering* 25: 1288–1293.

66 Mok, J.H., Choi, W., Park, S.H. et al. (2015). Emerging pulsed electric field (PEF) and static magnetic field (SMF) combination technology for food freezing. *International Journal of Refrigeration* 50: 137–145.

67 Higashi, T., Yamagishi, A., Takeuchi, T., and Kawaguchi, N. (1993). Orientation of erythrocytes in a strong static magnetic field. *Blood* 82: 1328–1334.

68 Schenck, J.F. (2005). Physical interactions of static magnetic fields with living tissues. *Progress in Biophysics and Molecular Biology* 87: 185–204.

69 Lin, C.Y., Wei, P.L., Chang, W.J. et al. (2013). Slow freezing couple static magnetic field exposure enhances cryopreservative efficiency – a study on human erythrocytes. *PLoS One* 8: e58988.

70 Kobayashi, A. and Kirschvink, J.L. (2015). Enhancement of electromagnetic freezing by stabilization and oscillation of biogenic magnetite particles. US20150037782A1, filed 10 July 2014 and issued 17 May 2016.

71 Cheng, X.F., Zhang, M., Xu, B.G. et al. (2015). The principles of ultrasound and its application in freezing related processes of food materials: a review. *Ultrasonics Sonochemistry* 27: 576–585.

72 Passot, S., Trelea, I.C., Marin, M. et al. (2009). Effect of controlled ice nucleation on primary drying stage and protein recovery in vials cooled in a modified freeze-dryer. *Journal of Biomechanical Engineering* 131: 074511.

73 Searles, J.A., Carpenter, J.F., and Randolph, T.W. (2001). The ice nucleation temperature determines the primary drying rate of lyophilization for samples frozen on a temperature-controlled shelf. *Journal of Pharmaceutical Sciences* 90: 860–871.

74 Pham, Q.T. (2012). Mathematical modelling of freezing processes. In: *Handbook of Frozen Food Processing and Packaging* (ed. D.-W. Sun), 147–184. Bosa Roca, US: CRC Press Taylor & Francis Group.

75 Awotwe-Otoo, D., Agarabi, C., Read, E.K. et al. (2013). Impact of controlled ice nucleation on process performance and quality attributes of a lyophilized monoclonal antibody. *International Journal of Pharmaceutics* 450: 70–78.

12

Desired Attributes and Requirements for Implementation

Howard Stamato[1] *and Jim Searles*[2]

[1] *Bridgewater, NJ 08807, USA*
[2] *Pfizer Global Supply, McPherson, KS 67460, USA*

12.1 Introduction

There are several promising next-generation drying technologies currently in development that are reviewed throughout the book. This chapter covers product and process attributes to be considered by anyone who is undertaking implementation of a new drying technology for pharmaceutical manufacturing. Since many of the technologies currently used in pharmaceuticals are adapted from other industries, some of the discussion and references are drawn from a broader view of industrial technology.

New technology often is measured in cost terms. There is a growing awareness that routine calculations of return on investment do not capture the complete valuation [1]. A broader evaluation including qualitative as well as quantitative measures is expected to be most effective [2, 3]. It is expected that a more successful approach will consider multiple aspects including the impact to product design, product quality, manufacturing flexibility, valuation, and stage of maturity.

In the pharmaceutical industry, there is an additional set of requirements related to standards and regulations known as current good manufacturing practice (cGMP). To provide a path for new technology in pharmaceuticals, it must be designed to meet the cGMP requirements, which cover all aspects of pharmaceutical manufacturing, testing, and quality control. Due to their importance for protecting patient safety, these practices are broadly discussed in books, professional journals, and trade magazines (e.g. *Journal of cGMP Compliance*), training courses (e.g. Pharmaceutical GMP Professional Certification offered by the American Society for Quality [www.asq.org]), and consultants. There are also cGMP guidance documents published by organizations such as the International Society for Pharmaceutical Engineering (ISPE) [4], World Health Organization (WHO) [5], and the International Council for Harmonization of Technical Requirements for Pharmaceuticals for Human Use (ICH) [6]. The evolving nature of what constitutes current practices and requirements dictates that early engagement with regulatory agencies and subject matter experts is important for smooth implementation of any new aspect of pharmaceutical

Drying Technologies for Biotechnology and Pharmaceutical Applications, First Edition.
Edited by Satoshi Ohtake, Ken-ichi Izutsu, and David Lechuga-Ballesteros.

manufacturing. Very often the written regulation, the interpretation in a written guidance, and the common understanding and practice around an issue are three separate representations and may be interpreted differently by different individuals and organizations. This very understandable communication challenge is all the more reason to discuss any novel developments early and thoroughly. Regulatory bodies such as the Food and Drug Administration (FDA) and European Medicines Agency (EMA) are fostering acceleration of new technology to realize the benefits it brings to patients. FDA has established an emerging technology program with its own laboratory and scientists along with a pathway for communication with regard to filing new technology [7, 8]. Similarly, the EMA has established an Innovation Network and Innovation Task Force [9, 10], which will be "Making the regulatory support available at national and EU level more visible and attractive to innovators since early stage" and "Establish a discussion platform for early dialogue with Applicants in particular SME's to proactively identify scientific, legal, and regulatory issues of emerging therapies and technologies" [11].

Successful implementation in pharmaceutical manufacturing requires clear identification of all relevant process parameters and the ability to control those parameters to consistently achieve all product quality attributes. cGMP requirements for quality control and process validation require the identification of the process parameters that impact the resulting quality attributes of the specifications.

Additional aspects of cGMP relating to manufacturing technologies include cleaning and, if applicable, sterilization, representative sampling and testing, equipment qualification, process and analytical method validation, process validation, product performance evaluation, and the container and closure requirements of the primary package.

A special note of caution is that regulations are evolving to apply additional requirements for pharmaceutical products that are coupled with medical devices to form a combination product [12, 13].

Drying is an essential step in many processes. At first assessment it may seem simple. However, there is an intricate overlap of heat transfer, mass transfer, flow, and material properties that must be considered so that the final product has the desired levels of residual solvent, structure, shape, uniformity, strength, and friability [14]. The design and operating parameters of drying equipment must be chosen so that the material is exposed to a controlled environment leading to the desired product attributes. Such an approach is consistent with the concept of Quality by Design, which has become an accepted practice in developing pharmaceutical processes [15]. Adopting a Quality by Design approach is expected to add value to the pharmaceutical development and commercialization process [16]. There are many examples of applying quality by design to various drying operations as well as discussion of the drying unit operation in general [14, 17, 18].

Methods of measuring material properties, concentrations, and bonding between solvent and product are needed to understand the input material, progression of changes during processing, and the final product. Physical, chemical, and spectroscopic methods are needed to assess micromeritic properties, the amount and position of the solvent and various components of the product, fluid and solid flows, and responses of the material to stress.

Applying an understanding of drying, and some measure of testing, dramatically reduces unexpected challenges and increases the likelihood of an efficient drying process producing the desired product attributes. This chapter gives a brief overview of the technology of drying so that the applications that follow can be assured success from awareness and use of drying technology principles.

12.2 Measuring Dryness

Because the drying process is most often focused on the removal of solvent from the product, much of the interest regarding drying processes is on the detection of solvent. As in any sensing method development, the specificity of the method used, accuracy, precision, and common errors need to be considered. Given the strong dependence of product properties on solvent level and inherent difficulties obtaining a representative sample, it may be necessary to use multiple types of determinations to assess the performance of the drying operation.

The simplest methods of detection subject samples to further drying under heating. The additional drying may be done with or without vacuum. The amount of solvent is directly, gravimetrically, determined by observing the weight loss over time. There are compendial standards for the loss-on-drying test [19].

While simple to use, these techniques are subject to variation in sampling, instrument configuration/performance, and end-point determination [20, 21]. For example, the performance of different devices using different heating units, radio-frequency (RF) radiation, or microwave (MW) radiation to heat the sample may yield different results or require selecting parameters to obtain the same results as the reference device [22].

Wet chemistry can be used to directly detect the level of moisture in samples. If the solvent is water, the Karl Fischer (KF) reaction is used to titrate a solution of the sample and determine the amount of moisture present. Where a gravimetric technique can be fine-tuned to show unbound and bound moisture, the KF technique will show only the total amount. Similar to loss on drying, the KF method is discussed in compendia [23].

Many methods measure the amount of residual solvent or moisture by a nondestructive technique where a secondary measurement is calibrated to the amount of solvent present [24]. Some devices pass a signal through the sample that is modulated by the dielectric properties of the moisture present. Passing an electrical current through the sample and measuring the resistivity, conductance, or capacitance and calibrating to moisture content is an effective nondestructive test. Similarly, transmission of RF or MW energy through a sample can be measured and correlated to the moisture or polar solvent content. Use of energy-based detection enters the realm of being able to detect solvent content during the process [25].

The most popular way of detecting composition during a process involves spectroscopic techniques. Near-infrared (NIR) and Raman spectroscopies are the most popular methods of determining content on or at line. It is necessary to consider the sampling aspect regarding penetration of the radiation, keeping the sampling window clear, and the amount of material the radiation sees. Some of the signal measured may be overlapped by absorption of the materials used, the depth of the component being measured, and the surface structure of the particles [26–28].

At the extreme end of this progression of measurements are techniques where more energetic radiation is used to determine sample properties. Moisture content has been measured using β-radiation [29–31] measured with γ-radiation [32, 33], X-ray [34, 35], or terahertz frequencies [36, 37].

In between these two extremes are other techniques with varying complexities. Analyzing the vapor in equilibrium with the sample has been used with gas chromatography [38], mass spectrometry [39], and tunable diode laser array spectrometry (TDLAS) [40].

It is also useful to consider the state of the solvent (moisture) being detected. Depending on the technique, whether the solvent is freely dispersed in the material, adsorbed on the surface, or trapped in a pore network, amorphous glass, or crystal structure will have an influence on the selection of the measurement technique, drying conditions, and product specifications. Moisture sorption analysis or thermogravimetric analysis is a more sensitive way than loss on drying for teasing out the solvent content and something about its binding to the substrate [41]. Measuring water activity provides understanding of the type of moisture present and its effect on stability or performance of the product [42–44].

12.3 Process Considerations

Understanding of the solvent distribution and its effects on the product are expected to increase with investment in improved sensing technology. A single sample point gives a measure of the material. However, variation in solvent content across the batch, within a particular section, or within a particle may lead to unacceptable product performance [45–48]. Interaction between the equipment and product is linked to the micromeritic structure, solvent distribution, and product quality [49–51].

While measurements of samples are important to understanding the particular condition of the solvent, material, and product performance, much can be gained by measurements of the process conditions or process streams. Detecting the humidity, temperature, gas/vapor flow, pressure, and vapor composition at various points in the process can be used to determine the state of the product [52–54]. Continued development of sensor technology leads to the ability to collect more data, at more points in the process, often with miniaturized devices. Where a large fixed temperature probe and similarly sized humidity sensor used to be the state of the art, environmental conditions can now be monitored with a device the size of a coin [55]. In another example, more pertinent to lyophilization, glass fibers are used to sense temperature in specific locations in the lyo-cake [56]. PAT can also have offline implementations such as nondestructive measurements of the lyo-cake pore structure using micro-CT [57].

The key to an efficient drying process is balancing effects. Flow patterns of gases, vapors, liquids, and solids are all important factors in considering the design and operating conditions in the equipment [58, 59]. Setting a condition at too low a target leads to inefficient drying and other undesirable effects such as product attrition. Setting conditions at too high a target can cause product damage due to heating and other undesirable effects such a lyophilized cake meltback [60, 61].

The rate of solvent removal is dependent on the system heat input, temperature, and solvent vapor content of the atmosphere (or system pressure for a vacuum system). The product position relative to the heat source, or in moving systems the mixing, and unit or particle structure also have an influence on the effectiveness of the processing and the final product quality. Too much mixing and the product may be subject to attrition [62]. Choosing conditions that homogenize product exposure to the desired drying conditions yields a uniform product performing to specifications.

Too low a pressure in a vacuum system or too low a gas flow will limit convective transfer of heat [63]. With adequate heating favoring rapid drying, the product may form a dry surface compared with a wet interior, reducing the mass transfer at the particle surface and increasing drying time. If the solvent measurement sees predominantly the product surface, a false reading could leave a high level of solvent in the product interior, leading to product failure. Understanding the material properties and product structure well enough, to choose values for the pressure or vapor pressure so that the solvent removal is efficient while preserving the desired product homogeneity and structure, leads to a successful drying process.

Similar balanced choices must be made with respect to heating. Convective, conductive, and radiant heat are all possible. However, if the heating surface in contact with the product is too hot or there are nodes where the MW or other irradiative techniques have a high local energy density, the product in this region could be destroyed [64]. While a high temperature of gas or vapor may have similar effects to direct heating, one of the product issues related to this condition is formation of a dry crust of material at the surface of the product with limited capacity for mass transfer [46].

By investing in sensors, local variation can be determined, and product quality preserved by managing the balance of effects including exceptions to the average condition. With detailed data across the geometry of the process and an understanding of the microstructure of the product, it is possible to model the drying process such that more efficient designs of equipment and process can be produced with less time and material [65].

12.4 Product Considerations

From the discussion of measurements and processing, it is clear that more attributes than just the solvent level are important in the drying operation and for the resulting product properties. The role each component of the material plays in the product performance and its motion due to mixing, the mass transfer effects in the drying process, the physical characteristics of the final product, and the level of any residual solvent present all have a role to play.

For the measurement of interactions with solvent, some methods of determining the solvent level give information regarding the state of interaction with the product. Measuring water activity, differential scanning calorimetry, nuclear magnetic resonance (NMR), or X-ray crystallography are a few of the analytical chemistry techniques that can probe solvent–product interaction, the transition between states, and the conditions in order to transition between states more thoroughly. This type of knowledge can be used to set the maximum temperature during a drying process in order to prevent product decomposition or to assure that the desired amount of a bound form of solvent remains in the product to assure product performance [50].

The microscopic structure of the product cake or particle will have a role to play in the removal of solvent and also in the product strength during further processing or use and in the performance of the material in its final use. An example is the applicable uses of a lyophilized product depending on the pore structure formed [66]. Another example from spray drying is as follows: if a dry crust of material is formed early in the process and the solvent is removed from the interior of the droplet, a hollow structure with good flow properties and very low density will be formed. Changing the drying rate in either direction has other outcomes. Slower drying could allow the shell to collapse, increasing density and reducing flow properties due to the irregular nature of the particle surface. At extremely fast drying conditions, the shell will shatter due to the internal pressure of solvent vapor, giving a very dense powder of very low particle size and poor flow properties [49].

Similar considerations apply to solids that can form pores in drying. Manipulating the drying such that there is adequate pore structure to assure solvent motion and efficient drying, also contributes to assurance that the product can be easily reconstituted. Too fine a structure or too few pores could result in longer drying times and more difficulty in reconstitution [67]. Pushing the process conditions too hard could cause the structure to collapse, adversely affecting both the process and product performance.

Measuring product structure and the content of that structure through various forms of microscopy/spectroscopy, controlled ablation, or radiation scanning techniques (X-ray tomography, terahertz) can help with understanding of the product response to various drying conditions and to select the desired final product confirmation.

The drying conditions can have an effect on the amount of amorphous material present. In some cases, an amorphous product has beneficial properties with regard to dissolution and bioavailability. A crystalline structure may be desired due to advantages in stability or measurement. In either case the effect of drying conditions on the amount of amorphous material or which crystal form is obtained should be considered [68].

Once the dry product has been formed, its mechanical properties have a role to play either in the process or in the proposed product use. For systems where the dried particles are mixed further in order to form the final product, a key question is whether the particle will stand up to various forces of impact and attrition [69]. These same forces are important to consider in shipping the product to its final destination and in use by the end user. Drying conditions will need to be adjusted so that the product will have the appropriate flow, size, strength, and appearance, yet suspend or dissolve as intended.

12.5 Scale-Up Considerations

The traditional approach for scale-up starts with geometric considerations and continues to process parameters. In doing those calculations and comparisons, it quickly becomes apparent that various factors scale at different rates. The simplest example is one of geometry. Where some factors scale linearly, factors of volume or area would scale in the cube or the square, and so a particular factor applied to the process will scale differently with regard to various factors. PAT applications afford us the opportunity to study process parameters and assure that qualities in the product such as porosity, component distribution, and mechanical properties can be measured and parameters found, which produce the same profile of attributes at two different scales. The expectation is that thoughtful selection of parameters and maintaining attribute values assure the product performs as designed. When there is an opportunity to innovate and redesign the process, there is a possibility to organize the material management to minimize the effect of scale. For example, designing a vacuum chamber for lyophilization such that each vial sees the same conditions or that the vial conditions can be adjusted more quickly would reduce the opportunity for variation as a result of changes in scale. Shortening distances for heat and mass transfer such as moving to particulates from a cake morphology reduces the opportunity to vary during a change in scale. Although a new technology can be designed for easier scale-up, the availability of new equipment of the appropriate scale may be a challenge in establishing confidence in a new technique. Technologies that have an early investment of commercial-scale equipment have a distinct advantage in adoption.

12.6 Implementation

In considering the type of technology applied to product drying operations, surveying similar processes, materials, sensors, and practices from other industries is helpful in identifying improvements and new techniques of high value. Knowledge of the materials involved and their interactions with each other and the solvents present is essential in determining the process, measurements, and desired final form of the product. Designing the product attributes essential to the product function such as shape, size, porosity, and strength in addition to the final solvent level will determine the measurement strategy and process parameters and assure the performance of the process and the desired product. The measurement techniques, process, and product perspectives presented in this chapter are expected to help choose effective process conditions, material measurements, and sensors, resulting in a product meeting the design criteria.

References

1 Corrado C, Hulten C, Sichel D, Measuring Capital and Technology: An Expanded Framework, Finance and Economics Discussion Series Divisions of Research & Statistics and Monetary Affairs Federal Reserve Board, Washington, D.C. ; 2004-65, https://www.federalreserve.gov/pubs/feds/2004/200465/200465pap.pdf (accessed October 7, 2019).

2 Schuh, G., Schubert, J., and Wellensiek, M. (2012). Model for the valuation of a technology established in a manufacturing system. *Procedia CIRP* 3: 602–607.

3 Ramasesh, R.V. and Jayakumar, M.D. (1991). Measurement of manufacturing flexibility: a value based approach. *Journal of Operations Management* 10 (4): 446–468.

4 International Society for Pharmaceutical Engineering (ISPE), www.ISPE.org (accessed 07 October 2019).

5 World Health Organization (WHO), www.WHO.org (accessed 07 October 2019).

6 International Council for Harmonization of Technical Requirements for Pharmaceuticals for Human Use (ICH), www.ICH.org (accessed 07 October 2019).

7 FDA. Emerging technology program. https://www.fda.gov/about-fda/center-drug-evaluation-and-research-cder/emerging-technology-program (accessed 07 October 2019).

8 FDA (September 2017). Advancement of Emerging Technology Applications for Pharmaceutical Innovation and Modernization Guidance for Industry. www.fda.gov/downloads/Drugs/GuidanceComplianceRegulatoryInformation/Guidances/UCM478821.pdf (accessed 05 February 2019).

9 EU innovation network. https://www.ema.europa.eu/en/human-regulatory/research-development/innovation-medicines#eu-innovation-network-section (accessed 07 October 2019).

10 Mandate of the European Innovation Network (6 September 2016). www.ema.europa.eu/documents/other/mandate-european-innovation-network_en.pdf (accessed 07 October 2019).

11 Mandate of the EMA innovation task force (ITF) (6 August 2014). www.ema.europa.eu/en/documents/other/mandate-european-medcines-agency-innovation-task-force-itf_en.pdf (accessed 07 October 2019).

12 Guidance for industry and FDA staff: current good manufacturing practice requirements for combination products. www.fda.gov/downloads/RegulatoryInformation/Guidances/UCM429304.pdf (accessed 24 June 2018).

13 European Medicines Agency (2016). Concept paper on developing a guideline on quality requirements of medicinal products containing a device component for delivery or use of the medicinal product. www.ema.europa.eu/docs/en_GB/document_library/Scientific_guideline/2017/02/WC500221747.pdf (accessed 24 June 2018).

14 Parikh, D.M. (2014). Solids drying: basics and applications. *Chemical Engineering* 121 (4): 42–45.

15 Yu, L.X., Amidon, G., Khan, M.A. et al. (2014). Understanding pharmaceutical quality by design. *AAPS Journal* 16 (4): 771–783.

16 Koeberle, M. and Schiemenz, W. (2017). QbD: improving pharmaceutical development and manufacturing workflows to deliver better patient outcomes. *Pharmaceutical Technology* (Supplement to Issue) 4 (9): s20–s23.

17 Troyankin, A., Kozlov, A., Voynovskiy, A., and Menshutina, N. (2009). Quality by design approach in drying process organization. *Computer Aided Chemical Engineering* 26: 291–296.

18 Jameel, F. and Khan, M. (2009). Quality-by-design as applied to the development and manufacturing of a lyophilized protein product. *American Pharmaceutical Review*. www.americanpharmaceuticalreview.com/Featured-Articles/117782-Quality-by-Design-as-Applied-to-the-Development-and-Manufacturing-of-a-Lyophilized-Protein-Product/ (accessed 11 July 2018).

19 USP41-NF 36 General Chapter 731 Loss on drying, The U.S. Pharmacopeial Convention USP-NF Online. www.uspnf.com (accessed 25 June 2018).

20 Ahn, J.Y., Kil, D.Y., Kong, C., and Kim, B.G. (2014). Comparison of oven-drying methods for determination of moisture content in feed ingredients. *Asian-Australasian Journal of Animal Sciences* 27 (11): 1615–1622.

21 Marjanovic-Balaban, Z., Jelic, D., Antunovic, V., and Gojkovic, V. (2014). Determination of water content in pharmaceutical substances. *Journal of Hygienic Engineering and Design* 6: 137–141.

22 Bizzi, C.A., Barin, J.S., Hermes, A.L. et al. (2011). A fast microwave-assisted procedure for loss on drying determination in saccharides. *Journal of the Brazilian Chemical Society* 11 (2): 376–381.

23 USP41-NF 36 General Chapter 921 Water determination, The U.S. Pharmacopeial Convention USP-NF Online. www.uspnf.com (accessed 25 June 2018).

24 Spitzlei, M. (2000). *Choosing a Method for Measuring your Material's Moisture Content*, vol. 4, 39–52. Powder and Bulk Engineering.

25 Hubner, C. and Kaatze, U. (2016). *Electromagnetic Moisture Measurement Principles and Applications*. Universitätsverlag Göttingen. http://univerlag.uni-goettingen.de. ISBN: 978-3-86395-260-0.

26 Berntsson, O., Burger, T., Folestad, S. et al. (1999). Effective sample size in diffuse reflectance near-IR spectrometry. *Analytical Chemistry* 71 (3): 617–623.

27 Fonti, S., Montanaro, S., Politi, R. et al. (2010). Infrared reflectance spectra of particulate mixtures. *Journal of Geophysical Research* 115: E06003. https://agupubs.onlinelibrary.wiley.com/doi/pdf/10.1029/2009JE003461 (accessed 3 July 2018).

28 Tamburini, E., Vincenzi, F., Costa, S. et al. (2017). Effects of moisture and particle size on quantitative determination of total organic carbon (TOC) in soils using near-infrared. *Spectroscopy* 17 (10): 2366. www.ncbi.nlm.nih.gov/pmc/articles/PMC5677457/ (accessed 11 July 2018).

29 Pattanashetti, I.I. and Galagali, M.N. (2017). Coefficient and water content determination of almond leaves using beta radiation attenuation. *International Journal of Innovative Science, Engineering and Technology* 3: 571–573.

30 Batra, R.K., Singh, B., and Singh, K. (1992). Determination of water content of plant leaves by beta attenuation. *International Journal of Radiation Applications and Instrumentation. Part A. Applied Radiation and Isotopes* 43 (10): 1235–1239.

31 Kirandeep, K., Bala, P., and Sharma, A. (2015). Determination of attenuation coefficient and water content of broccoli leaves using beta particles. *International Journal of Computer Applications*, JCA Proceedings on International Conference on Advancements in Engineering and Technology ICAET 2: 25–28.

32 Hatcher, J.D. (1964). The use of gamma radiation to measure moisture distribution during drying processes. Master's thesis in Mechanical Engineering. Georgia Institute of Technology.

33 Nielsen, A.F. (1972). Gamma-ray-attenuation used for measuring the moisture content and homogeneity of porous concrete. *Building Science* 7 (4): 257–263.

34 Holubeka, M. and Koronthalyova, O. (2017). Comparison of TDR and X-ray method for determining moisture transport parameters. *Energy Procedia* 132: 723–728.

35 Bunaciu, A.A., Udristioiu, E.G., and Aboul-Enein, H.Y. (2015). X-ray diffraction: instrumentation and applications. *Critical Reviews in Analytical Chemistry* 45 (40): 289–299.

36 Banerjee, D., von Spiegel, W., Thomson, M.D. et al. (2008). Diagnosing water content in paper by terahertz radiation. *Optics Express* 16 (12): 9060–9066.

37 Malinowski, P., Pałka, N., Opoka, S. et al. (2015). Moisture detection in composites by terahertz spectroscopy. *Journal of Physics: Conference Series* 628: 012100.

38 Degg, B. (2014). Analyzing water content in solid pharmaceuticals. *The Column* 10 (7). www.chromatographyonline.com/analyzing-water-content-solid-pharmaceuticals (accessed 14 July 2018).

39 Merriman, D. (February 2015). PAT implementation: removing solvents from the process. www.pharmpro.com/article/2016/02/pat-implementation-removing-solvents-process (accessed 14 July 2018).

40 Schneid, S.C., Gieseler, H., Kessler, W.J. et al. (2011). Optimization of the secondary drying step in freeze drying using TDLAS technology. *AAPS PharmSciTech* 12 (1): 379–387. www.ncbi.nlm.nih.gov/pmc/articles/PMC3066362/ (accessed 14 July 2018).

41 Kargosha, K. and Shirazi, Z. (2015). Determination of water content of crystalline pharmaceutical solids under different percentages of relative humidity. *Pharmaceutical Sciences* 21 (Suppl 1): 127–135.

42 Fontana, A.J. (1999). Pharmaceutical applications for water activity. *Pharmaceutical Online* (29 April). www.pharmaceuticalonline.com/doc/pharmaceutical-applications-for-water-activit-0001 (accessed 14 July 2018).

43 Angamuthu, M., Shankar, V.K., and Murthy, N.S. (2018). Water activity and its significance in topical dosage forms. *Journal of Pharmaceutical Sciences* 107: 1656–1666.

44 Waterman, K.C., Chen, L., Waterman, P. et al. Modeling of in-use stability for tablets and powders in bottles. *Drug Development and Industrial Pharmacy* 42 (10): 1571–1578.

45 Webster, S. (2011). How Biopharma Technology is using laser-based headspace moisture analysis for moisture determination. *Manufacturing Chemist* (14 October). www.manufacturingchemist.com/news/article_page/Moisture_analysis/55599 (accessed 14 July 2018).

46 Parikh, D. (2011). Transferring tray drying to fluid bed drying. *Powder and Bulk Solids* (8 February). http://www.powderbulksolids.com/article/transferring-tray-drying-fluid-bed-drying (accessed 15 July 2018).

47 Xue Liu, X., Muzzio, F.J., Khinast, J.G., and Glasser, B.J. (2013). Fluidized bed drying of pharmaceutical materials: moisture measurement and effects of particle size. *American Pharmaceutical Review*. www.americanpharmaceuticalreview.com/Featured-Articles/134043-Fluidized-Bed-Drying-of-Pharmaceutical-Materials-Moisture-Measurement-and-Effects-of-Particle-Size/ (accessed 15 July 2018).

48 Zoglio, M.A., Streng, W.H., and Carstensen, J.T. (1975). Diffusion model for fluidized-bed drying. *Journal of Pharmaceutical Sciences* 64 (11): 1869–1873.

49 Paluch, K.J., Tajber, L., Corrigan, O.I., and Healy, A.M. (2012). Impact of process variables on the micromeritic and physicochemical properties of spray-dried porous microparticles, part I: introduction of a new morphology classification system. *Journal of Pharmacy and Pharmacology* 64 (11): 1570–1582.

50 Römer, M., Heinämäki, J., Miroshnyk, I. et al. (2008). Phase transformation of erythromycin A dihydrate during fluid bed drying. *Journal of Pharmaceutical Sciences* 97 (9): 4020–4029.

51 Yu, J. and Anchordoquy, T.J. (2009). Effects of moisture content on the storage stability of dried lipoplex formulations. *Journal of Pharmaceutical Sciences* 98 (9): 3278–3289.

52 Petersen, L.N., Poulsen, N.K., Niemann, H.H. et al. (2017). Comparison of three control strategies for optimization of spray dryer operation. *Journal of Process Control* 57: 1–14.

53 Alkeev, N., Averin, S., and Gratowski, S. (2015). New method for monitoring the process of freeze drying of biological materials. *AAPS PharmSciTech* 16 (6): 1474–1479.

54 Nail, S., Tchessalov, S., Shalaev, E. et al. (2017). Recommended best practices for process monitoring instrumentation in pharmaceutical freeze drying—2017. *AAPS PharmSciTech* 18 (7): 2379–2393.

55 Pandey, P., Ji, J., Subramanian, G. et al. Understanding the thermodynamic micro-environment inside a pan coater using a data logging device. *Drug Development and Industrial Pharmacy* 40 (4): 542–548.

56 Horn, J. and Friess, W. (2018). Detection of collapse and crystallization of saccharide, protein, and mannitol formulations by optical fibers in lyophilization. *Frontiers in Chemistry*. www.frontiersin.org/articles/10.3389/fchem.2018.00004/full (accessed 16 July 2018).

57 Izutsu, K., Yonemochi, E., Yomota, C. et al. (2014). Studying the morphology of lyophilized protein solids using X-ray micro-CT: effect of post-freeze annealing and controlled nucleation. *AAPS PharmSciTech* 15 (5): 1181–1188.

58 Southwell, D.B. and Langrish, T.A.G. (2000). Observations of flow patterns in a spray dryer. *Drying Technology* 18 (3): 661–685.

59 Langrish, T.A.G. and Fletcher, D.F. (2003). Prospects for the modelling and design of spray dryers in the 21st century. *Drying Technology* 21 (2): 197–215.

60 Patel, M.S., Nail, S.L., Pikal, M.J. et al. (2017). Lyophilized drug product cake appearance: what is acceptable? *International Journal of Pharmaceutics* 106 (7): 1706–1721.

61 Ohori, R. and Yamashita, C. (2017). Effects of temperature ramp rate during the primary drying process on the properties of amorphous-based lyophilized cake, Part 1: Cake characterization, collapse temperature and drying behavior. *Journal of Drug Delivery Science and Technology* 39: 131–139.

62 Lee, T. and Lee, J. (2003). Particle attrition by particle–surface friction in dryers. *Pharmaceutical Technology*: 64–72. www.pharmtech.com/pharmaceutical-technology-05-02-2003 (accessed 15 July 2018).

63 Ganguly, A., Nail, S.L., and Alexeenko, A.A. (2010). *Experimental Determination of the Key Heat Transfer Mechanisms in Pharmaceutical Freeze Drying*. School of Aeronautics and Astronautics Faculty Publications. Paper 27. http://dx.doi.org/10.2514/6.2010-4654 (accessed 16 July 2018).

64 Waters, L.J., Bedford, S., and Parkes, G.M.B. (2011). Controlled microwave processing applied to the pharmaceutical formulation of ibuprofen. *AAPS PharmSciTech* 12 (4): 1038–1043.

65 Tchessalov, S., Dassu, D., Latshaw, D., and Nulu, S. (2017). An industry perspective on the application of modeling to lyophilization process scale up and transfer. *American Pharmaceutical Review*. www.americanpharmaceuticalreview.com/Featured-Articles/335416-An-Industry-Perspective-on-the-Application-of-Modeling-to-Lyophilization-Process-Scale-up-and-Transfer/ (accessed 16 July 2018).

66 Angulo, D.E.L. and do Amaral Sobral, P.J. (2016). The effect of processing parameters and solid concentration on the microstructure and pore architecture of gelatin–chitosan scaffolds. *Materials Research* 19 (4): 839–845.

67 Beech, K.E., Biddlecombe, J.G., van der Walle, C.F. et al. (2015). Insights into the influence of the cooling profile on the reconstitution times of amorphous lyophilized protein formulations. *European Journal of Pharmaceutics and Biopharmaceutics* 96: 247–254.

68 Baghel, S., Cathcart, H., and O'Reilly, N.J. (2016). Polymeric amorphous solid dispersions: a review of amorphization, crystallization, stabilization, solid-state characterization, and aqueous solubilization of biopharmaceutical classification system class II drugs. *Journal of Pharmaceutical Sciences* 105: 2527–2544.

69 DeLeersnyder, F., Vanhoorne, V., Bekaert, H. et al. (2018). Breakage and drying behaviour of granules in a continuous fluid bed dryer: influence of process parameters and wet granule transfer. *European Journal of Pharmaceutical Sciences* 115: 223–232.

Part IV

Formulation Considerations for Solid Dosage Preparation

13

The Roles of Acid–Base Relationships, Interfaces, and Molecular Mobility in Stabilization During Drying and in the Solid State

Danforth P. Miller[1], *Evgenyi Shalaev*[2], *and Jim Barnard*[2]

[1] *Respira Therapeutics, 1828 El Camino Real, Suite 806, Burlingame, CA 94010, USA*
[2] *Allergan, Irvine, CA 92612, USA*

13.1 Introduction

The primary motivation for development of a drying process is the need to transform an inherently labile molecule into a more stable dosage form. While formulation and process development will depend to some extent on the type of dosage form and the nature of the drying process, there are some common themes that emerge in formulation and stabilization of small molecules and macromolecules. These themes are important in addressing physicochemical degradation induced during processing and long-term storage. First, control of pH is important during formulation development of both macromolecules and small molecule therapeutics. Understanding acid–base relationships and the change in ionization state during freezing and drying informs selection of excipients and formulation composition. Second, the interfaces formed during freeze drying, spray drying, and other drying processes create a high specific surface area milieu for physical (e.g. adsorption) and chemical processes. The influence of these interfaces on drug stability has become a key area in understanding and controlling process-induced degradation. Third, because many drying processes yield an amorphous or partially amorphous product, the long-term physicochemical stability of dried materials is a particular concern. Degradation during storage requires molecules to have sufficient energy and the proper orientation to undergo chemical reaction. Thus, understanding structure and the types of molecular mobility can be important to development of stable, dried products. This chapter will explore these concepts, all of which have relevance to the myriad drying technologies in use today as well as those yet to be invented.

Given that the majority of dried products on the market today are manufactured using freeze drying (lyophilization) or spray drying, many of the examples provided below will pertain to these processes. However, in many cases, the concepts described will be relevant to materials dried using other process.

Drying Technologies for Biotechnology and Pharmaceutical Applications, First Edition.
Edited by Satoshi Ohtake, Ken-ichi Izutsu, and David Lechuga-Ballesteros.

13.2 Acid–Base Relationships and Change in Ionization During Freezing and Drying

To ensure stability and bioavailability, many pharmaceutical dosage forms require pH control during manufacture, storage, and use. This section is focused predominantly on biopharmaceuticals, although the same considerations are applicable to other types of drug molecules. Most proteins are sensitive to pH, and any significant changes in proton concentration and/or activity could result in protein destabilization and degradation. Changes in the acid–base relationships can destabilize protein molecules either directly, via specific acid–base catalysis, or indirectly, by changing the ionization state of the protein and thus making it potentially more susceptible to both physical (e.g. aggregation) and chemical (e.g. oxidation) degradation pathways. The most commonly recognized root cause for change in the acidity during freeze drying is crystallization of buffer components. It is widely known, for example, that freezing of sodium phosphate buffer solutions could lead to crystallization of disodium hydrogen dodecahydrate ($Na_2HPO_4{\cdot}12H_2O$), resulting in a pronounced acidic pH shift in the freeze concentrate [1–3]. Succinate buffer is another example of a crystallizable buffer, for which a “pH swing,” with pH initially increasing from 4 to 8 followed by a precipitous drop to 2, was observed during freezing. The pH swing was attributed to sequential crystallization of the buffer components [4]. Furthermore, significant changes in the apparent acidity[1] could be observed even in completely amorphous systems for which buffer components do not crystallize. Water crystallization (ice formation) during freezing significantly increases the solutes’ concentration in the solution coexisting with ice crystals, with a corresponding decrease in polarity. Freezing of an aqueous sucrose solution, for example, would decrease the dielectric constant by more than 20 units, from approximately 76 in 10% (w/w) solution to approximately 50 in the frozen concentrate [5]. Such a decrease in the dielectric constant could lead to a major pK_a change; for example, the apparent pK_a of acetic acid increases significantly with decreases in polarity, from 4.76 in water (dielectric constant 78.3) to 10.32 in ethanol (dielectric constant 24.3) [6]. Changes in pH with a reduction in water content were directly monitored in two different buffers in the presence of sugars and sugar alcohols [7]. It was observed that pH depended on both the buffer type (phosphate vs. citrate) and the water activity/dielectric constant, with up to 0.7 pH unit difference reported between dilute and more concentrated solutions. To further illustrate the relationships between dielectric constant of a solution and its acidity, Figure 13.1 presents several different acidity functions in the water–ethanol system [6, 8]. These data illustrate two important points. First, acidity depends on the water content, and therefore, relatively large changes in the acidity can be expected with changes in water content. This occurs even in the absence of buffer crystallization. Second, there is no absolute acidity scale in systems other than dilute aqueous solutions. To emphasize the latter point, Paul and Long wrote: “ …there is no single, unique good measure of

1 Term “apparent acidity” is used because the proton activity scale, which can be considered as the true acidity, is established only in dilute aqueous solutions.

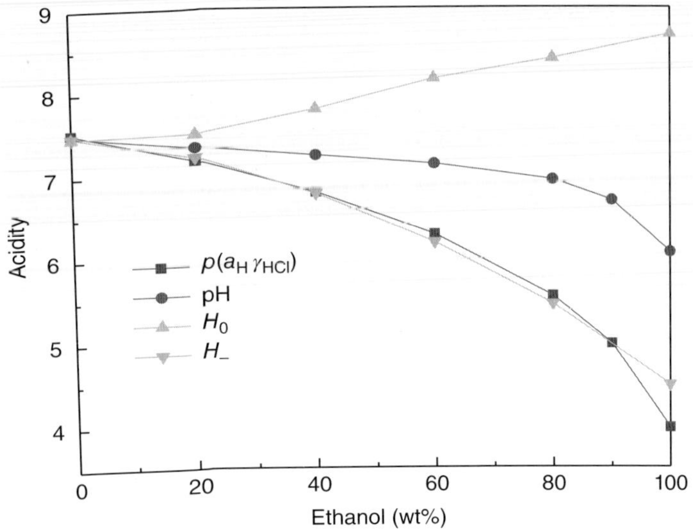

Figure 13.1 Acidity functions in ethanol–water solvents with 4 mM triethanolammonium chloride and 2 mM triethanolamine. pH = $-\log a_H$; a_H is proton activity. γ_{HCl} is the activity coefficient of HCl. H_0 and H_- refer to the Hammett acidity function with different indicators. H_0 indicator: *N,N′*-diethyl-toluidine; H_- indicator: *p*-nitrophenol. Source: Data from Bates 1973 [6] and Bates 1955 [8].

acidity. There are a variety of them, and any preference depends on such things as ease of measurement and ultimate application" [9].

There are several different ways to measure the acidity of frozen aqueous solutions. In pioneering studies of Van Den Berg [1], the unfrozen portion of the sample was physically separated from the solid phase at sub-zero temperature. The pH of the unfrozen solution was measured with a pH electrode. More recently, low-temperature pH electrodes have been developed, with measurements performed directly in the frozen sample, without physical separation of the freeze-concentrated phase from ice. The temperature range of these pH electrodes has been extended from −20 °C in earlier [10] versions to −30 °C more recently. Finally, the apparent acidity during freezing can also be measured with probe molecules. These molecules change their extent of protonation (and therefore their spectral properties) as a function of the local acidity of the given medium. Common pH indicators have been used as such probe molecules, and the change in the apparent acidity can be detected either visually by observing a color change [11] or more quantitatively by using diffuse reflectance (DR) spectroscopy to measure the ratio of the concentrations of deprotonated to protonated indicator species [12]. In the latter case, the apparent acidity can be expressed as the Hammett acidity function via Eq. (13.1):

$$H_x = pK_a + \log_{10}\frac{C_d}{C_p} = pK_a + \log_{10}\left(\frac{F(R)_d\varepsilon'_p}{F(R)_p\varepsilon'_d}\right) \tag{13.1}$$

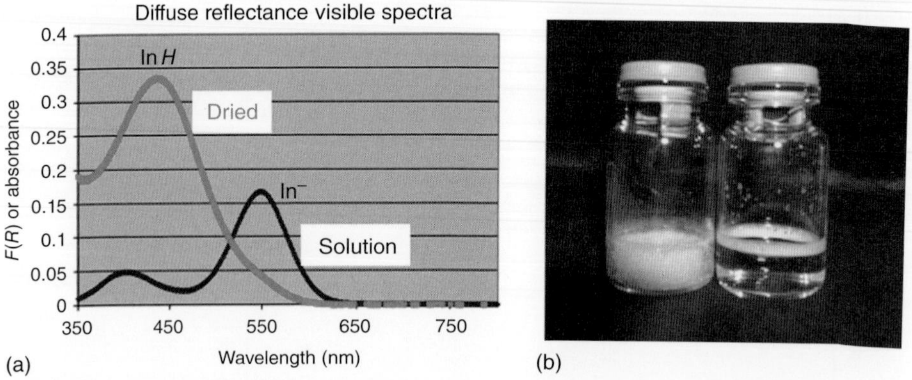

Figure 13.2 Change in the apparent acidity from solution to lyophile, as qualitatively measured via visual change of the color of an indicator (a), quantified by measuring the ionization extent of the indicator in solution and in the lyophile (diffuse reflectance visible spectra), and expressed as the Hammett acidity function, H_x (b) (Eq. (13.1)). Subscript x corresponds to the charge of the basic form of the given probe molecule; for sulfonephthalein pH indicators in typical pharmaceutical materials, x is equal to either −2 or −1. The change in color from solution to the lyophile reflects a significant change in the extent of protonation of the indicator and therefore a major shift in the apparent acidity during freeze drying. Visible diffuse reflectance spectra of solution and freeze-dried formulations show a major shift in the protonation of an indicator, from partially protonated in solution (pH 3.2) to completely protonated in the freeze-dried state ($H_- < 1.0$). (see online version for color figure)

Here, C is the indicator concentration, and the subscripts C_p and C_d refer to the protonated and deprotonated indicator species, respectively. K_a is the ionization constant of the indicator, $F(R)C_d/F(R)C_p$ is the ratio of the peak signals of the deprotonated to the protonated indicator forms determined from the DR spectra, and $\varepsilon'_p/\varepsilon'_d$ is the ratio of the extinction coefficients of the two species in the lyophiles.

A key advantage of the probe molecules is that they can also be used in the solid state [13], as exemplified in Figure 13.2. The change in color from solution to lyophile reflects a significant change in the extent of protonation of the indicator and therefore a major shift in the apparent acidity during freeze drying. Visible diffuse reflectance spectra of solution and freeze-dried formulations show a major shift in the protonation of an indicator, from partially protonated in solution (pH 3.2) to completely protonated in the freeze-dried state ($H_- < 1.0$). The subscript x corresponds to the charge of the basic form of the given probe molecule; for sulfonephthalein pH indicators in typical pharmaceutical materials, x is usually equal to −2.

When the ionization extent of a probe molecule is determined, the apparent acidity can be expressed as either the Hammett acidity function or the pH equivalent [14]. Note that other types of probe molecules and corresponding detection methods have been used as well; for example, ^{13}C-labeled probes with solid-state nuclear magnetic resonance (NMR) detection have been applied to monitor changes in the apparent acidity during freeze drying [15].

It has been shown that freeze drying could result in a significant change in the ionization of a probe molecule, i.e. a change in the apparent acidity, as illustrated

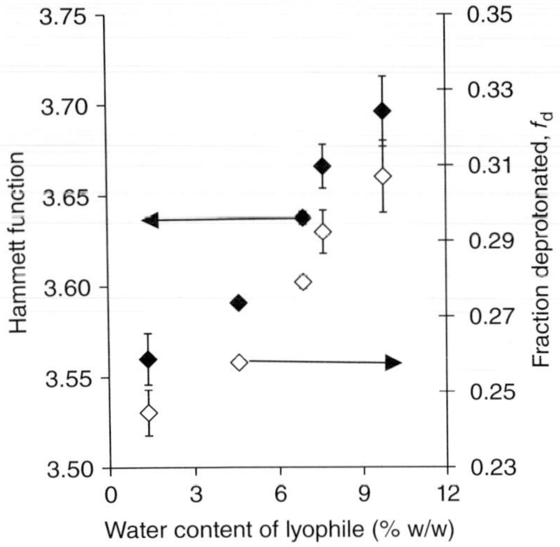

Figure 13.3 The effect of water content on the ionization of bromophenol blue in amorphous freeze-dried trehalose–citrate mixtures. The pH of the aqueous solution prior to lyophilization was 3.79. The fraction deprotonated, f_d, was calculated as $f_d = (c_d/(c_d + c_p))$, where c_d and c_p are concentrations of deprotonated and protonated indicator species, respectively. Source: Govindarajan et al. 2006 [14]. Reproduced with permission of Elsevier.

in Figure 13.2. This decrease in ionization (i.e. increase in the extent of protonation) indicates an increase in the apparent acidity of the lyophile matrix. Note that a change in the pK_a of the indicator could also be a contributing factor.

It should also be noted that proton mobility, and therefore the ionization extent, is not "arrested" in freeze-dried materials even well below the T_g and can change on a practical experimental time scale (hours or days). Govindarajan et al. [14] report one example of direct experimental observation of change in the ionization of an amorphous solid upon exposure to water vapor. In that study, freeze-dried powder was rehydrated via the vapor phase, and ionization of a probe molecule was measured by UV/vis diffuse reflectance spectroscopy both before and after rehydration (Figure 13.3). An increase in water content from 1.4% to 9.8% (w/w) increased the deprotonated fraction from 0.25 to 0.31, with a corresponding increase of approximately 0.15 units in the Hammett acidity function (i.e. a decrease in the acidity).

To illustrate the practical importance of the Hammett acidity function for development of pharmaceutical formulations, multiple studies have highlighted correlations between the Hammett acidity function (or an equivalent expression of the solid-state acidity called pH_{eq}) and solid-state degradation of a number of acid-sensitive compounds including acetylsalicylic acid [16], sucrose [17], quinapril hydrochloride [18], cefotaxime sodium [19], cefovecin [20], an enzyme (hydrolytic haloalkane dehalogenase) [12], and atorvastatin Ca [21].

Furthermore, application of the Hammett acidity function to freeze-dried formulations provides insight into the role of a critical excipient (i.e. lyoprotector) in stabilization. For example, while the pre-lyophilization solution pH strongly influences the apparent acidity in the lyophilized state, the type of lyoprotector also plays a role in the apparent solid-state acidity and therefore the stability of an acid-sensitive active pharmaceutical ingredient. This effect was demonstrated in studies that used sucrose as a model of an acid-sensitive compound that was lyophilized using several different lyoprotectors [22, 23]. These formulations contained sucrose and a co-solute (lactose and polyvinylpyrrolidone [PVP]

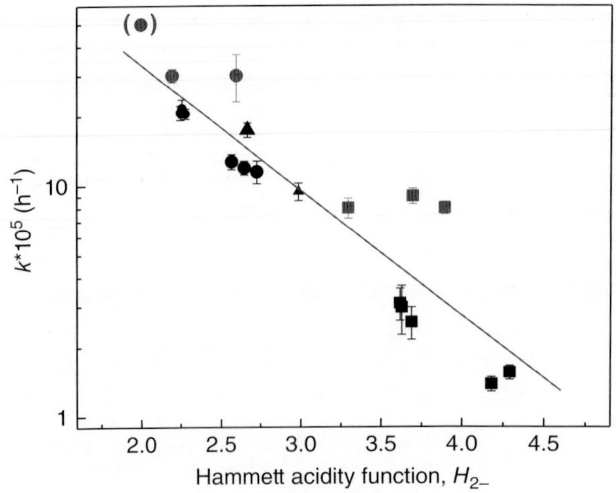

Figure 13.4 Pseudo-first-order rate constants of sucrose inversion in PVP (squares), lactose (triangles), and dextran (circles) lyophiles as a function of Hammett acidity function. The line reflects the correlation between the rate constant (logarithmic scale) and the Hammett acidity function. Source: Light gray symbols are data from Chatterjee et al. 2008 [22] and black symbols are data from Lu et al. 2009 [23].

and dextran of different molecular weights) at a 1 : 10 weight ratio. All were formulated using a citrate buffer and had an identical pH before lyophilization. The rate of acid-catalyzed sucrose inversion was determined during storage of the lyophiles. The apparent acidity of the freeze-dried formulations was determined using sulfonephthalein indicators and expressed as the Hammett acidity function. The relationships between the sucrose inversion rate (to form glucose and fructose) and the Hammett acidity function are shown in Figure 13.4. A significant difference in the H_{2-} was observed between formulations, with dextran-based formulations determined to be the most acidic and PVP-based formulations to be least acidic. Accordingly, the rate of acid-catalyzed sucrose inversion was highest in the dextran formulations followed by lactose- and then PVP-containing formulations (Figure 13.4). Interestingly, the least stable formulations also had the *highest* glass transition temperatures, whereas other physical properties including residual water content, amorphous structure, and rate of enthalpy relaxation were similar among the formulations studied.

Note that the phenomena discussed in this section are relevant to processes besides freeze drying. For example, other freezing processes (spray freeze drying) could cause a "pH swing" due to crystallization of buffer components or freeze concentration of dissolved solutes. Also, the Hammett acidity function is a useful tool to quantify the extent of ionization in the solid state, regardless of the drying process used.

To conclude, the Hammett acidity function can be used to predict the relative stability of an acid-sensitive molecule in different formulations and has been proven to be a useful tool in developing stable freeze-dried formulations. It should be noted, however, that the Hammett acidity function does not represent an absolute measure of proton activity. Therefore, any correlations of the Hammett acidity function with solid-state chemical stability should be considered as empirical relationships, which limit their predictive power. Govindarajan et al. [14] discuss in greater detail the limitations of the acidity scale based on sulfonephthalein probes. Finally, there are other physical properties of the amorphous state that could also strongly influence solid-state stability, as discussed below.

13.3 Role of Interfaces in Instability During Freeze Drying and Spray Drying

During freeze-drying or spray-drying processes, proteins are exposed to a variety of interfaces such as air–water, ice–solution, glass–solution, etc. It is well established with numerous proteins that encounters with various interfaces likely result in some degree of protein adsorption [24]. For example, Burke et al. [25] performed experiments on 20 different proteins that ranged from 6.5 to 670 kDa in molecular weight and from 4.3 to 10.5 in isoelectric point. These proteins, representing a broad range of physicochemical properties, were exposed to a variety of pharmaceutically relevant contact materials such as glass, treated glass, or several different polymers. In nearly all protein interface combinations evaluated, some level of protein adsorption (in the $\mu g/cm^2$ range) was observed.

Although protein adsorption to a variety of surfaces is common, the nature of the adsorption can be complex and depend on the physicochemical properties of both the surface material and the protein itself. In addition, the properties of the formulation such as pH, ionic strength, presence of surfactant, etc. can affect the extent and nature of adsorption. In most cases, protein adsorption occurs because of favorable entropy. However, charge–charge interactions, van der Waals interactions, and hydrogen bonding between a given protein and surface can influence the rate or nature of adsorption (i.e. packing density, reorientation, etc.) [26]. The rate of adsorption is often limited by the transport of protein molecules to the surface by simple diffusion. Electrostatic parameters (charge–charge interactions and charge shielding) are thought to play a larger role in the orientation, monolayer packing efficiency, reversibility, or whether multiple layers of adsorbed protein molecules will attach to a given surface.

Protein adsorption at interfaces can be an acute problem in cases where a low protein concentration is required (e.g. <100 μg/ml) since measurable losses in protein concentration from the bulk become more likely. But even for higher protein concentration formulations, where losses in protein concentration due to adsorption are often below the limit of detection, adsorption to interfaces can still be problematic. This is because adsorption can lead to structural changes (partial unfolding on the interface) and potential desorption of the partially unfolded protein. Partially unfolded species can lead to further instability such as aggregation or particulate formation [27, 28].

Freeze drying presents both an air–solution interface when solution is filled into vials and an ice–solution interface during the freezing process. Proteins have been shown to adsorb to air–solution interfaces and can continue to accumulate until a gel layer forms (as measured by interfacial shear rheology) [29]. The formation of a gel layer due to adsorption of protein at the air–solution interface can occur over relatively short time scales (e.g. <10 minutes). In the same study, it was shown that the addition of surfactant (Polysorbate 80) completely prevented protein adsorption at the air–solution interface, likely via a competitive adsorption effect.

It is established that freeze/thaw cycling can damage proteins. Freezing presents several destabilizing stresses such as pH shifts arising from crystallization of buffer components or cryo-concentration of excipients. A prominent destabilizing stress during freezing, however, is the formation of the ice crystal surface. Protein can adsorb to the ice interface (similar to other surfaces discussed), with evidence of partially unfolded proteins at ice interfaces having been observed by infrared microscopy [30]. When a solution is rapidly frozen, smaller and more numerous ice crystals are formed, thus presenting a larger surface area for protein–ice interaction to occur [31]. On the microscopic level, protein molecules could predominantly partition into the quasi-liquid layer, rather than be directly sorbed to the ice crystals, as was indeed indicated in a recent study [32]. The quasi-liquid layer (also known as liquid-like layer) is a thin film of liquid water on the surface of ice crystals, which exists well below the ice melting temperature, even in pure water [33]. Protein molecules in the quasi-liquid layer could be exposed to destabilizing stresses, such as an increased local acidity due to the negative charge on the surface of ice crystals [34]. The ice surface has been shown to carry negative charge when in equilibrium with a solution at pH values higher than 4; the negative charge is balanced by an elevated local concentration of cations, including protons, in the quasi-liquid layer next to the ice surface, resulting in a corresponding increase in the local acidity.

In addition to the ice–solution interface and the adjacent quasi-liquid layer, freezing could create an additional pathway for surface-related protein instability due to newly formed solution–air interface, as suggested by Salnikova et al. [35]. It was shown that the growth of ice crystals increased the local concentrations of oxygen and nitrogen in the freeze-concentrated solution, resulting in formation of air bubbles and therefore additional solution–air interface [36]. While sorption of protein on these freezing-induced air bubbles could lead to protein destabilization, the contribution of this potential mechanism to overall protein destabilization has not been quantitatively studied. Finally, additional interfaces could be created in the maximally freeze-concentrated solution when it is cooled below the glass transition temperature, as suggested in a recent study of a model sorbitol–water system [37]. In that study, a sorbitol–water mixture with a composition representative of the maximally freeze-concentrated solution was studied by small-angle neutron scattering (SANS). Cooling of the sample below its calorimetric T_g (approximately 210 K) resulted in development of domains with well-defined and sharp interfaces on the sub-micrometer length scale, likely as a result of the appearance and growth of microscopic voids in the glassy matrix. These voids and interfaces probably reflect an intrinsic property of amorphous solids, i.e. their heterogeneous structure consisting of cooperative domains and interfaces separating the domains, although a contribution from dissolved gases to the emergence of these voids cannot be ruled out at this point. Importantly, these interfaces persisted even when the sample was heated to temperatures above T_g; therefore, they could represent an additional source of protein surface-related instability during freeze-thawing and freeze drying/reconstitution.

In freeze-dried cakes, protein molecules are not distributed homogeneously. A higher protein concentration has been observed at the surface of the cake (i.e. at the air–surface interface), with the surface protein concentration 1–2 orders of magnitude higher than the bulk concentration [38]. In this case, the secondary structure of the surface protein was found to be disrupted. In addition, it was suggested that the surface protein molecules would have much higher rates (more than 2 orders of magnitude) of chemical reactivity and aggregation than bulk molecules [38–40].

Additional exposure of protein molecules to air–solution interfaces can also occur during reconstitution. Recent research has shown that reconstitution of amorphous cakes containing saccharides such as sucrose and trehalose can lead to the formation of stable nanobubbles upon reconstitution [41]. It has also been demonstrated that these nanobubbles can contribute to protein aggregation and particulate formation following reconstitution of a lyophilized protein sample [42]. Other research has found that the formation of such bubbles can be minimized by annealing during lyophilization [40]. This was attributed to Ostwald ripening of the pores in the lyophilized solid during annealing, with larger pores resulting in larger but fewer bubbles upon reconstitution.

Although exposure to different interfaces during bioprocessing is inevitable, protein adsorption to these interfaces can be reduced. The most common excipients used to prevent adsorption are nonionic surfactants such as polysorbates and poloxamers. These have been used in spray drying, for example. Although the exposure of protein to the air–solution interface is transient (<100 ms) when compared with freeze drying, spray drying presents an enormous air–solution interface. In a spray-dried formulation of human growth hormone, the addition of 0.1% (w/v) Polysorbate 20 reduced the formation of soluble and insoluble aggregates by approximately 70% and 85%, respectively [43]. This and other nonionic surfactants primarily prevent protein adsorption by occupying and competing with protein molecules for available surfaces. In some cases, the surfactant can interact with the protein molecule itself to form protein–surfactant complexes that have less adsorption affinity [44]. Polysorbates are typically formulated above the critical micelle concentration (CMC). The CMC is the point at which all available surface adsorption sites are occupied and excess surfactant molecules are confined to the bulk solution and form thermodynamically favorable micelles. Although formulating above the CMC ensures occupation of available adsorption sites, excess surfactant has been shown to structurally destabilize proteins in some cases [45].

While this section has focused on biologicals, these concepts could also be relevant to adsorption of some small molecule drugs at interfaces, with a corresponding change in their stability [46].

13.4 Influence of Molecular Mobility on Physicochemical Stability

The primary motivation for using a drying process is to transform an inherently labile molecule into a stable, solid dosage form. In many cases, the dried solid product is amorphous. Even when the dried product is highly crystalline, a fraction of the material may be amorphous, arising either from the starting material or induced during the manufacturing process. A key differentiator between amorphous and crystalline solids is that the molecules in amorphous materials are not in fixed positions. The molecular motions in an amorphous solid are significant when compared with those of its crystalline counterpart. This term comprises long-range motions related to molecular diffusion as well as local motions such as bond rotations. These motions are collectively referred to as "molecular mobility" and play a role in processes important to physical and chemical stability, such as crystallization, protein aggregation, and myriad chemical reaction pathways. For example, crystallization requires nucleation and crystal growth, the latter of which depends on molecular diffusion. And, for a chemical reaction to occur, collision theory states that molecules must have sufficient energy and the proper orientation. Both are related to molecular mobility. The central principle in solid-state stabilization of amorphous materials is that molecular mobility leads to undesirable physical and chemical changes. Therefore, formulation strategies for amorphous materials include characterization and suppression of molecular mobility. Although stabilization of amorphous formulations is oftentimes an empirical exercise, understanding the basic principles of molecular mobility will help a formulator rationally develop stable solid-state formulations.

The existence of a relationship between molecular mobility and undesirable physicochemical processes is intuitive. However, to be useful, the catchall term of "molecular mobility" must be carefully defined and understood in terms of the types of motions present. Before discussing dynamics in more detail, it is helpful to understand the formation of a glass because the structure and dynamics of a glass depend on its history. Most importantly, there is not a single glassy state. The physical properties and dynamics of a glassy material depend upon its structure, which, in turn, depends on how it was made [47–50]. Thus, there can be practically meaningful differences in the properties of glasses of the same composition made using different processes (e.g. freeze drying, vacuum drying, spray drying, quench cooling, milling, etc.). Although drying processes are the topic of this volume, it is oftentimes conceptually easier to understand glass formation in terms of a cooling process (i.e. where temperature is the only variable and composition does not change). In this case, a glass can be formed by cooling a liquid sufficiently fast to avoid nucleation and crystallization. This liquid could be either a melt of a pure compound or a solution. At slow cooling rates, molecular rearrangements enable some materials to follow the path of a supercooled liquid (Figure 13.5), with a volume and enthalpy that are extrapolated from the properties above the melting point, T_m. As this liquid is cooled further, its viscosity increases and its molecular motions start to slow. At sufficiently low temperatures, the characteristic time scale for these molecular rearrangements becomes comparable to the cooling rate. At this point, the supercooled liquid becomes a "glass" and exhibits solid-like properties. This is defined as "the" glass transition temperature, T_g. Because this depends on a crossing of time scales for observation and molecular rearrangement, T_g depends on the cooling rate and is a kinetic parameter. Thus, T_g does not represent a thermodynamic phase transition. Although Figure 13.5 was developed in terms of a cooling process, analogous diagrams could be constructed for glasses formed by other routes as well (e.g. a drying process).

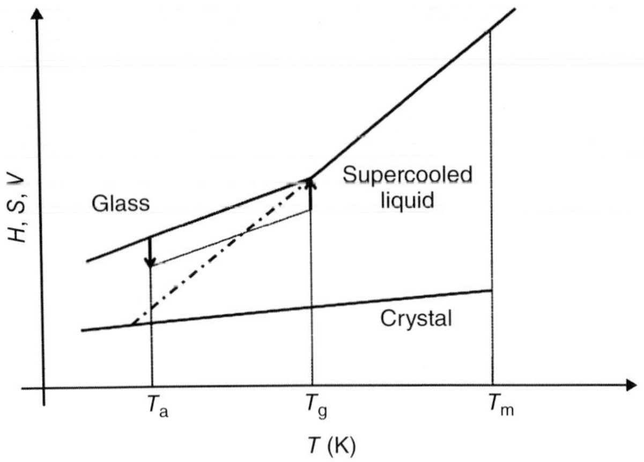

Figure 13.5 A glass can be viewed as a nonequilibrium supercooled liquid. Source: Janssens and Van den Mooter 2009 [51]. Reproduced with permission of John Wiley & Sons.

Cooling a glass to a temperature further below T_g results in a material with a volume (and enthalpy and entropy) that is greater than that of the so-called "equilibrium" supercooled liquid. During storage at a given temperature, molecular rearrangements will decrease the volume and enthalpy of the glassy material toward that of the (hypothetical) supercooled liquid. These rearrangements are termed "structural relaxation," also known as α-relaxation. These long-range molecular motions are cooperative in nature, as the reorientation of a given molecule will require some reorientations of surrounding molecules. The time scale for such motions increases markedly as temperature decreases below T_g (or, conversely, as the T_g is raised at a fixed observation temperature). Because stabilization of a molecule in a glass limits its long-range molecular mobility, this has become the most common formulation strategy for solid-state stabilization of amorphous drugs.

While control of the α or "primary" motions through formulation or storage below T_g has received widespread attention, the importance of other types of molecular motions has become increasingly recognized in the pharmaceutical literature [52–54]. The nomenclature (α, β, etc.) used to designate the types of molecular motions originates from broadband dielectric spectroscopy. Dielectric relaxation spectra are conventionally plotted on a frequency scale. When interpreting these spectra, the dielectric loss peaks at the lowest frequencies are designated as α motions, the higher frequency (shorter time scale) motions as β motions, then γ, and so forth (Figure 13.6). Thus, β and other motions that occur at higher frequencies are referred to as "secondary" motions. These are often ascribed to intramolecular motions of different molecular moieties (e.g. side chains of a protein). However, even rigid molecules undergo these motions [56]. Fast local reorientations of entire molecules are termed Johari–Goldstein relaxations. In a simplistic physical picture, the β motions are sometimes described as random "cage rattling" of a species trapped among its nearest neighbors. At some point, the local motions of the nearest neighbors provide sufficient free volume to enable a diffusive jump of the trapped species. This jump represents an α motion. Thus, the local β motions can lead to global relaxation (α motions),

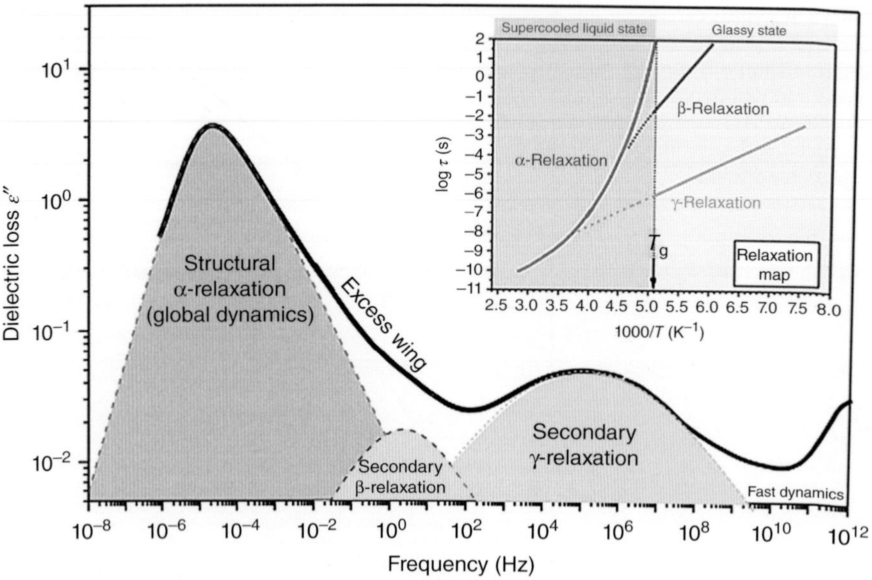

Figure 13.6 Illustration of dielectric spectra obtained in the broad frequency range after subtraction of the DC conduction contribution and the corresponding relaxation map (inset). Note that α-relaxations below T_g are not shown here because dielectric analysis is not well suited in this region (i.e. measurements are extremely time consuming). Source: Grzybowska et al. 2016 [55]. Reproduced with permission of Elsevier.

a concept proposed and developed in the extended mode coupling theory of Ngai [57].

Beyond theoretical interest, these local motions are an area of applied research from a practical perspective. The inset of Figure 13.6 shows an example of the temperature dependence of several processes measured using dielectric relaxation spectroscopy. The time scales of the α motions are much stronger functions of temperature than those of the β motions. Thus, while storage at low temperatures can strongly suppress α-relaxation, secondary motions can still persist at such temperatures. The practical significance is that slowing α mobility by raising T_g or reducing the storage temperature does not necessarily ensure long-term physicochemical stability.

With an understanding of the fundamentals of the molecular mobility of glassy materials, a formulator is faced with practical questions regarding how to characterize and control these motions. The glass transition temperature, T_g, provides the simplest measure of molecular mobility. Being a single quantity and measurable using equipment found in most physical characterization laboratories, T_g is one of the most basic descriptors of an amorphous material. For pharmaceuticals, T_g is most often determined using differential scanning calorimetry (DSC). The calorimetric T_g represents a relaxation time on the order of 100 seconds [58] – a period over which the relaxation time is commensurate with the observation time of a DSC measurement (usually at a heating rate between about 2 and 10 °C/min). Although T_g is most often measured calorimetrically, it can be determined using spectroscopic, mechanical, or volumetric methods that interrogate a sample as a function of temperature. These techniques include thermomechanical analysis, dynamic mechanical analysis, inverse gas chromatography, NMR, and dielectric relaxation spectroscopy. These and other emerging technologies (e.g. oscillatory squeezing flow, thermal mechanical compression test, positron annihilation lifetime spectroscopy [PALS], thermally stimulated depolarization current, and atomic force microscopy) are described in a review by Abiad et al. [59] and references therein. In the absence of T_g data, the glass transition temperature can be estimated using an empirical rule based on the melting temperature, T_m. For example, based on a linear regression of measured T_g and T_m values of 70 different amorphous small molecule pharmaceuticals, T_g/T_m was found to be 0.73 ± 0.01 [60]. This value is similar to the central value measured for crystallizable polymers, $T_g/T_m \approx 0.66$.

Knowledge of T_g helps delineate temperature regimes. Qualitatively, an amorphous material below its T_g is a glass with the mechanical properties of a solid. At temperatures just above T_g, a glassy material begins to soften and is sometimes designated as a "rubber" or a supercooled liquid. At even higher temperatures (e.g. 10 or 20 K above T_g), viscous flow occurs, resulting in macroscopic changes to an amorphous material over practical time scales. In lyophilized materials, viscous flow can lead to unacceptable changes in product appearance or in product performance attributes (e.g. longer reconstitution time due to a loss of surface area). In some spray-dried powders for inhalation, this can sometimes lead to stickiness and irreversible sintering of amorphous particles, ultimately affecting particle size and aerosol performance. In some cases, a drug could crystallize, leading to changes in its bioavailability. Likewise, crystallization of excipients could affect not only the physical properties but also the chemical stability of the drug itself.

Because viscous flow can result in gross changes in appearance or performance, knowledge of T_g provides a formulator and process development engineer a rational approach to developing formulations and processes to avoid viscous flow during product manufacturing, storage, and use [61]. Enhancement of physicochemical stability is based upon a simple concept of raising T_g by formulating a drug with one or more excipients that have a higher T_g. However, the use of high-T_g excipients is not necessarily sufficient, as formation of an amorphous solid dispersion requires miscibility of the drug and glass-forming agent(s) on a molecular scale [62]. Solid-state miscibility with the drug is a necessary condition when using any glass former to stabilize an amorphous drug. On a molecular level, such a mixture is often described as a solid solution or an amorphous solid dispersion (in some cases, this latter term is reserved for mixtures of polymer and drug). A number of models have been developed to predict the T_g of such mixtures based on the T_g values of the individual components [63]. All of these models assume that the drug and excipient comprise a single amorphous phase. Although T_g values of mixtures can be predicted with reasonable accuracy, it is more difficult to predict a priori the miscibility of an excipient and drug. Greenhalgh et al. [64] developed an approach based on Hildebrand solubility parameters. Although this is an attractive approach because these parameters can be calculated using group contribution methods, its predictive ability is limited. In the absence of accurate predictive methods, miscibility is usually assessed empirically using a number of different approaches, including vibrational spectroscopy, X-ray powder diffraction, and thermal analysis (see, for example, the overview provided by Van Eerdenbrugh et al. [65]).

Approaches to identify suitable glass formers often begin with a simple screening to select materials with high T_g values. Although such an approach will help identify many molecules with T_g values well above 100 °C, concerns will remain with respect to miscibility with drug, biocompatibility, and hygroscopicity. For example, many polymers tend to have high T_g values. However, due to the large differences in size between polymers and small molecule drugs, some polymeric molecules tend to be poorly miscible with drugs or have a limited composition range over which they form amorphous solid dispersions.

Molecular mobility persists at temperatures below T_g; physicochemical processes continue, albeit at reduced rates. Crystallization over pharmaceutically relevant time scales has been shown to occur even at temperatures nearly 50 °C below T_g [66]. And, for compositions and storage conditions for which crystallization is effectively inhibited, chemical degradation reactions still occur. Over the last 20 years, numerous studies have investigated whether T_g is a predictor of stability [59, 67–69]. Despite some evidence of positive correlations, a simple relationship between T_g and long-term stability does not exist. Materials with similar T_g values sometimes have different propensities to crystallize [70]. Also, formulations with lower T_g values can have even greater stability than those with elevated T_g values [71]. Although T_g is not necessarily predictive, it has value in defining the regime for viscous flow (typically at temperatures at least 10–20 °C above T_g) and for its use in scaling relationships (e.g. time–temperature superposition [72]).

The limited predictive ability of T_g has driven the evolution of the field from T_g measurements and the use of simple rules of thumb (e.g. storage at temperatures at least 50 K below T_g) [73] toward more specific and direct assessments of molecular mobility. Structural (α) relaxation requires molecular mobility and reduces the enthalpy and volume of an amorphous material. Thus, it can be assessed using calorimetry [74] (e.g. high-sensitivity DSC, isothermal microcalorimetry) or high-precision density measurements [75], for example. Structural relaxation data are fit to a model, the most common being the Kohlrausch–Williams–Watts (KWW) stretched exponential function [76–78]:

$$\varphi = \exp\left(-\left(\frac{t}{\tau}\right)^{\beta}\right) \tag{13.2}$$

where τ is a characteristic relaxation time and β is the degree of non-exponentiality. This "stretching" parameter, β, is also considered to be a measure of the width of the distribution of relaxation times and the fragility of the glass; lower β values denote a broad distribution of relaxation times. Thus, a glass with a given composition and thermal history will have a characteristic relaxation time and "stretching" parameter. Because τ increases and β tends to decrease during structural relaxation measurement, practitioners suggest that τ^{β} tends to be a more robust parameter than τ alone [79].

When considering the use of structural relaxation time as a predictive tool, one must consider whether the molecular motions involved in the rate-limiting step of a chemical reaction or in recrystallization are the same as those involved in long-range (α) molecular mobility. Strong correlations have been reported between chemical reaction rates and structural relaxation time for low molecular weight drugs [80] as well as for peptides and proteins [81]. Studies of the relationship between molecular mobility and reaction rates below T_g include examples in which degradation is "coupled" to some extent with α molecular mobility [82–84]. Yoshioka et al. published a series of papers [80, 85–88] in which they investigated the relationship between (α) molecular mobility and the chemical stability of insulin formulations. The extent of coupling varied widely and depended strongly on the excipient used. Shamblin et al. studied the coupling between chemical reactivity and structural relaxation for two drug formulations [84]. Coupling was incomplete and was different in each case. This is not surprising, given that coupling represents the relevance of the molecular motions involved in structural relaxation to those in the rate-limiting steps of chemical degradation processes. Sadrzadeh et al. [89] compared reaction rate constants of an amorphous spray-dried insulin powder formulation to those estimated from structural relaxation experiments, showing moderate coupling of the solid-state degradation pathways with the molecular motions involved in structural relaxation. Grzybowska et al. [55] reviewed the extent of correlation between relaxation time and the characteristic time scale for crystallization of small molecules at temperatures both above and below T_g. For the limited number of compounds studied below T_g, the extent of correlation varied widely. This is perhaps not surprising given the different types of molecular motions involved and the molecular mechanisms that govern crystal nucleation and growth.

Although structural relaxation tends to provide better correlations with stability than simple measures like T_g, there are examples where neither metric is predictive. Figure 13.7 shows an example of protein aggregation rate in lyophilized IgG1 antibody/sucrose formulations [90]. Based on the T_g data alone, one would erroneously predict that higher sucrose concentrations would decrease protein stability. The structural relaxation data show different trends depending on the sucrose concentration. Below a sucrose weight fraction of 0.5, protein stability increases with structural relaxation time, as would be expected. However, the opposite trend is observed at higher sucrose contents. These data illustrate that the extent of coupling between long-range molecular mobility and stability depends on the formulation.

Incomplete or poor coupling might be explained in part by the importance of secondary motions. Reactions that require long-range molecular mobility will be more strongly coupled than those that only require, for example, diffusion of small species such as oxygen and H_2O. Given the small size and high molecular diffusivity of oxygen, oxidation could occur even when the long-range molecular mobility of a drug is limited. In such cases, the oxygen mobility would be considered to be independent (or decoupled) from that of the structural relaxation of the amorphous matrix. Water is another example of a small molecule reactant. That amorphous materials can be dried at temperatures

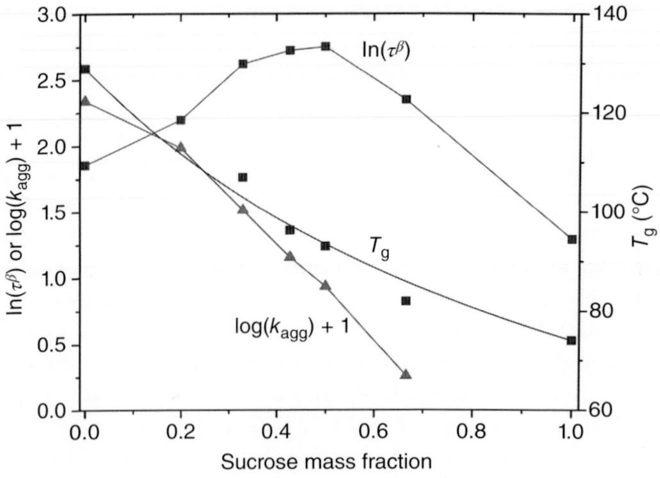

Figure 13.7 Correlations between T_g, structural relaxation time (τ^{β}), and protein aggregation rate at 40 °C (k_{agg}) in lyophilized formulations of an IgG1 antibody and sucrose. Source: Cicerone et al. 2015 [90]. Adapted with permission of Elsevier.

far below their T_g is an indication of the significant mobility of water within a glassy matrix. However, other moieties beyond small molecular species play a role in protein stability. Protein formulators have recognized the importance of controlling intramolecular secondary motions [87]. Yoshioka et al. examined the influence of the mobility of insulin side chains (β motions) on chemical degradation of lyophilized formulations containing trehalose or dextran. Based on relaxation times measured using NMR, they concluded that β motions were more critical than matrix mobility (α-relaxation) in chemical degradation of lyophilized formulations containing trehalose. The authors deemed their findings related to β-relaxation to be intuitive, given that insulin degradation via a cyclic intermediate would not be expected to require long-range molecular mobility. As another example, crystallization of small molecules near T_g has been suspected to arise from β motions [91, 92].

13.5 Fast β-Relaxation in Practice

Although secondary motions have been studied for several decades in solid-state physics, they are not routinely measured in the food science and pharmaceutical fields. This likely arises from either the lack of commercially available instrumentation to measure these motions or the slow adoption of techniques pioneered in other fields. Measurement often requires specialized instrumentation or techniques that can be prone to artifacts and experimental difficulties (e.g. inelastic neutron scattering, solid-state NMR, and thermally stimulated current spectroscopy). While there are commercially available broadband dielectric spectrometers that cover a broad frequency "window," this technique has made only modest inroads into the pharmaceutical laboratory. More recently, terahertz time domain spectroscopy (THz-TDS) has been used to characterize crystalline materials and, more recently, amorphous materials [93–97]. While this and other spectroscopies probe molecular motions across a range of time domains, a challenge lies in interpretation of the spectral features and attribution to rotational, vibrational, and relaxational motions.

Complementary to dynamics and molecular motions, assessment of structure can provide insight into the mechanisms. Free volume is a key concept in understanding local motions. Molecules do not pack perfectly. As one example, the increase in volume due to thermal expansion arises from increases in free volume. While this is an intuitive concept, measurement can require sophisticated equipment. Perhaps the most widely used technique to probe free volume is PALS. PALS can be used to measure the dimensions of free volume holes, the fractional free volume, and the average free volume hole size in amorphous materials [98, 99]. The technique relies upon the use of positrons – positively charged electrons. These short-lifetime particles undergo annihilation to form γ-rays. This requires enough annihilation events to produce a statistically smooth decay curve. A model is used to correlate ortho-positronium (o-PS) lifetime and the hole dimension. Note that although PALS is a useful tool with a strong theoretical underpinning, it requires safety considerations with respect to handling of radioactive materials and specialized equipment not available in ordinary labs.

The free volume concept provides a useful mental model for formulation approaches: molecular filling of free volume holes. Suppression of β motions in amorphous formulations is typically done with the addition of low molecular weight organic excipients, such as glycerol [100], mannitol, sorbitol [90], and dimethyl sulfoxide. Although these are the most frequently reported excipients to suppress β motions, other organic molecules could serve this purpose (e.g. buffer salts, counterions, oligomers of simple sugars). These excipients are hypothesized to suppress motions of high-mobility domains by raising the local viscosity. To the reader familiar with the vast literature on glassy stabilization, the use of such excipients might seem counterintuitive. While these diluents reduce free volume, these and most other low molecular weight materials have low T_g values and will reduce the T_g of a formulation, a phenomenon known as plasticization [101]. However, these excipients can also diminish secondary motions. Thus, they are referred to as antiplasticizers or sometimes as plasticizers, depending on the point of reference; although they plasticize the α motions, they antiplasticize the β motions and other secondary motions. Note that this terminology is a potential source of confusion in the literature; the designation of a material as a plasticizer or an antiplasticizer depends on whether one's point of reference is the α motions or the secondary motions.

Because solid-state stabilization of proteins requires formulation of a glassy matrix, the contributions of α and secondary motions are of particular interest. Although the literature has numerous references of using glass-forming agents to stabilize proteins [102–104], until recently, there have been few specific references to the influence of these agents on local motions [100, 105]. Although the glass transition temperatures of proteins are difficult to measure, most data suggest that $T_g > 150\,°C$ [106]. Thus, the excipients (e.g. disaccharides such as sucrose or trehalose) most commonly used to stabilize proteins will also plasticize the α motions in the protein (and antiplasticize secondary motions). The then-prevailing hypotheses (e.g. vitrification and water replacement) that explain the protective mechanisms of these excipients were quantitatively explored in the work of Cicerone and Douglas [107]. In elegantly designed experiments, Douglas and Cicerone used dielectric relaxation spectroscopy and neutron backscattering to probe the local motions in a diverse range of proteins formulated in sugar glasses. Figure 13.8a shows how the sugar mass fraction influences the mean-squared displacement ($\langle u^2 \rangle$) of hydrogen atoms in globular proteins formulated in freeze-dried sugar glasses. These motions depend on sugar mass fraction in an approximately linear fashion. Douglas and Cicerone then reviewed stability studies of nearly 20 pharmaceutically important proteins for which aggregation or chemical degradation rates were reported as a function of sugar (sucrose or trehalose) concentration. Using the linear relationship shown in Figure 13.8a, they expressed aggregation or chemical degradation rates in terms of mean-squared displacement (Figure 13.8b). This and other supporting work demonstrate that β motions either largely or entirely govern the stability of proteins in sugar glasses (i.e. β-relaxation times are correlated with degradation time constants). Thus, disaccharides likely antiplasticize β motions in protein formulations.

In practice, an empirical approach is often used to control secondary motions, oftentimes relying on product-relevant measures (e.g. stability testing; see Figure 13.9) rather than direct measurement of structure and dynamics. Using this approach, one determines the antiplasticizer concentrations needed to reduce secondary motions while not adversely affecting the long-range molecular (α) mobility. Typically, the concentration of an antiplasticizer is systematically varied, and the physicochemical stability of the formulation is assessed. Of course, this can only be done when the excipient forms a single-phase molecular dispersion with the drug. Generally, high antiplasticizer concentrations are avoided because they can excessively plasticize the α motions (lowering the T_g) or can result in crystallization of the antiplasticizer itself. As an example, this approach was used to develop the marketed formulation of Exubera, an inhalable insulin. This spray-dried formulation contained small amounts of low molecular weight excipients (mannitol and glycine) that enabled development of the first room-temperature stable protein powder for inhalation [108].

While the preceding discussion has focused on molecular mobility as a bulk phenomenon in amorphous solids, recent work demonstrates that molecules near the surface can have a higher molecular mobility than that in the bulk [109, 110]. The diffusion constant of molecules at a surface can be several orders of magnitude higher than that in the interior [111]. Enhanced surface diffusion has potential implications for materials dried using different processes, as the specific surface area of a dried material can depend strongly on the process (e.g. spray dried > freeze dried > film dried [112]). Although most studies to date have focused on the relationship between surface mobility and crystallization [113], it is likely that this mobility can also lead to other modes of physicochemical instability.

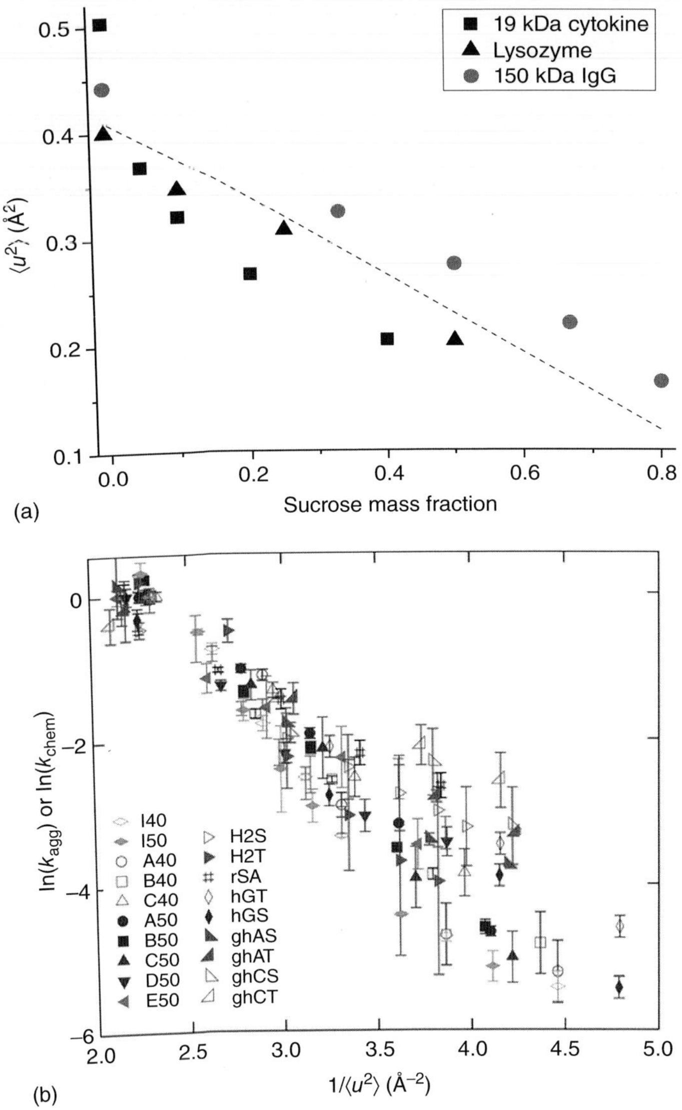

Figure 13.8 The influence of β motions on protein stability. (a) Greater sugar concentrations reduce the mean-squared displacement ($\langle u^2 \rangle$) of hydrogen atoms in globular proteins of a range of molecular weight (19–150 kDa) formulated in freeze-dried sugar glasses (cytokine [squares], lysozyme [triangles], and IgG [circles]). (b) The aggregation or chemical degradation rates of nearly 20 pharmaceutically important proteins formulated in sugar glasses, expressed in terms of (reciprocal) mean-squared displacement of hydrogen atoms. Source: Cicerone and Douglas 2012 [107]. Reproduced with permission of Royal Society of Chemistry.

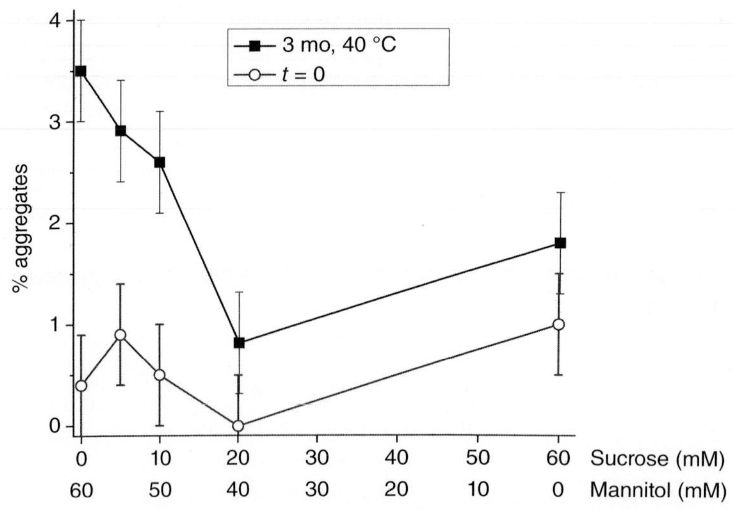

Figure 13.9 Aggregation of a monoclonal antibody human epidermal growth factor receptor 2 (HER2) formulated in mannitol–sucrose formulations. The existence of an optimum mannitol–sucrose ratio suggests that suppressing both long-range (α) and local (β) motions is critical to physicochemical stability. Samples were analyzed in duplicate (CV ±5%). Source: Cleland et al. 2001 [104]. Adapted with permission of John Wiley & Sons.

13.6 Conclusions and Advice to the Formulator

The overall goal of any drying process is to develop a stable dosage form that meets all product performance quality attributes. Here, this broadly encompasses all aspects of a product, from a molecule to the finished dosage form. At a molecular level, the formulator must understand the pathways for physicochemical degradation. This can be the stresses due to pH and the interfaces formed, both during manufacturing and over long-term storage. Product appearance goes beyond cosmetic considerations, as shape and morphology can have a bearing on performance attributes (dry powder aerosols, reconstitution of lyophilized "cakes," etc.).

Process-induced degradation can be studied by evaluating the effects of individual processing steps. Forced degradation studies or the known degradation chemistry of structurally similar compounds can provide insight into the mechanism(s) of physicochemical degradation during long-term storage. This can be supplemented with characterization of the structure and dynamics of the material formulated in a "platform formulation."

The concepts discussed in this chapter provide a framework for rational development of stable, dried dosage forms:

- *Acid–base relationships*: Select a buffer composition and pH to ensure stability during processing and storage, as well as to ensure physiological tolerability. Note that changes in freezing and drying can change the dielectric constant of water, the pK_a of buffer species, and the apparent acidity. Thus, the apparent pH or acidity function of a dried material can differ markedly from that of the "parent" aqueous solution.

- *Interfaces*: Use of excipients (e.g. nonionic surfactants) that can occupy available surfaces can reduce or prevent protein adsorption and associated surface-induced degradation. In addition, the surface area of ice crystals and, consequently, the specific surface area of freeze-dried cakes can be reduced during manufacturing by application of a controlled ice nucleation technique or using annealing during the freezing step of the freeze-drying process.
- *Glass former*: Use of a glass former with a sufficient T_g can increase physical stability during manufacturing, handling, and storage. The properties of an ideal glass former are a biocompatible material with a high glass transition temperature that is miscible with the drug, forming a single amorphous phase that is only weakly plasticized by water.

The concepts related to molecular mobility discussed here are relevant to glassy materials made using any drying process. We emphasize that the structure and dynamics of a glass will depend on how the glass was prepared and its history (e.g. aging or annealing after manufacture). Given that different drying processes can impart different structures on both a molecular and macroscopic level, the drying process can influence molecular mobility:

- α *Motions*: Structural relaxation time is a useful measure of stability when degradation pathways are known *and* there is evidence that these pathways require long-range molecular mobility (i.e. they are strongly coupled with α mobility).
- *Secondary motions*: Given that there is strong evidence that β motions either largely or entirely govern the stability of proteins in sugar glasses, these motions should be addressed in formulation design. Although these secondary motions can be characterized by a number of techniques, they currently require highly specialized equipment not available in most pharmaceutical labs. For this reason, fast β-relaxations are often addressed empirically through the use of low molecular weight antiplasticizers. Using this approach, a protein is formulated with a range of antiplasticizer concentrations, and its stability is assessed through accelerated stability studies. This is typically an optimization effort – use of sufficient antiplasticizer to ensure physicochemical stability, yet not compromise physical stability of the dosage form.

While this chapter is focused on three specific themes, these practical recommendations would not be complete without mentioning the need to stabilize secondary, ternary, and, when applicable, tertiary structure of protein molecules. This subject is addressed in multiple publications - see, for example, Chang et al. (2005) [83].

References

1 Van Den Berg, L. (1966). pH changes in buffers and foods during freezing and subsequent storage. *Cryobiology* 3 (3): 236–242.

2 Gomez, G., Pikal, M.J., and Rodriguez-Hornedo, N. (2001). Effect of initial buffer composition on pH changes during far-from-equilibrium freezing of sodium phosphate buffer solutions. *Pharmaceutical Research* 18 (1): 90–97.

3 Pikal-Cleland, K.A., Cleland, J.L., Anchordoquy, T.J., and Carpenter, J.F. (2002). Effect of glycine on pH changes and protein stability during freeze-thawing in phosphate buffer systems. *Journal of Pharmaceutical Sciences* 91 (9): 1969–1979.

4 Sundaramurthi, P., Shalaev, E., and Suryanarayanan, R. (2010). "pH swing" in frozen solutions – consequence of sequential crystallization of buffer components. *Journal of Physical Chemistry Letters* 1 (1): 265–268.

5 Mathlouthi, M. and Reiser, P. (eds.) (1995). *Sucrose: Properties and Applications*. Springer Publishing.

6 Bates, R. (1973). *Determination of pH: Theory and Practice*. New York/London/Sydney/Toronto: Wiley.

7 Bell, L.N. and Labuza, T.P. (1992). Compositional influence on the pH of reduced-moisture solutions. *Journal of Food Science* 57 (3): 732–734.

8 Bates, R.G. and Schwarzenbach, G. (1955). Uber pH-werte nichtwasseriger losungen. *Helvetica Chimica Acta* 38: 699–716.

9 Paul, M.A. and Long, F.A. (1957). H_0 and related indicator acidity functions. *Chemical Reviews* 57 (1): 1–45.

10 Larsen, S.S. (1973). Stability of drugs in frozen systems. VI. Effect of freezing upon pH for buffered aqueous solutions. *Archiv for Pharmaci og Chemi, Scientific Edition*. 1: 41–53.

11 Orii, Y. and Morita, M. (1977). Measurement of the pH of frozen buffer solutions by using pH indicators. *Journal of Biochemistry* 81: 163–168.

12 Krauskova, L., Prochazkova, J., Klaskova, M. et al. (2016). Suppression of protein inactivation during freezing by minimizing pH changes using ionic cryoprotectants. *International Journal of Pharmaceutics* 509 (1–2): 41–49.

13 Li, J.J., Chatterjee, K., Medek, A. et al. (2004). Acid–base characteristics of bromophenol blue–citrate buffer systems in the amorphous state. *Journal of Pharmaceutical Sciences* 93 (3): 697–712.

14 Govindarajan, R., Chatterjee, K., Gatlin, L. et al. (2006). Impact of freeze-drying on ionization of sulfonephthalein probe molecules in trehalose–citrate systems. *Journal of Pharmaceutical Sciences* 95 (7): 1498–1510.

15 Lay, A., Yuan, X., Delaney, S., et al. (2017). Assessing solid state acidity of lyophilized formulations by monitoring butyric acid ionization. American Association of Pharmaceutical Scientists Annual Meeting, San Diego, CA (November 2017).

16 Glombitza, B.W. and Schmidt, P.C. (1995). Surface-acidity of solid pharmaceutical excipients. 2: Effect of the surface-acidity on the decomposition rate of acetylsalicylic-acid. *European Journal of Pharmaceutics and Biopharmaceutics* 41 (2): 114–119.

17 Alkhamis, K.A. (2008). Influence of solid-state acidity on the decomposition of sucrose in amorphous systems. I. *International Journal of Pharmaceutics* 362 (1–2): 74–80.

18 Hailu, S.A. and Bogner, R.H. (2010). Solid-state surface acidity and pH-stability profiles of amorphous quinapril hydrochloride and silicate formulations. *Journal of Pharmaceutical Sciences* 99 (6): 2786–2799.

19 Gana, F.Z., Rashid, I., Badwan, A., and Alkhamis, K.A. (2012). Determination of solid-state acidity of chitin–metal silicates and their effect on the degradation of cephalosporin antibiotics. *Journal of Pharmaceutical Sciences* 101 (7): 2398–2407.

20 Wu, C., Shamblin, S., Varshney, D., and Shalaev, E. (2015). Advance understanding of buffer behavior during lyophilization. In: *Lyophilized Biologics and Vaccines: Modality-Based Approaches* (eds. D. Varshney and M. Singh), 25–41. Springer.

21 Govindarajan, R., Landis, M., Hancock, B. et al. (2015). Surface acidity and solid-state compatibility of excipients with an acid-sensitive API: case study of atorvastatin calcium. *AAPS PharmSciTech* 16 (2): 354–363.

22 Chatterjee, K., Shalaev, E.Y., Suryanarayanan, R., and Govindarajan, R. (2008). Correlation between chemical reactivity and the Hammett acidity function in amorphous solids using inversion of sucrose as a model reaction. *Journal of Pharmaceutical Sciences* 97 (1): 274–286.

23 Lu, E.X., Ewing, S., Gatlin, L. et al. (2009). The effect of bulking agents on the chemical stability of acid-sensitive compounds in freeze-dried formulations: sucrose inversion study. *Journal of Pharmaceutical Sciences* 98 (9): 3387–3396.

24 Bee, J.S., Chiu, D., Sawicki, S. et al. (2009). Monoclonal antibody interactions with micro- and nanoparticles: adsorption, aggregation, and accelerated stress studies. *Journal of Pharmaceutical Sciences* 98 (9): 3218–3238.

25 Burke, C.J., Steadman, B.L., Volkin, D.B. et al. (1992). The adsorption of proteins to pharmaceutical container surfaces. *International Journal of Pharmaceutics* 86 (1): 89–93.

26 Rabe, M., Verdes, D., and Seeger, S. (2011). Understanding protein adsorption phenomena at solid surfaces. *Advances in Colloid and Interface Science* 162 (1–2): 87–106.

27 Fink, A.L. (1998). Protein aggregation: folding aggregates, inclusion bodies and amyloid. *Folding and Design* 3 (1): R9–R23.

28 Chi, E.Y., Krishnan, S., Randolph, T.W., and Carpenter, J.F. (2003). Physical stability of proteins in aqueous solution: mechanism and driving forces in nonnative protein aggregation. *Pharmaceutical Research* 20 (9): 1325–1336.

29 Liu, L., Qi, W., Schwartz, D.K. et al. (2013). The effects of excipients on protein aggregation during agitation: an interfacial shear rheology study. *Journal of Pharmaceutical Sciences* 102 (8): 2460–2470.

30 Schwegman, J.J., Carpenter, J.F., and Nail, S.L. (2009). Evidence of partial unfolding of proteins at the ice/freeze-concentrate interface by infrared microscopy. *Journal of Pharmaceutical Sciences* 98 (9): 3239–3246.

31 Cao, E.H., Chen, Y.H., Cui, Z.F., and Foster, P.R. (2003). Effect of freezing and thawing rates on denaturation of proteins in aqueous solutions. *Biotechnology and Bioengineering* 82 (6): 684–690.

32 Zakharov, B., Fisyuk, A., Fitch, A. et al. (2016). Ice recrystallization in a solution of a cryoprotector and its inhibition by a protein: synchrotron X-ray diffraction study. *Journal of Pharmaceutical Sciences* 105 (7): 2129–2138.

33 Petrenko, V.F. and Whitworth, R.W. (1999). *Physics of Ice*. Oxford University Press.

34 Kallay, N. and Cakara, D. (2000). Reversible charging of the ice–water interface: I. Measurement of the surface potential. *Journal of Colloid and Interface Science* 232 (1): 81–85.

35 Salnikova, M., Varshney, D., and Shalaev, E. (2015). *Heterogeneity of Protein Environments in Frozen Solutions and in the Dried State*. Springer.

36 Korber, C. (1988). Phenomena at the advancing ice liquid interface – solutes, particles and biological cells. *Quarterly Reviews of Biophysics* 21 (2): 229–298.

37 Chou, S.G., Soper, A.K., Khodadadi, S. et al. (2012). Pronounced micro-heterogeneity in a sorbitol–water mixture observed through variable temperature neutron scattering. *Journal of Physical Chemistry B* 116 (15): 4439–4447.

38 Xu, Y.M., Grobelny, P., Von Allmen, A. et al. (2014). Protein quantity on the air–solid interface determines degradation rates of human growth hormone in lyophilized samples. *Journal of Pharmaceutical Sciences* 103 (5): 1356–1366.

39 Devineni, D., Gonschorek, C., Cicerone, M.T. et al. (2014). Storage stability of keratinocyte growth factor-2 in lyophilized formulations: effects of formulation physical properties and protein fraction at the solid–air interface. *European Journal of Pharmaceutics and Biopharmaceutics* 88 (2): 332–341.

40 Webb, S.D., Cleland, J.L., Carpenter, J.F., and Randolph, T.W. (2003). Effects of annealing lyophilized and spray-lyophilized formulations of recombinant human interferon-γ. *Journal of Pharmaceutical Sciences* 92 (4): 715–729.

41 Zhou, C., Cleland, D., Snell, J. et al. (2016). Formation of stable nanobubbles on reconstituting lyophilized formulations containing trehalose. *Journal of Pharmaceutical Sciences* 105 (7): 2249–2253.

42 Snell, J.R., Zhou, C., Carpenter, J.F., and Randolph, T.W. (2016). Particle formation and aggregation of a therapeutic protein in nanobubble suspensions. *Journal of Pharmaceutical Sciences* 105 (10): 3057–3063.

43 Mumenthaler, M., Hsu, C.C., and Pearlman, R. (1994). Feasibility study on spray-drying protein pharmaceuticals: recombinant human growth hormone and tissue-type plasminogen activator. *Pharmaceutical Research* 11 (1): 12–20.

44 Kim, H.L., McAuley, A., Livesay, B. et al. (2014). Modulation of protein adsorption by poloxamer 188 in relation to Polysorbates 80 and 20 at solid surfaces. *Journal of Pharmaceutical Sciences* 103 (4): 1043–1049.

45 Deechongkit, S., Wen, J., Narhi, L.O. et al. (2009). Physical and biophysical effects of Polysorbate 20 and 80 on darbepoetin alfa. *Journal of Pharmaceutical Sciences* 98 (9): 3200–3217.

46 Teagarden, D.L., Anderson, B.D., and Petre, W.J. (1989). Dehydration kinetics of prostaglandin-E1 in a lipid emulsion. *Pharmaceutical Research* 6 (3): 210–215.

47 Tropin, T.V., Schmelzer, J.W.P., and Schick, C. (2011). On the dependence of the properties of glasses on cooling and heating rates I. Entropy, entropy production, and glass transition temperature. *Journal of Non-Crystalline Solids* 357 (4): 1291–1302.

48 Crowley, K.J. and Zografi, G. (2002). Cryogenic grinding of indomethacin polymorphs and solvates: assessment of amorphous phase formation and amorphous phase physical stability. *Journal of Pharmaceutical Sciences* 91 (2): 492–507.

49 Einfal, T., Planinsek, O., and Hrovat, K. (2013). Methods of amorphization and investigation of the amorphous state. *Acta Pharmaceutica* 63 (3): 305–334.

50 Zografi, G. and Newman, A. (2017). Interrelationships between structure and the properties of amorphous solids of pharmaceutical interest. *Journal of Pharmaceutical Sciences* 106 (1): 5–27.

51 Janssens, S. and Van den Mooter, G. (2009). Review: physical chemistry of solid dispersions. *Journal of Pharmacy and Pharmacology* 61 (12): 1571–1586.

52 Bras, A.R., Noronha, J.P., Antunes, A.M.M. et al. (2008). Molecular motions in amorphous ibuprofen as studied by broadband dielectric spectroscopy. *Journal of Physical Chemistry B* 112 (35): 11087–11099.

53 Bhattacharya, S. and Suryanarayanan, R. (2009). Local mobility in amorphous pharmaceuticals – characterization and implications on stability. *Journal of Pharmaceutical Sciences* 98 (9): 2935–2953.

54 Dranca, I., Bhattacharya, S., Vyazovkin, S., and Suryanarayanan, R. (2009). Implications of global and local mobility in amorphous sucrose and trehalose as determined by differential scanning calorimetry. *Pharmaceutical Research* 26 (5): 1064–1072.

55 Grzybowska, K., Capaccioli, S., and Paluch, M. (2016). Recent developments in the experimental investigations of relaxations in pharmaceuticals by dielectric techniques at ambient and elevated pressure. *Advanced Drug Delivery Reviews* 100: 158–182.

56 Johari, G.P. and Goldstein, M. (1970). Viscous liquids and the glass transition. *Journal of Chemical Physics* 53: 2372–2388.

57 Ngai, K.L. (2003). An extended coupling model description of the evolution of dynamics with time in supercooled liquids and ionic conductors. *Journal of Physics: Condensed Matter* 15 (11): S1107–S1125.

58 Angell, C.A. (1995). Formation of glasses from liquids and biopolymers. *Science* 267 (5206): 1924–1935.

59 Abiad, M.G., Carvajal, M.T., and Campanella, O.H. (2009). A review on methods and theories to describe the glass transition phenomenon: applications in food and pharmaceutical products. *Food Engineering Reviews* 1 (2): 105–132.

60 Kerc, J. and Srcic, S. (1995). Thermal analysis of glassy pharmaceuticals. *Thermochimica Acta* 248: 81–95.

61 Miller, D.P., Tan, T., Nakamura, J. et al. (2017). Physical characterization of tobramycin inhalation powder: II. State diagram of an amorphous engineered particle formulation. *Molecular Pharmaceutics* 14 (6): 1950–1960.

62 Mensink, M.A., Nethercott, M.J., Hinrichs, W.L. et al. (2016). Influence of miscibility of protein-sugar lyophilizates on their storage stability. *AAPS Journal* 18 (5): 1225–1232.

63 Roos, Y.H. (1995). *Phase Transitions in Foods*. San Diego, CA: Academic Press.

64 Greenhalgh, D.J., Williams, A.C., Timmins, P., and York, P. (1999). Solubility parameters as predictors of miscibility in solid dispersions. *Journal of Pharmaceutical Sciences* 88 (11): 1182–1190.

65 Van Eerdenbrugh, B., Lo, M., Kjoller, K. et al. (2012). Nanoscale mid-infrared evaluation of the miscibility behavior of blends of dextran or maltodextrin with poly(vinylpyrrolidone). *Molecular Pharmaceutics* 9 (5): 1459–1469.

66 Aso, Y., Yoshioka, S., and Kojima, S. (2000). Relationship between the crystallization rates of amorphous nifedipine, phenobarbital, and flopropione, and their molecular mobility as measured by their enthalpy relaxation and H-1 NMR relaxation times. *Journal of Pharmaceutical Sciences* 89 (3): 408–416.

67 Duddu, S.P. and DalMonte, P.R. (1997). Effect of glass transition temperature on the stability of lyophilized formulations containing a chimeric therapeutic monoclonal antibody. *Pharmaceutical Research* 14 (5): 591–595.

68 Hancock, B.C. and Zografi, G. (1997). Characteristics and significance of the amorphous state in pharmaceutical systems. *Journal of Pharmaceutical Sciences* 86 (1): 1–12.

69 Slade, L. and Levine, H. (1995). Glass transitions and water-food structure interactions. *Advances in Food and Nutrition Research* 38: 103–269.

70 Marsac, P.J., Konno, H., and Taylor, L.S. (2006). A comparison of the physical stability of amorphous felodipine and nifedipine systems. *Pharmaceutical Research* 23 (10): 2306–2316.

71 Duddu, S.P., Zhang, G.Z., and DalMonte, P.R. (1997). The relationship between protein aggregation and molecular mobility below the glass transition temperature of lyophilized formulations containing a monoclonal antibody. *Pharmaceutical Research* 14 (5): 596–600.

72 Angell, C.A., Ngai, K.L., McKenna, G.B. et al. (2000). Relaxation in glass-forming liquids and amorphous solids. *Journal of Applied Physics* 88 (6): 3113.

73 Hancock, B.C., Shamblin, S.L., and Zografi, G. (1995). Molecular mobility of amorphous pharmaceutical solids below their glass-transition temperatures. *Pharmaceutical Research* 12 (6): 799–806.

74 Kawakami, K. and Pikal, M.J. (2005). Calorimetric investigation of the structural relaxation of amorphous materials: evaluating validity of the methodologies. *Journal of Pharmaceutical Sciences* 94 (5): 948–965.

75 Haruyama, O., Yokoyama, Y., and Inoue, A. (2007). Precise measurement of density in the isothermal relaxation processes of $Pd_{42.5}Cu_{30}Ni_{7.5}P_{20}$ and $Zr_{50}Cu_{40}Al_{10}$ glasses. *Materials Transactions* 48 (7): 1708–1710.

76 Kohlrausch, F. (1863). Ueber die elastische Nachwirkung bei der Torsion. *Annalen der physik* 195 (7): 337–368.

77 Williams, G. and Watts, D.C. (1970). Non-symmetrical dielectric relaxation behaviour arising from a simple empirical decay function. *Transactions of the Faraday Society* 66 (565P): 80–85.

78 Yoshioka, S., Aso, Y., and Kojima, S. (2001). Usefulness of the Kohlrausch–Williams–Watts stretched exponential function to describe protein aggregation in lyophilized formulations and the temperature dependence near the glass transition temperature. *Pharmaceutical Research* 18 (3): 256–260.

79 Peyron, M., Pierens, G.K., Lucas, A.J. et al. (1996). The modified stretched-exponential model for characterization of NMR relaxation in porous media. *Journal of Magnetic Resonance Series A* 118 (2): 214–220.

80 Yoshioka, S., Aso, Y., and Kojima, S. (2004). Temperature- and glass transition temperature-dependence of bimolecular reaction rates in lyophilized formulations described by the Adam–Gibbs–Vogel equation. *Journal of Pharmaceutical Sciences* 93 (4): 1062–1069.

81 Roy, M.L., Pikal, M.J., Rickard, E.C., and Maloney, A.M. (1992). The effects of formulation and moisture on the stability of a freeze-dried monoclonal antibody-vinca conjugate: a test of the WLF glass transition theory. *Developments in Biological Standardization* 74: 323–340.

82 Guo, Y.S., Bryn, S.R., and Zografi, G. (2000). Physical characteristics and chemical degradation of amorphous quinapril hydrochloride. *Journal of Pharmaceutical Sciences* 89 (1): 128–143.

83 Chang, L.Q., Shepherd, D., Sun, J. et al. (2005). Mechanism of protein stabilization by sugars during freeze-drying and storage: native structure preservation, specific interaction, and/or immobilization in a glassy matrix? *Journal of Pharmaceutical Sciences* 94 (7): 1427–1444.

84 Shamblin, S.L., Hancock, B.C., and Pikal, M.J. (2006). Coupling between chemical reactivity and structural relaxation in pharmaceutical glasses. *Pharmaceutical Research* 23 (10): 2254–2268.

85 Yoshioka, S., Miyazaki, T., and Aso, Y. (2006). Degradation rate of lyophilized insulin, exhibiting an apparent Arrhenius behavior around glass transition temperature regardless of significant contribution of molecular mobility. *Journal of Pharmaceutical Sciences* 95 (12): 2684–2691.

86 Yoshioka, S. and Aso, Y. (2005). A quantitative assessment of the significance of molecular mobility as a determinant for the stability of lyophilized insulin formulations. *Pharmaceutical Research* 22 (8): 1358–1364.

87 Yoshioka, S., Miyazaki, T., and Aso, Y. (2006). Beta-relaxation of insulin molecule in lyophilized formulations containing trehalose or dextran as a determinant of chemical reactivity. *Pharmaceutical Research* 23 (5): 961–966.

88 Yoshioka, S., Aso, Y., and Miyazaki, T. (2006). Negligible contribution of molecular mobility to the degradation rate of insulin lyophilized with poly(vinylpyrrolidone). *Journal of Pharmaceutical Sciences* 95 (4): 939–943.

89 Sadrzadeh, N., Miller, D.P., Lechuga-Ballesteros, D. et al. (2010). Solid-state stability of spray-dried insulin powder for inhalation: chemical kinetics and structural relaxation modeling of Exubera above and below the glass transition temperature. *Journal of Pharmaceutical Sciences* 99 (9): 3698–3710.

90 Cicerone, M.T., Pikal, M.J., and Qian, K.K. (2015). Stabilization of proteins in solid form. *Advanced Drug Delivery Reviews* 93: 14–24.

91 Sun, Y., Xi, H., Ediger, M.D., and Yu, L. (2008). Diffusionless crystal growth from glass has precursor in equilibrium liquid. *Journal of Physical Chemistry B* 112 (3): 661–664.

92 Alie, J., Menegotto, J., Cardon, P. et al. (2004). Dielectric study of the molecular mobility and the isothermal crystallization kinetics of an amorphous pharmaceutical drug substance. *Journal of Pharmaceutical Sciences* 93 (1): 218–233.

93 Jepsen, P.U., Cooke, D.G., and Koch, M. (2011). Terahertz spectroscopy and imaging – modern techniques and applications. *Laser & Photonics Reviews* 5 (1): 124–166.

94 Parrott, E.P.J. and Zeitler, J.A. (2015). Terahertz time-domain and low-frequency Raman spectroscopy of organic materials. *Applied Spectroscopy* 69 (1): 1–25.

95 Sibik, J. and Zeitler, J.A. (2015). Terahertz response of organic amorphous systems: experimental concerns and perspectives. *Philosophical Magazine* 96 (7–9): 842–853.

96 Sibik, J., Lobmann, K., Rades, T., and Zeitler, J.A. (2015). Predicting crystallization of amorphous drugs with terahertz spectroscopy. *Molecular Pharmaceutics* 12 (8): 3062–3068.

97 Sibik, J. and Zeitler, J.A. (2016). Direct measurement of molecular mobility and crystallisation of amorphous pharmaceuticals using terahertz spectroscopy. *Advanced Drug Delivery Reviews* 100: 147–157.

98 Jean, Y.C. (1990). Positron annihilation spectroscopy for chemical analysis: a novel probe for microstructural analysis of polymers. *Microchemical Journal* 42 (1): 72–102.

99 Bigg, D.M. (1996). A review of positron annihilation lifetime spectroscopy as applied to the physical aging of polymers. *Polymer Engineering and Science* 36 (6): 737–743.

100 Cicerone, M.T. and Soles, C.L. (2004). Fast dynamics and stabilization of proteins: binary glasses of trehalose and glycerol. *Biophysical Journal* 86: 3836–3845.

101 Ubbink, J. (2016). Structural and thermodynamic aspects of plasticization and antiplasticization in glassy encapsulation and biostabilization matrices. *Advanced Drug Delivery Reviews* 100: 10–26.

102 Carpenter, J.F., Pikal, M.J., Chang, B.S., and Randolph, T.W. (1997). Rational design of stable lyophilized protein formulations: some practical advice. *Pharmaceutical Research* 14 (8): 969–975.

103 Chan, H.K., Clark, A.R., Feeley, J.C. et al. (2004). Physical stability of salmon calcitonin spray-dried powders for inhalation. *Journal of Pharmaceutical Sciences* 93 (3): 792–804.

104 Cleland, J.L., Lam, X., Kendrick, B. et al. (2001). A specific molar ratio of stabilizer to protein is required for storage stability of a lyophilized monoclonal antibody. *Journal of Pharmaceutical Sciences* 90 (3): 310–321.

105 Cicerone, M.T., Tellington, A., Trost, L., and Sokolov, A. (2003). Substantially improved stability of biological agents in dried form. *BioProcess International* 1: 36–47.

106 Matveev, Y.I., Grinberg, V.Y., Sochava, I.V., and Tolstoguzov, V.B. (1997). Glass transition temperature of proteins. Calculation based on the additive contribution method and experimental data. *Food Hydrocolloids* 11 (2): 125–133.

107 Cicerone, M.T. and Douglas, J.F. (2012). β-Relaxation governs protein stability in sugar-glass matrices. *Soft Matter* 8 (10): 2983.

108 White, S., Bennett, D.B., Cheu, S. et al. (2005). Exubera: pharmaceutical development of a novel product for pulmonary delivery of insulin. *Diabetes Technology & Therapeutics* 7 (6): 896–906.

109 Zhu, L., Brian, C.W., Swallen, S.F. et al. (2011). Surface self-diffusion of an organic glass. *Physical Review Letters* 106 (25): 256103.

110 Daley, C.R., Fakhraai, Z., Ediger, M.D., and Forrest, J.A. (2012). Comparing surface and bulk flow of a molecular glass former. *Soft Matter* 8 (7): 2206–2212.

111 Brian, C.W. and Yu, L. (2013). Surface self-diffusion of organic glasses. *Journal of Physical Chemistry A* 117 (50): 13303–13309.

112 Abdul-Fattah, A.M., Lechuga-Ballesteros, D., Kalonia, D.S., and Pikal, M.J. (2008). The impact of drying method and formulation on the physical properties and stability of methionyl human growth hormone in the amorphous solid state. *Journal of Pharmaceutical Sciences* 97 (1): 163–184.

113 Sun, Y., Zhu, L., Kearns, K.L. et al. (2011). Glasses crystallize rapidly at free surfaces by growing crystals upward. *Proceedings of the National Academy of Sciences* 108 (15): 5990–5995.

Part V

Implementation

14

Challenges and Considerations for New Technology Implementation and Synergy with Development of Process Analytical Technologies (PAT)

Howard Stamato[1] and Jim Searles[2]

[1] *Bridgewater,, NJ 08807, USA*
[2] *Pfizer Global Supply, McPherson, KS 67460, USA*

Introducing a new technology to an organization entails two sets of activities. When adopting any change there is an expenditure of energy necessary to inform, engage, and train participants in the new paradigm. Layered on this is the justification, investment, and mastery of the new technology proposed. Either of these is a significant challenge on its own. Managing organizational expectations is key to maintaining the consistent momentum necessary to harvest the value of new technology.

There are many works discussing the culture change aspects of something new, so this discussion will focus on aspects of developing the technology and managing organizational expectations to provide consistent support and reaching clear decisions based on the authors' experience. Different explanations of the stages of understanding or approaches to successfully achieving a culture change depend on the style and data of those describing the observations and methods. It is certain that there are multiple approaches to change management and many types of organizational cultures, as well as many challenges that may have different drivers in an organization's life. These factors suggest that tailoring an approach to the organization and the particular situation to be addressed will yield the desired outcome [1–3].

A typical response to new technology from the prospective champion is often overly optimistic regarding the timelines of implementation and capability. This is often followed by undue pessimism from those effected by the culture change at the first challenge in its implementation. If the program survives, there can be many cycles, eventually leading to the true valuation at maturity. Along the way each downturn is an opportunity for the resistance stage of culture change to stop the program. While the pace of technology adoption is increasing, many factors can affect the time it takes to adoption that is measured in years [4].

There are situations where a senior manager with adequate resources can identify enough benefit to the business to drive technology in a rapid, yet painful, top-down approach. A robust evaluation process and defined budget for innovation may also speed adoption as there is a common language for expectation setting and more collegiality and stakeholder engagement in this approach. If

Drying Technologies for Biotechnology and Pharmaceutical Applications, First Edition.
Edited by Satoshi Ohtake, Ken-ichi Izutsu, and David Lechuga-Ballesteros.

there is a scenario where there is high development cost and low maturity, a risk impeded situation, then spreading the cost and risk in a consortium or collaboration approach can lower barriers to adoption. A collaborative development must leverage the talent, resources, and speed characteristics of each contributing organization. For example, a large pharmaceutical company may have the funding but needs a start-up company to execute at the speed necessary to realize the value. Both may have to combine forces or join in a consortium approach in order to demonstrate understanding and robustness of the innovation to regulators. Common language, extensive communication, common standards, and shared commitment to a common benefit, either within or external to an organization, help to reduce the cost of change management and speed adoption.

The appetite for new technology has intrinsic value. Managing the process of exploring new technology to harvest value at each stage of development assures the good use of investments and mitigates the negative effects from the cycle of enthusiasm. Valuation should include the typical return on investment (ROI) calculation. This is only one dimension in which the exploration of technology has a positive effect and other measures help in choosing the appropriate actions.

While exposure to a new idea is exhilarating, putting that idea into the context of other methods of achieving the result supports a rational choice of which ideas to pursue and at what resource levels. While an ROI is often applied to determine the value of a technology and is a key factor in deciding to implement, many stages of the process yield value in ways that are difficult to measure but may be more than the differential efficiency calculated by ROI. Accounting for softer measures of value is more complex but has been done in the evaluation of technological improvements [5–7]. Regardless of the implementation of the initial idea, exploring new technology is a great way of evaluating and potentially improving existing technology, developing a lifecycle view of strategy, and gaining knowledge to feed the next cycle of innovation.

It is an easy decision to push innovation into the future. There is always a reason to lower organizational stress by avoiding change management, delay expenses in favor of today's profit, or simply wait for a broader, more mature implementation of technology before deciding to adopt it. Falling behind in technology adoption could be more costly than keeping a stable, manageable investment until adoption. The use of technology requires both expertise and an adjustment in culture. Racing to adopt something, even if expertise is hired from the outside, will be difficult to integrate into the existing technical community culture, practices, and documentation. The consequences could be dire for an organization that is seen as out of compliance due to a lack of understanding of current practices or is eclipsed by competitors who have steadily accumulated incremental advantage due to their investment in technology.

Mastery of a new technology can be divided into interim milestones to reap value prior to full implementation. Discovery of a new key parameter, providing a second method to verify results, and reducing the time to prototype are all potential benefits of testing new technology, whether or not it is eventually selected to produce the product at commercial scale. Each stage of a new technology program structured in this way has modest goals and investment seeking to overcome the next manageable challenge in the direction of implementation.

Value from the learnings at each stage may be applied immediately, helping to overcome smaller challenges while the overall system is designed. With segmented goals, the level of resource justification and energy to adopt change become easier to manage and more focused on the task at hand.

Basic research is often funded without connection to ROI and has the luxury of time to develop technology. Mature technology has demonstrated important value drivers and ROI so that it is readily applied to commercial production. It is between inception and maturity when technology has a barrier to entry where the time available and funding for it are lean. This stage is often encountered when the technology must be applied to a development project with fast-moving timelines and limited materials to work with [8].

While pharmaceuticals are often viewed as a conservative industry, the rapid advance of the effectiveness and types of therapies offered suggest that innovation is at the core of the industry. Further encouragement can be derived from ongoing calls for modernization and innovation from health authorities and active discussion at industry forums. For example, the Food and Drug Administration (FDA) [9] and European Medicines Agency (EMA) [10] have programs devoted to new approaches and technology. Industry forums such as the International Consortium for Innovation and Quality in Pharmaceutical Development (IQ) [11], Advanced Mammalian Bioprocessing Innovation Center (AMBIC) [12], and National Institute for Innovation in Manufacturing Biopharmaceuticals (NIIMBL) [13] are organizations in which the industry, academe, and government support development of new technology.

New drying technology goes beyond the need for efficiency and provides the opportunity to tune product characteristics suitable for new uses or create product structures that could revolutionize the handling and delivery to patients [14]. Each advance in drying technology opens a new design space for which our standard concepts and expectations no longer apply. Given the complexity of drying when all factors are considered, and a new design space to explore, extensive measurement of materials and sensing of the process is essential. With a growing number of process analytical techniques (PAT) achieving a routine practical application, reasonable cost, and acceptance as reliable, the inclusion of PAT is expected to lead to the success of these endeavors. "When a technology is immediately enabling, and allows for new medicines, that would otherwise fail in development, to reach the market, the business case for the extra initial investment to enable success is clear" [15].

PAT will be needed to efficiently achieve product and process understanding and control. It is easier to include PAT with a new process than retrofit for an existing one as there is no culture to change to manage, equipment to modify, or additional regulatory filing to make if the PAT is part of the original design. Therefore, a new process has the easiest path to include PAT and, because large amounts of data improve understanding the new process design space, derives the largest value from implementation.

PAT does not have to be exotic technology to serve the purpose. The value is in obtaining data that is necessary for product or process characterization. This may be accomplished by a very simple sensor put in the right place. Temperature, pressure, and humidity are all valuable measurements in drying and are more valuable as the number of locations these measurements are taken increases. Whether offline, at-line, or in-line, technology that can be used to understand and control a process has value. Because the batch could and would fail without this control, the technology can be viewed as having a value comparable with a significant portion of the material being processed cumulative over the life of the instrument. A full valuation of process analytical technology considers the savings in testing, reduction in excursions, investigations, etc. [16].

When developing an understanding of the materials and process space, it is advantageous to make many measurements early in development. Extensive testing with PAT and traditional methods can generate the data necessary for product and process understanding. With that understanding and a control strategy, the number of data streams can be reduced to those needed to control the process as it is commercialized. PAT is not something that should be "bolted on" once the process equipment and parameters are defined, but earlier is better so that entire benefits can be realized. Many PAT techniques are designed to measure scale-independent attributes of the material. These types of measurements are invaluable in assuring product quality. Many process parameters have contributions from multiple factors, which may scale at different rates and cause product attributes to vary at the new scale in an unexpected manner. Having a scale-independent PAT measure enables the study of parameter space with attribute-based product qualities as the metric to assure the product performs as intended.

Managing stakeholder expectations is key to both the new technology and measurements being developed. Correlation with current standards and studies showing the specificity, accuracy, and precision of methods will be needed. Understanding the design space via development experiments, perhaps assisted by modeling and simulation, and both method and process validation will need to occur before commercialization of product from the new technology is accepted. Early communication with stakeholders at both the operating and decision-making levels helps to align quality, production, business unit, and health authority stakeholders with the value of the new technology being developed. This alignment is key to developing momentum that will "pull" the technology forward into implementation and smooth the path to approval as questions have been answered as the technology progressed.

The road to implementation for most new technology can be measured in years if not decades. Taking the time to survey the technology landscape and making clear choices about which candidates will be given resources helps to assure that the value of one of the candidates will eventually be implemented. Segmented goals where the amount of resources committed, milestone to be met, and change adopted are manageable help to sustain the momentum of technology development. Interim milestones that celebrate the value derived from the progress made, rather than waiting until final implementation, assure that resources are well spent.

An example of an alternate route to introducing new technology is the post-market adoption of new processes, sensors, or information management. This approach ensures that new chemical entities in development are not burdened with additional risk related to manufacturing technology. In this case the product goes quickly to launch with the most basic knowledge necessary. In parallel or immediately afterward, efficiency and robustness are considered, so that on a timeline where more time-consuming application of technology and in-depth analysis can be tolerated, a second version of the manufacture can be filed. Several iterations of chemical synthesis are often crafted before and after the regulatory filing. The same approach can realize the value of new technology and make funding decisions easier as there is a revenue stream to tap into and to compare the value of the change with.

Whether for the initial launch, or a supplemental process, early communication to assure questions are answered and stakeholders are prepared, or even excited to receive the technology, smooths the path to adoption. Stakeholder engagement is enhanced by incorporating measurements and sensors early in the process development cycle, which coupled with process and product understanding form the basis for PAT. The knowledge generated help to explain the design, performance, and validation of the methods, process, and assurance of the product performance. Following these principles in the new drying technologies discussed in this book is expected to lead to more efficient, rapid, and smooth adoption of these exciting technologies.

References

1 Nguyen, H., Groth, M., Ng, J.L. et al. (2016). Time to change: a review of organizational culture change in health care organisations. *Journal of Organizational Effectiveness: People and Performance* 3 (3): 265–288.

2 Scott, T., Mannion, R., Davies, H.T.O., and Marshall, M.N. (2003). Implementing culture change in health care: theory and practice. *International Journal for Quality in Health Care* 15 (2): 111–118.

3 Mallinger, M., Goodwin, D., and O'Hara, T. (2009). Recognizing organizational culture in managing change. *Graziadio Business Review* 12 (1): 1–10. https://gbr.pepperdine.edu/2010/08/recognizing-organizational-culture-in-managing-change/.

4 Comin, D. and Mestieri, M. (2014). Technology diffusion: measurement, causes and consequences. In: *Handbook of Economic Growth* (Chapter 2), 1e, vol. 2 (eds. P. Aghion and S. Durlauf). North Holland: Elsevier.

5 Schuh, G., Schubert, J., and Wellensiek, M. (2012). Model for the valuation of a technology established in a manufacturing system. *Procedia CIRP* 3: 602–607.

6 Bloch, M. and Hoyos-Gomez, A. (2009). How CIO's should think about business value. Mckinsey and Company. www.mckinsey.com/business-functions/digital-mckinsey/our-insights/how-cios-should-think-about-business-value (accessed 18 July 2018).

7 Ramasesh, R. and Jayakumar, M.D. (1991). Measurement of manufacturing flexibility: a value based approach. *Journal of Operations Management* 10 (4): 446–468.

8 Dacey, J. (2014) Navigating the Valley of Death, Physics World, http://live.iop-pp01.agh.sleek.net/2014/10/27/navigating-the-valley-of-death/ (accessed 07 October 2019.

9 Emerging Technology Program, www.fda.gov/aboutfda/cetersoffices/officeofmedicalproductsandtobacco/cder/ucm523228.htm (accessed 07 October 2019).

10 European Medicines Agency. Innovation in medicines. https://www.ema.europa.eu/en/human-regulatory/research-development/innovation-medicines (accessed 07 October 2019).

11 International Consortium for Innovations and Quality for Pharmaceutical Development, Iqconsortium.org (accessed 18 July 2018).

12 Advanced Mammalian Biomanufacturing Innovation Center, www.ambic.org (accessed 18 July 2018).

13 National Institute for Innovation in Manufacturing Biopharmaceuticals, www.niimbl.org (accessed 18 July 2018).

14 Angulo, D.E.L. and do Amaral Sobral, P.J. (2016). The effect of processing parameters and solid concentration on the microstructure and pore architecture of gelatin-chitosan scaffolds produced by freeze-drying. *Materials Research* 19 (4): 839–845.

15 O'Connor, T.F., Yu, L.X., and Lee, S.L. (2016). Emerging technology: a key enabler for modernizing pharmaceutical manufacturing and advancing product quality. *International Journal of Pharmaceutics* 509 (1–2): 492–298.

16 Valporsson, H. (2006). PAT implementation in pharmaceutical manufacturing and its economical impact. Inauguraldissertation. University of Basel. edoc.unibas.ch/722/1/DissB_8178.pdf (accessed 18 July 2018).

Part VI

Future Perspectives

15

Future Directions: Lyophilization Technology Roadmap to 2025 and Beyond

Alina Alexeenko[1,2] *and Elizabeth Topp*[3,4]

[1] *Purdue University, Davidson School of Chemical Engineering, 480 W. Stadium Ave, West Lafayette, IN 47907, USA*
[2] *Birck Nanotechnology Center, 1205 W State St, West Lafayette, IN 47907, USA*
[3] *Purdue University, Department of Industrial and Physical Pharmacy, West Lafayette, IN 47907, USA*
[4] *National Institute for Bioprocessing Research and Training, Dublin A94 X099, Ireland*

15.1 Introduction

Lyophilization/freeze drying removes water by sublimation at low temperature in vacuum and is used in the biotech and pharmaceutical industries to preserve sensitive materials such as protein drugs, diagnostic reagents, live virus vaccines, and bacterial cultures.

The worldwide market for lyophilized foods and pharmaceuticals is approximately US$16 billion per year, a value equaled by the market for lyophilization equipment and services. Many food and pharmaceutical products could not be commercially viable without lyophilization. However, lyophilization is among the most time-consuming and expensive unit operations, with an energy efficiency of less than 5%, batch mode operation, open-loop processing, and lack of in-line quality monitoring.

To address these issues and to develop improved drying technologies for current and future products, an industry-led consortium – LyoHUB – was formed in 2014 with the support from NIST Advanced Manufacturing Technology Consortia program. LyoHUB's member companies span the value chain for lyophilization and include manufacturers of lyophilization equipment, instrument manufacturers, software providers, and end users in the food and pharmaceutical industries. The long-term goals of LyoHUB are to advance lyophilization technology through workforce training and industry-led pre-competitive research and development. LyoHUB's current activities include formulating and disseminating "best practices" papers on various aspects of lyophilization technology, hosting meetings and training workshops on topics of interest to the members, providing online access to information and simulation tools through an interactive website, and maintaining a pilot-scale technology demonstration facility where the latest lyophilization instrumentation technologies are presented and innovative new approaches are tested and developed.

A critical activity in the early years of LyoHUB has been the development of a technology roadmap for lyophilization. Generally speaking, a technology

Drying Technologies for Biotechnology and Pharmaceutical Applications, First Edition.
Edited by Satoshi Ohtake, Ken-ichi Izutsu, and David Lechuga-Ballesteros.

roadmap is a planning tool that connects the societal trends and pressures facing a product or industry with the technologies needed to address them. Technology roadmapping can identify gaps in broad areas such as fundamental science, technology, communication, logistics, and regulatory interactions, pointing a group toward their most impactful efforts over a particular time horizon. For LyoHUB, technology roadmapping has involved conducting a comprehensive survey of the current uses of lyophilization, projecting future needs and new product types, identifying critical gaps in current lyophilization practices and barriers to implementation of new technologies, and defining goals for the development of new lyophilization methods. The LyoHUB roadmap addresses a 10+ year timeframe, embracing both current and projected needs.

This chapter presents a summary of the lyophilization technology roadmap. We first describe the process used to construct the roadmap and present the resulting roadmap in overview form. Subsequent sections then describe the five major areas of the roadmap in greater detail, identifying the advances that are needed in (15.4) lyophilized products, (15.5) lyophilization processes, (15.6) lyophilization equipment, (15.7) the regulatory interface, and (15.8) workforce training and education. While the roadmap is focused on lyophilization and related technologies, we hope that the needs identified will be broadly applicable to other drying technologies as well. For example, many of the needs for product-related technologies in lyophilization (Figure 15.1) also apply to other drying methods, the need for disruptive lyophilization methods (Figure 15.2) may inspire the development of new drying processes that are not lyophilization based, and the overarching needs for education and workforce training (Figure 15.3) probably reflect broader needs of the industry.

15.2 Overview of the Roadmapping Process

The process to develop the initial LyoHUB technology roadmap began with a structured workshop, and the roadmap proceeded to refine and focus industry feedback through a series of meetings, workshops, and discussions. The efforts progressed through three broadly defined stages as summarized below in Section 15.2.1 as (i) development of roadmap taxonomy; (ii) workshop to gather input over a broad range of topics in the taxonomy; (iii) concluding series of webinars and surveys to finalize the content and timelines of the roadmap.

15.2.1 Roadmap Framework and Development

The original roadmap format included long-term, broad strategic objectives (key area topics) that would be achieved via medium-term research actions. In turn, the medium-term research actions would consist of short-term focused projects. These efforts would be guided by an impact matrix intended to capture roadmap stakeholder expectations.

A core team, consisting of industry and academic members, was formed to develop the roadmap taxonomy. To help guide the early efforts, the team engaged the Institute for Manufacturing (IfM) at the University of Cambridge for assistance in developing the roadmap structure and to facilitate the first workshop. The workshop followed IfM's S-Plan process, a well-established process to collect

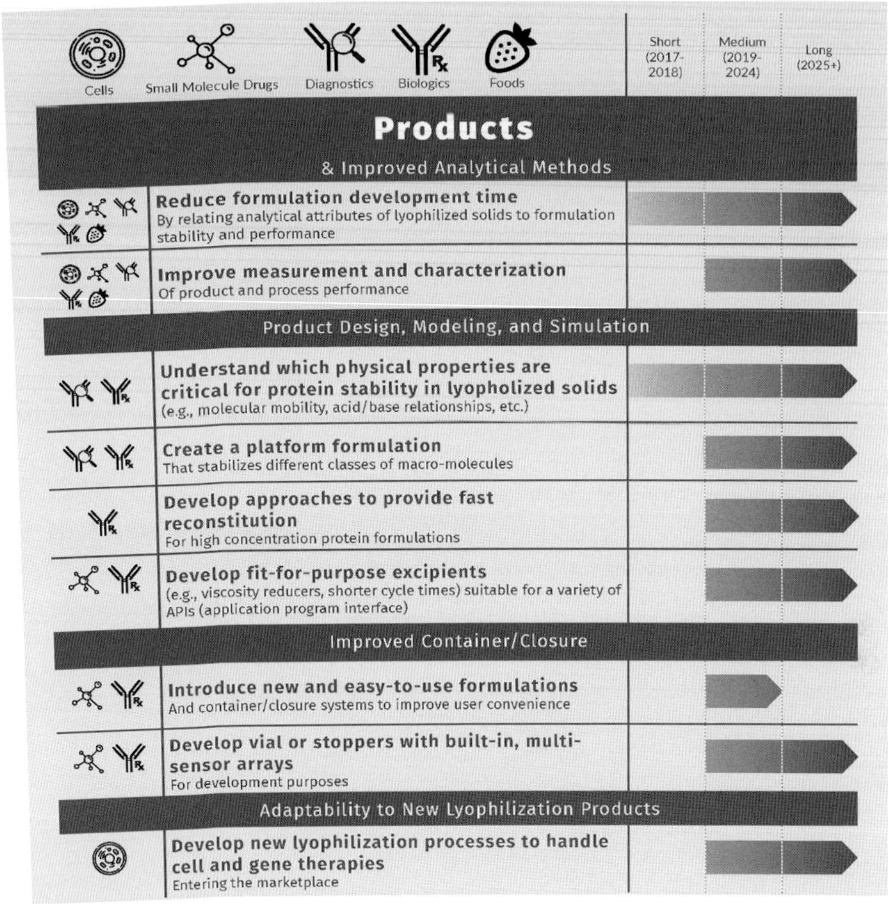

Figure 15.1 Product-related technology roadmap.

information covering a broad scope of topics that were defined through a series of core team meetings prior to the workshop. Topics were grouped in three interconnected layers: (i) trends and drivers, (ii) product families, and (iii) technologies and other capabilities. Participants were invited to provide their input on the predefined layer topics, which were then aggregated into topical groups. Approximately 350 issues formed the basis for 20 trend and driver groups, 15 product family groups, and 15 technologies and other capabilities groups. Multi-voting was used to prioritize the groups, and in turn, the prioritized groups were subsequently revised and refined in stage 2 and 3 activities.

Input from LyoHUB members and other subject matter experts was solicited through subsequent meetings, conference participation, and calls. That input ultimately led to a roadmap framework with two overarching focus areas with associated categories and subcategories. The focus areas and categories are (i) advancing lyophilization technologies and techniques and (ii) strengthening the industry foundation. A concluding series of webinars with accompanying surveys was held to finalize the content and timelines for the initial roadmap. The webinars focused on a single category with in-depth discussions on each topic and its corresponding timeline.

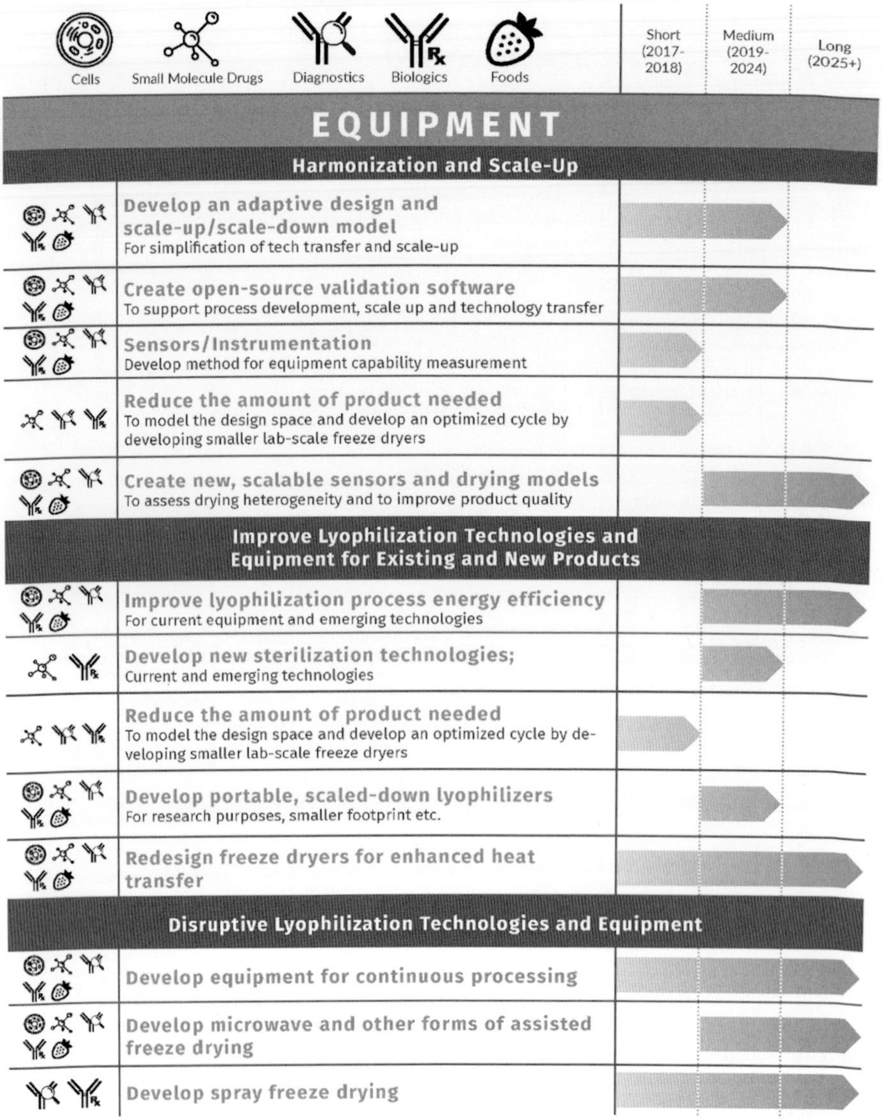

Figure 15.2 Equipment-related technology roadmap.

15.2.2 Roadmap Summary

The technology roadmap for advancing lyophilization is summarized in the roadmap summary table (Figure 15.4). The overall goal of innovation in lyophilization is high quality, lower cost, and more readily available lyophilized products. The roadmap identifies two broad areas of effort needed to move toward this goal: (i) advancing lyophilization technologies and techniques and (ii) strengthening the industry foundation. Technical innovations will be required in areas related to lyophilized products, the lyophilization process, and

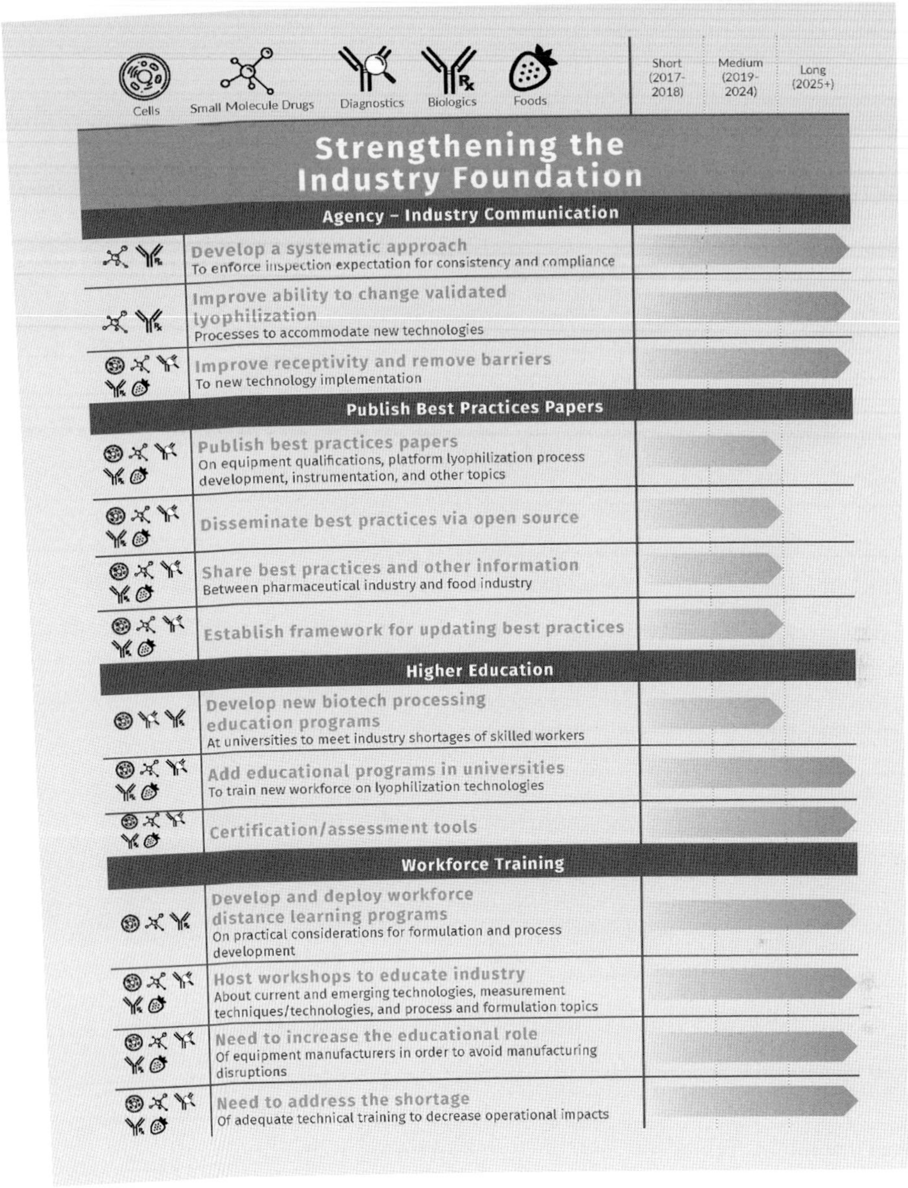

Figure 15.3 Industry foundation roadmap.

lyophilization equipment. The full implementation of these technical innovations will depend on a strong industry foundation. This in turn will require that the interface between the industry and regulatory agencies be strengthened and that a well-trained workforce be developed and maintained.

The remainder of this chapter provides additional details in each of the five key areas of the roadmap: lyophilized products, the lyophilization process, lyophilization equipment, the regulatory interface, and workforce development

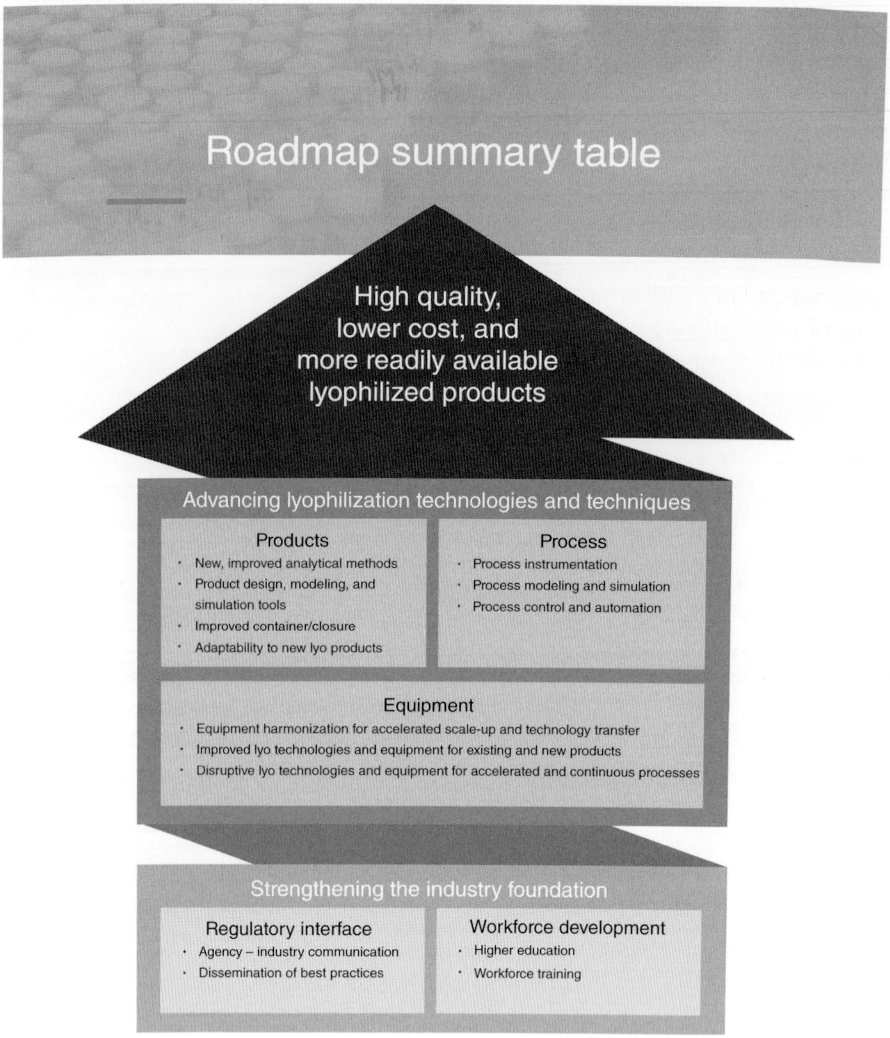

Figure 15.4 Lyophilization roadmap summary table.

(overview table). Tables for each area expand on the bulleted items listed in the overview table, giving specific objectives as well as the anticipated timeframe for their completion (short, medium, and/or long term).

Lyophilization can be applied to a number of different types of products, and not all of the innovations are expected to be useful for all product types. Accordingly, icons in the area tables identify the lyophilized products most likely to be affected by achieving each objective. The product types are cells (including cell-based therapies), small molecule drugs, diagnostics, biologics (including peptides, recombinant proteins, and vaccines), and foods. Each of the roadmap tables also indicates the lyophilized product development lifetime stage that the specific technology topic is relevant to. Drug product development stages are

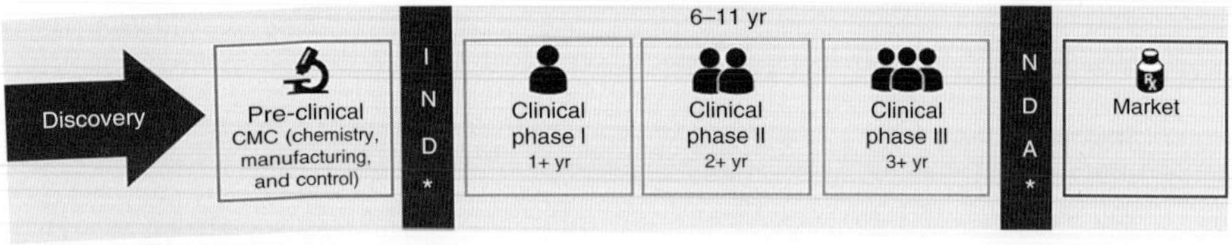

Figure 15.5 Pharmaceutical product lifetime stages. IND, Investigational New Drug application; NDA, New Drug Application.

summarized in Figure 15.5. The preclinical stage spans from the initial investigation of promising agents to *in vivo* animal testing and results in Investigational New Drug Application that requires (i) animal pharmacology and toxicology studies; (ii) manufacturing information related to composition, stability, and controls of drug substance and the drug product; (iii) clinical protocols and investigator information for proposed clinical studies with a rationale for testing a new compound in humans, strategies for protection of human volunteers, and a clinical testing plan. Phase 1 clinical studies focus on the safety and pharmacology and involve the compound being administered initially at very low doses to a few dozen healthy volunteers. Phase 2 studies consider efficacy and typically involve a few hundred patients suffering from the condition the new drug is designed to treat. Effective dosage, delivery method, and additional product safety issues are further addressed in this stage. Phase 3 studies are designed to test previous findings on larger populations often involving thousands of patients and multiple sites. After successful completion of phase 3 studies, a New Drug Application can be filed. Upon approval of the New Drug Application (NDA), the marketing and production of the new pharmaceutical product commences. Some of the technological topics are relevant to all five stages as reflected in the roadmap tables.

15.3 Trends and Drivers

The lyophilized pharmaceutical sector is encountering and will need to continue to adapt to an increasing number of patient-driven trends and drivers. These factors include single-use technologies, self-administered medical devices, and an increased globalization of manufacturing facilities to decrease the time and distance to end consumers. In turn, more indirect trends and drivers (viewed from a patient perspective) include reducing manufacturing process time, simplifying changes to processes, and increasing process efficiency. The industry's ability to respond to these trends and drivers is constrained by a number of factors, not least of which is the paramount importance of ensuring patient safety and maintaining uniformly high product quality. Since lyophilized products are usually intended for parenteral use, the need to maintain aseptic conditions adds to the level of scrutiny of innovative technologies. All of these trends and drivers, when addressed with full consideration of the constraints, will enable manufacturers to provide patients with cost-effective, efficacious treatments.

A major driver for innovation in lyophilization technologies is the growth in the number of newly approved pharmaceutical products that are manufactured

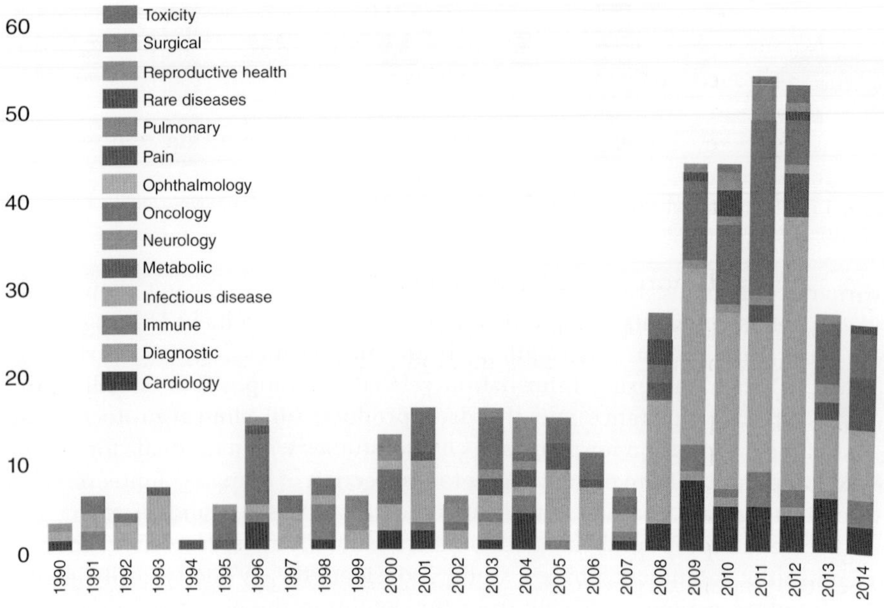

Figure 15.6 Lyophilized drug approvals by FDA from 1990 to 2014. Source: IMA Life.

in a lyophilized dosage form. Figure 15.6 shows the data from 1990 to 2014 for new Food and Drug Administration (FDA) approvals of lyophilized drugs by year and indication. The fast increase since 2008 has been spurred by many new products for infectious diseases and oncology. Of the 472 lyophilized drug products approved since 1990, 107 and 100 are in infectious disease and oncology categories, respectively. Additionally, from 1990 to 1998 the share of newly approved lyophilized drugs as a share of all injectable/infusible drugs was 11.9%. In 2011, it was 41%, and in 2013–2015 injectable/infusible drugs requiring reconstitution made up half of all new approvals [1].

15.4 Lyophilized Products

Foods and pharmaceuticals together account for more than 95% of the global market for lyophilized end products, strong justification for a focus on these industries. While the largest end-product market is lyophilized foods, the greatest compound annual growth rate (CAGR) (11–13%) among all lyophilized products is for lyophilized biologics, the sector of the pharmaceutical industry that includes recombinant protein drugs, vaccines, and blood products.

The strong growth for lyophilized forms of these products is attributable to the overall rapid growth of this drug class and to the fact that lyophilized forms are frequently needed to ensure adequate shelf stability. It is estimated that, without the use of lyophilization, 60% of current pharmaceutical biologics could not be commercially viable.

Through technology roadmapping, LyoHUB participants have identified several broad areas of need for lyophilized products, including the need for new and improved analytical methods to characterize lyophilized solids, the need for modeling and simulation tools to support the design of lyophilized products, the need for improved container/closure systems, and the need to adapt lyophilization to entirely new types of end products. Each of these areas is discussed in greater detail below.

15.4.1 New and Improved Analytical Methods

Currently, lyophilized pharmaceuticals are characterized using a number of chemical, physical, and biophysical methods. The attributes measured include moisture content (e.g. by Karl Fisher titration), glass transition temperature (T_g, e.g. by differential scanning calorimetry), chemical integrity of the drug molecule (e.g. by high-performance liquid chromatography and/or mass spectrometry), and, for proteins and other biologics, the secondary and higher order structure of the drug molecule in the solid powder (e.g. by Fourier transform infrared [IR] spectroscopy). Often, these properties are weakly correlated to the storage stability of the lyophilized product, if at all, so that the development and selection of an optimally stable formulation is largely a matter of trial and error. Additionally, lyophilized drug products are typically administered to patients after reconstitution, i.e. not directly as a dried solid. Hence, it is also important to assess the stability of the lyophilized drug product post-reconstitution, which is potentially affected by the reconstitution procedure and associated time. Roadmapping participants thus identified a need to reduce formulation development time by relating the analytical attributes of lyophilized solids to formulation stability and performance. Similarly, participants felt there was a need for improved solid-state analytical methods that would offer improved characterization of frozen and freeze-dried solids that better predicted storage stability and other performance attributes (e.g. reconstitution time). Since excipients are critical to the properties of lyophilized solids, participants suggested that the design, development, and clinical evaluation of new excipients could help to expand formulation options and improve product performance.

15.4.2 Improved Container/Closure Systems

Roadmapping participants also identified a need for new and improved container/closure systems. Currently, most lyophilized pharmaceuticals undergo lyophilization in individual glass vials with rubber stoppers, which also serve as the container/closure system for the final product, although some are supplied in dual-chamber syringes.

Participants identified the need for new and easy-to-use container/closure systems, perhaps involving needle-free systems. The possible advantages of replacing glass containers with plastics were also discussed, together with the need to better characterize chemical and physical interactions between the formulation and the container. Participants also identified a need for lyophilization vials or stoppers with built-in multisensor arrays, which would allow the conditions experienced by an individual vial (e.g. temperature, pressure) to be monitored during lyophilization, shipping, and storage. Vials with built-in sensors would enable out-of-range conditions to be identified for single vials. As a result, lyophilization cycles could be better controlled, valuable information could be provided to inform lyophilizer design, and, in production, out-of-range vials could be discarded without compromising all of the vials in the lot.

15.4.3 Adapt Lyophilization to New Product Types

As noted above, foods and pharmaceuticals account for more than 95% of current lyophilized end products. During technology roadmapping, participants identified a need for new lyophilization processes that can handle the entirely different types of products now entering the marketplace. These products include gene therapies, cell-based therapies, and diagnostics, all of which may require dried forms produced without heating to ensure shelf stability. Participants noted that there is little to no information on lyophilizing these materials in the open literature.

15.5 Process

Current lyophilization practice uses open-loop controls with predetermined settings for process input parameters, such as heat transfer fluid temperature and chamber pressure, with some monitoring of process output parameters. Product attributes such as product temperature, drying rate, and residual moisture content are rarely monitored directly in the manufacturing setting. Process deviations from the approved settings require evaluation, investigation, and response according to regulatory agency requirements. Process automation, on the other hand, uses a network of process sensors and actuators that are analyzed and controlled by computerized process software. Similar to its effect in the chemical industry, process automation is likely to bring about a significant increase in productivity and efficiency of lyophilization processes. For example, monitoring both heat flow to the product and product temperature while varying heat transfer fluid input has been shown to accelerate primary drying by 50%. (1LyoPAT™: Real-Time Monitoring and Control of the Freezing and Primary Drying Stages During Freeze-drying for Improved Product Quality and Reduced Cycle Times) [2].

The transition from the current open-loop processes to more efficient automated closed-loop control in lyophilization will require better scientific understanding of the process as well as technology development.

The LyoHUB roadmapping participants identified three major areas for future technology development related to lyophilization process: (i) process monitoring instrumentation, (ii) process modeling and simulation, and (iii) process control and automation (Figure 15.7).

15.5.1 Process Monitoring Instrumentation

Process monitoring instrumentation during lyophilization in a good manufacturing practices (GMPs) production setting is very limited due to the harsh vacuum environment and strict sterility requirements. The roadmap participants identified several areas of technology development that would have high impact for process improvement. The current practice in process development mainly involves wired temperature probes for product temperature monitoring. Whereas such wired probes are widely used in process development at laboratory and pilot scale, they are typically not compatible with the automatic loading systems used in the production environment. Wireless, noninvasive product temperature sensors that could be used in a GMP setting are a high priority for future technology development. Real-time spectroscopic measurements of product residual moisture content and vapor flow rates are desirable technologies that would enable direct monitoring of product attributes and process uniformity.

15.5.2 Process Modeling and Simulation

Mathematical modeling of heat and mass transfer processes in freeze drying is widely recognized as an important tool for developing robust lyophilization processes. Reliable models of quasi-steady-state primary drying stage are currently widely used by the industry. The roadmapping participants recognized the need for advancing the mathematical modeling tools for freezing and secondary drying stages. Additionally, there is a need to develop models and simulations that quantify the impact of process variations, such as chamber pressure, variation in product loads, and equipment modifications on product quality attributes, using physics-based and statistical approaches. Development and broader adoption of computational fluid dynamics and coupled fluid–thermal–structural simulations for analysis and design of lyophilization processes is needed for accelerated lyophilization process development and closed-loop control.

15.5.3 Process Control and Automation

The consensus of roadmapping participants was that there are two major areas of future technology development for process control: (i) control of the freezing process at all scales from laboratory to production and (ii) closed-loop control of the primary drying stage. Controlled ice nucleation in the freezing stage is needed for consistent ice crystal structure and, as a consequence, uniform mass transfer resistance and drying rates across the product batch. The primary drying stage is typically the longest and most energy-intensive stage of freeze drying. Currently, only the end of primary drying is monitored in production by monitoring residual moisture content in the chamber through comparative pressure measurement. The closed-loop control of primary drying can bring about significant process acceleration and efficiency improvement and will require development of process analytical technologies for the monitoring and controlling of heat flow and product temperature in real time.

15.6 Equipment

Because of the high capital costs for production-scale pharmaceutical lyophilization systems and the lengthy regulatory approval process, the pace of innovation

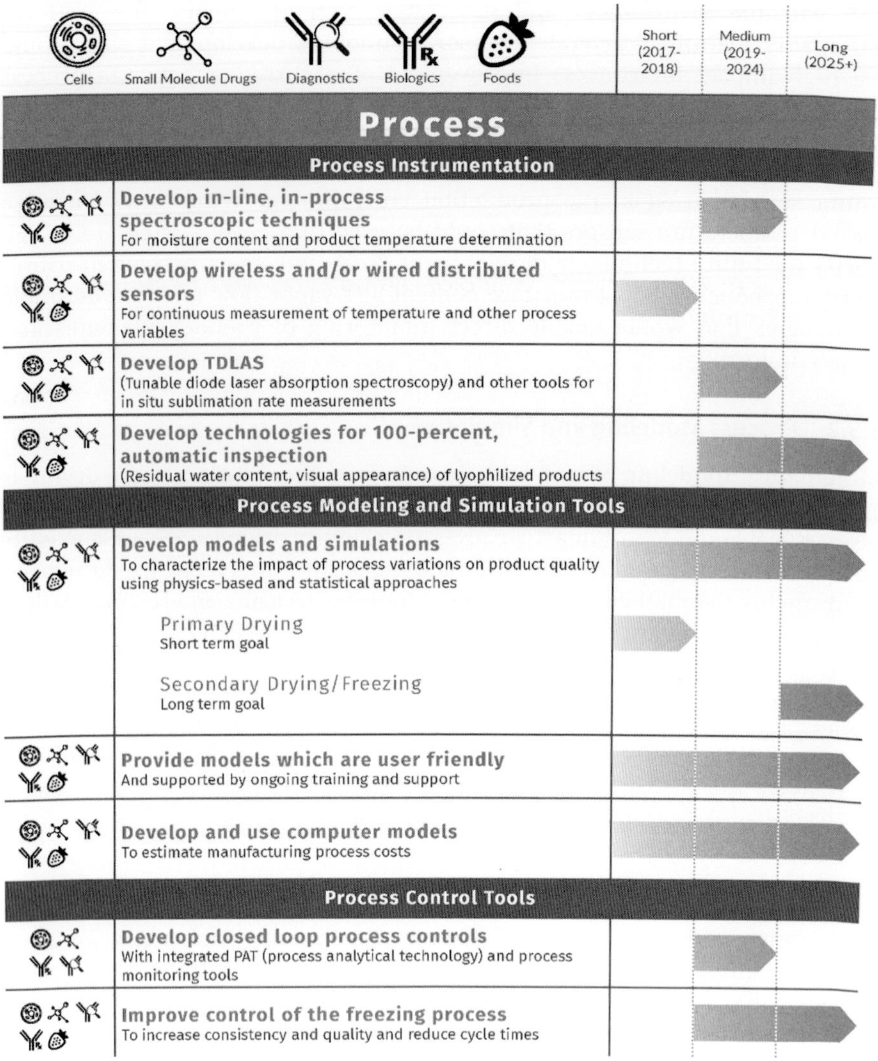

Figure 15.7 Process-related technology roadmap.

in lyophilization equipment has been slow. The essential design of lyophilizers has not changed appreciably in the decades since the first tray-style lyophilizers were introduced. However, changes in the design of lyophilizer components, such as the size and location of the duct between the product chamber and condenser, can increase vapor removal capacity, shorten cycle times, and increase overall energy efficiency. LyoHUB roadmap participants have identified several technologies that are likely to improve current lyophilization equipment and may lead to disruptive new technological alternatives to lyophilization.

15.6.1 Equipment Harmonization and Scale-Up

There is consensus in the lyophilization community regarding the need for harmonization of performance characterization of lyophilization equipment.

Such harmonization can significantly shorten the equipment and installation validation time and accelerate process development and technology transfer between different lyophilizer systems. As an initial step in this direction, LyoHUB is preparing a publication of recommended best practices in lyophilization equipment performance characterization. A unified approach for testing and reporting is needed for equipment characteristics, such as minimum controllable pressure, temperature, and pressure uniformity under various loads.

15.6.2 Improve Lyophilized Technologies and Equipment for Existing and New Products

Current production lyophilizers have very low energy efficiency. Improvement of both process and equipment is needed to achieve highly efficient and robust lyophilization. The major directions for current equipment improvement include:

(1) More efficient heat transfer to the product.
(2) Improved transport of sublimed vapor from chamber to condenser through changes in the design of chamber-to-condenser interface and valves.
(3) Optimized configuration and operating conditions of icing condensers.

An additional area of major improvement for current lyophilization equipment is the sterilization methods. Pharmaceutical lyophilization systems are sterilized to eliminate microorganisms and inactivate viruses, and typically a sterility assurance level of 10^{-6} needs to be demonstrated. The current sterilization methods are time consuming and costly. The most widely used sterilization is achieved by exposure to saturated steam at a temperature of 121–125 °C. Steam sterilization involves heating and recooling the entire lyophilization system, producing undesirable thermal stresses that accelerate equipment wear and aging. Due to the large thermal mass of production-scale equipment, a typical sterilization cycle takes more than six hours. There is a need for low-temperature sterilization methods and associated technologies. Alternatives to steam sterilization include vaporized hydrogen peroxide (VHP) sterilization [3] and cold plasma sterilization [4].

15.6.3 Disruptive Lyophilization/Drying Technologies and Equipment

The use of electromagnetic radiation in the form of infrared (IR) heaters or volumetric heating by microwave- or radio-frequency dielectric heating can significantly accelerate the freeze-drying process. Technology development is needed to adapt electromagnetic heating methods to the scale and operating requirements of pharmaceutical lyophilization systems. The use of electromagnetic fields to induce ice nucleation in freezing and assist in drying is considered in detail in Chapter 11 [5]. The main advantages of electromagnetic heating are the extremely fast response and greater tunability, including local temperature control, as compared with the currently used heating methods based on circulating heat transfer fluids. Such highly tunable and responsive heat inputs are advantageous for closed-loop, automated lyophilization processes.

Spray freeze drying can be used to produce bulk lyophilized drug substance much faster than freeze drying in trays and vials [6]. This is due to the large surface area available for sublimation because of small particle size and faster heat transfer by forced convection or high-temperature radiant heating instead of low-temperature conduction and radiation in traditional freeze drying. An in-depth consideration of dynamic spray freeze drying and related technologies is presented in Chapter 8 [7].

A critical step in advancing spray freeze-drying technology for pharmaceutical manufacturing is achieving better process understanding and development of mathematical models of spray freeze drying that could be used for process design. Additionally, sterile powder filling technology needs to be more readily available for spray freeze drying to be applicable for manufacturing unit dosage forms of lyophilized products.

In current practice, the lyophilization of pharmaceutical and biological products is performed as a batch-type operation. The starting liquid solutions are filled in vials, syringes, or trays and then lyophilized as a single batch. Batch uniformity remains a serious issue, especially for large-scale production lyophilizers. Food freeze drying has seen a shift over the last few decades to semicontinuous and even completely continuous operations. The progression from batch to continuous processing typically brings about increased productivity and uniformity in product attributes. Various approaches for semicontinuous and continuous lyophilization are being explored by industry and academic researchers [8]. Examples include semicontinuous processes based on spray freezing and agitated vacuum drying, atmospheric spray freeze drying, foam drying, rotary shell freeze drying in vials, and electrospinning, some of which are covered in the book. The roadmapping participants identified continuous lyophilization as a high-priority technology development area for pharmaceutical manufacturing.

15.7 Regulatory Interface

In addition to the technical innovations described above, progress in lyophilization is critically dependent on the interface between the industry and various regulatory agencies, including the US FDA. Together with workforce education and training, the regulatory interface provides the foundation on which any technical innovations must rest.

Participants in technology roadmapping identified several strategies for improving the regulatory interface for lyophilization and related technologies. At a broad level, they saw opportunities to improve communication between regulatory agencies and the industry. Specific strategies suggested by the participants included developing a systematic approach to setting inspection expectations to ensure consistency and compliance and improving the industry's ability to change validated lyophilization processes to accommodate new technologies. Similarly, participants felt that improving the receptivity of regulatory agencies to new technologies through various means of communication would help reduce the barriers to implementation of new technologies. A specific form of communication embraced by the roadmapping participants is the creation and dissemination of "best practices" papers.

A best practices paper summarizes the views of industry and academic researchers at a given time regarding the most preferred and/or accepted methods or techniques, as well as identifying areas for improvement. In the pharmaceutical industry, best practices papers serve as a form of communication among industry members and with regulatory agencies. For lyophilization, participants in technology roadmapping felt that best practices papers on equipment qualification, platform lyophilization process development, instrumentation, and other topics were needed. They recommended that the documents be disseminated via open access, though they did not preclude publication in scientific or trade journals. The participants further recommended that best practices information be shared between the food and pharmaceutical industries and that a framework or set of criteria for updating best practices be established.

Recently, the first best practices efforts have commenced to address several challenging aspects of lyophilization in need of harmonization. Recommended best practices for process monitoring instrumentation in pharmaceutical freeze drying have been published in early 2017 [9]. Another paper [10] presented harmonized nomenclature and description for variations in cake appearance for lyophilized products and proposed acceptance criteria. Additionally, the Biophorum Operations Group (BPOG), a collaboration of major pharmaceutical companies recently published a paper summarizing an industry perspective on the application of modeling in lyophilization process scale-up and transfer [11]. It is expected that in the near future such harmonization efforts will lead to establishment of recognized consensus standards in lyophilization as applied to manufacture of pharmaceutical and biopharmaceutical products.

15.8 Workforce Development

Effective implementation of new and existing lyophilization technologies will require a skilled workforce across all education levels. In technology roadmapping, participants identified a need for new educational programs in biotechnology processing at the university level to meet the industry shortages of skilled workers. They suggested that content related to lyophilization technologies be included in such programs and that universities develop certification and assessment tools that would be recognized by the industry. For continuing education of both technical and operational workers, roadmapping participants felt that distance learning programs related to practical considerations for lyophilization formulation and process development should be developed and deployed. Similarly, participants also recognized the need for workshops to educate industry about current and emerging lyophilization technologies, process and formulation topics, and measurement techniques. A need to expand the educational role of equipment manufacturers was also identified and thought to be important in avoiding manufacturing disruptions. At the operator level, there is a need to address the shortage of technical training in lyophilization to decrease operational impacts.

References

1 Arduini, M. (2016). *Aseptic Processing Symposium*, Buffalo, NY (12–14 September 2016).

2 Thompson, T.N. (2013). LyoPAT™: Real-time monitoring and control of the freezing and primary drying stages during freeze-drying for improved product quality and reduced cycle times. *American Pharmaceutical Review* 16 (7): 68–74.

3 Johnson, J.W., Nail, S.L., and Renzi, E. (1992). Vaporized hydrogen peroxide sterilization of freeze dryers. *PDA Journal of Pharmaceutical Science and Technology* 46 (6): 215–225.

4 Denis, B., Steves, S., Semmler, E. et al. (2012). Plasma sterilization of pharmaceutical products: from basics to production. *Plasma Processes and Polymers* 9 (6): 619–629.

5 Woo, M. and Mujumdar, A.S. (2020). Effects of electric and magnetic field on freezing. In: *Drying Technologies for Biotechnology and Pharmaceutical Applications* (Chapter 11) (eds. S. Ohtake, K. Izutsu and D. Lechuga-Ballesteros), 283–302, Wiley.

6 Wanning, S., Süverkrüp, R., and Lamprecht, A. (2015). Pharmaceutical spray freeze drying. *International Journal of Pharmaceutics* 488 (1): 136–153.

7 Luy, B. and Stamato, H. (2020). Spray freeze drying. In: *Drying Technologies for Biotechnology and Pharmaceutical Applications* (Chapter 8) (eds. S. Ohtake, K. Izutsu and D. Lechuga-Ballesteros), 219–238, Wiley.

8 Walters, R.H., Bhatnagar, B., Tchessalov, S. et al. (2014). Next generation drying technologies for pharmaceutical applications. *Journal of Pharmaceutical Sciences* 103 (9): 2673–2695.

9 Nail, S., Tchessalov, S., Shalaev, E. et al. (2017). Recommended best practices for process monitoring instrumentation in pharmaceutical freeze drying-2017. *AAPS PharmSciTech* 18: 2379–2393.

10 Patel, S.M., Nail, S.L., Pikal, M.J. et al. (2017). Lyophilized drug product cake appearance: what is acceptable? *Journal of Pharmaceutical Sciences* 106 (7): 1706–1721.

11 Tchessalov, S., Dassu, D., Latshaw, D., and Nulu, S. (2017). An industry perspective on the application of modeling to lyophilization process scale up and transfer. *American Pharmaceutical Review* 20.

Index

Drying Technologies for Biotechnology and Pharmaceutical Applications, First Edition.
Edited by Satoshi Ohtake, Ken-ichi Izutsu, and David Lechuga-Ballesteros.

e

f

t